ALLE · ZEIT · WACH · 1842

Drugs and Aging

Edited by Dieter Platt

With 105 Figures and 49 Tables

Springer-Verlag
Berlin Heidelberg New York Tokyo

Professor Dr. med. DIETER PLATT
Direktor des Instituts für Gerontologie
der Universität Erlangen-Nürnberg
und der 2. Medizinischen Klinik
Klinikum Nürnberg, Flurstraße 17
D-8500 Nürnberg, FRG

ISBN-13: 978-3-642-70790-2 e-ISBN-13: 978-3-642-70788-9
DOI: 10.1007/978-3-642-70788-

Library of Congress Cataloging in Publication Data. Main entry under title: Drugs and aging. Articles based on lectures and discussions held at the 2nd International Erlangen-Nuremberg Symposium on Experimental Gerontology, Nov. 28-Dec. 1, 1984. Bibliography: p. Includes index. 1. Geriatric pharmacology – Congresses. I. Platt, Dieter. II. International Erlangen-Nuremberg Symposium on Experimental Gerontology (2nd: 1984) RC953.7.D777 1985 615.5'47 85-22228 ISBN 0-387-15913-4 (U.S.)

List of Contributors

You will find the addresses at the beginning of the respective contribution

Preface

Experimental gerontological research is necessary to obtain optimal information and thus ensure proper drug therapy for the elderly. Most older persons acquire multiple diseases, first of all chronic diseases. They involve complex problems of a physical, social, and psychological nature. The multimorbidity of the elderly raises many questions in drug therapy. By contrast with our extensive knowledge of pharmacokinetics and pharmacodynamics in younger age groups, few facts are available in respect of the elderly. A variety of factors may influence drug therapy. Physiological and pathological age-related changes of molecules, cells, organs, and the total organism may interact to enhance or inhibit drug therapy in higher age groups. It is well known that elderly patients are overmedicated and therefore the incidence of adverse drug reactions increases with age.

Elderly patients with multimorbidity often have a diminished body clearance of drugs; age-related changes of the kidney seems to be one of the most important factors in this regard. Far less important than the elimination of drugs through the kidney is their excretion in the bile. So far results have disclosed that oxidative steps in drug clearance are more likely to be disturbed than phase II reactions. Furthermore, changes in distribution volume and age-related alterations in receptor sensitivity also influence the clearance of drugs in the elderly.

The contributions compiled in this book cover drug actions and interactions at the molecular, cellular, organ, and organism level. They are based on the lectures and discussions of the 2nd International Erlangen-Nuremberg Symposium on Experimental Gerontology (November 28–December 1, 1984) in which many distinguished scientists in the fields of biology, biochemistry, pharmacology, pathology, and medicine participated. This book will expand the knowledge of drug therapy in the elderly and will provide a firm foundation for future work on clinical and experimental pharmacology in the aged.

I wish to thank Albert-Roussell, Wiesbaden, Boehringer Mannheim GmbH, Mannheim, Hoechst AG, Frankfurt, ICI-Pharma, Plankstadt, Lipha Arzneimittel GmbH, Essen, Luitpold-Werk, Munich, Dr. Madaus and Co., Cologne, Röhm Pharma GmbH, Darmstadt, Schaper & Brümmer, Salzgitter, and Zyma GmbH, Munich, for the financial assistance they have provided for the meeting in Nuremberg.

Erlangen-Nuremberg DIETER PLATT

Contents

Age-Related Changes of Transcription and RNA Processing

Z. A. Medvedev [1]

Introduction

Among the three main groups of biological macromolecules uniquely linked by transfer and expression of genetic information: (DNA – RNA – Proteins), the RNA stage is the least studied for possible age-related changes. There have been many recent reviews about age-related changes of DNA and proteins, or DNA–protein complexes in chromatin. Recently however, there has been only one review on the role of RNA and RNA metabolism in aging (Rothstein 1982), and a brief supplement to it (Eichhorn 1983) which summarizes the available experimental data up to 1980 on the age-related changes of the synthesis of different types of RNA (rRNA, mRNA, and tRNA). The authors have not linked factual information with several relevant theories of aging [genetic program theory, codon-restriction theory, loss of rRNA genes theory, loss of gene repression theory (dysdifferentiation), general error theory, and others which cannot be proved without special study of transcription and RNA] simply because the information about the age-related changes of RNA is very limited and too general. There have recently been two reviews on the age-related changes of chromatin (Thakur 1984; Medvedev 1984), which also included attempts to cover the connected problems of age-related changes of DNA and the pattern of transcription. Here we would like to select the role of RNA in the aging process for more detailed analysis. The amount of knowledge in this field has not increased dramatically during the last 3–4 years, although there have been many quite interesting studies of changes of RNA in aging tissues which could be added to the list of studies covered by previous reviews. However, we would like to use a different approach which may prove useful. Rothstein (1982) and Eichhorn (1983) have discussed the problem of age-related changes of RNA directly and tried to show what is really known about RNA and transcription in old tissues and cells. We want to look at the same problem from current knowledge of RNA synthesis in general and to expose some gaps in age-related studies of RNA. It is often important to describe not only the information which is *known,* but also the potential in widening a research net. There were many authors in the 1950s and 1960s who studied the age-related changes of the content of different RNAs in tissues and the activity of RNA synthesis and were convinced that the synthesis of RNA is a one-step process which needs only one RNA polymerase. The discovery of the "multi-cistrone" RNA

[1] Genetic Division, National Institute for Medical Research, Mill Hill, London NW7 1AA, Great Britain

Drugs and Aging
Ed. by D. Platt

(hnRNA), RNA processing, splicing, introns, post-transcriptional modification, separate polymerases for ribosomal, transfer, and messenger RNAs, polyadenylation of mRNA, the selectivity of nuclear–cytoplasmic transfer of RNA, and some other intermediate processes which divide initial transcripts from their complex function in protein synthesis have rapidly made our knowledge on the role of RNA in aging very obsolete. Therefore, an attempt to compare what is known about RNA synthesis and about RNA aging could still be useful, even if it does not add much to existing knowledge about the role of RNA in the aging process, already considered by Rothstein (1982). We also speculate about the possible role of RNA processing in the elimination of the alterations of DNA which cannot be removed by the DNA repair systems.

Taking into account the special interest of this symposium in the problem of drug effects related to the molecular and cellular level of aging, we shall make some comments about the attempts to use RNA, ribonucleotides, and some RNA synthesis stimulating drugs for different geriatric treatments.

Age-Related Changes of RNA Content and RNA Synthesis

Most studies show the age-related decrease of RNA content and RNA synthesis in tissues and per diploid cell. (For review see: Medvedev 1964; Berdyshev 1970; Rothstein 1982). Some results on the incorporation of labeled nucleotides into nuclei which originally indicated the possibility of a steady increase of RNA turnover in old tissues (Wulff et al. 1962, 1964, 1966) and stimulated the formulation, by the authors, of a theory of increased synthesis of nonfunctional defective RNA (Wulff et al. 1962; Wulff 1966) were later shown to be artifacts. The authors used labeled nucleotide precursors with high specific activity and tested their incorporation after short intervals. They did not take into consideration the sharp reduction of the free nucleotide pool in aging tissues which made the labeled precursors much less diluted (before incorporation) (Bucher and Swarfield 1966; Davi et al. 1966). Current studies of the age changes of the pool of free nucleotide monophospates and nucleotide bases in liver nuclei (Bolla and Miller 1980) have found an almost eight- to tenfold reduction in their concentration.

The age-related decrease of RNA synthesis (usually in liver and muscles from rats) has been shown with different RNA precursors – [^{32}P] (Shereshevskaya 1963; Nikitin and Shereshevskaya 1962), [^{3}H] uridine (Soriero and Talbert 1975), and [^{14}C] uracil (Kanungo et al. 1970) and by other methods (Schneider and Shorr 1975; Macieira-Coeho and Loria 1976). Some authors have incubated isolated nuclei in vitro with labeled nucleotides (Devi et al. 1966; Mainwaring 1968; Britton et al. 1972; Castle et al. 1978) and confirmed the same tendency. However, it would be more interesting to find out how this general conclusion about the age-related reduction of RNA synthesis and nucleotide metabolism (size of nucleotide pool) is reflected in the synthesis and turnover rates of functionally specific groups of RNA.

Ribosomal RNA

The largest proportion of cellular RNA is represented by ribosomal RNA (rRNA). rRNAs are the final gene products and they make an important structural element of several million ribosomes in each cell. The proliferating tissues and particularly developing tissues need a very active synthesis of rRNAs. The proper supply of rRNA is possible only because each cell normally contains multiple, highly redundant copies of ribosomal genes. The level of this redundancy is species specific. Human cells contain about 200 rRNA genes per haploid genome, but this figure could reach 1000 or higher in some amphibian species. The high level of the redundancy of rDNA is necessary for critical development stages. Adult tissues, and particularly those which have no mitotic activity, do not need so many ribosomal genes. It is not yet clearly established whether the rate of transcription of ribosomal genes is sharply reduced in differentiated cells, or whether most rRNA genes remain idle and inactive while a few continue to be transcribed at a high rate. The ribosomal genes are transcribed by RNA polymerase I. The original transcript is a precursor (45S RNA) and its post-transcriptional processing includes a cleavage which produces one copy each of 28S rRNA, 18S rRNA, and 5.8S rRNA, which are assembled into ribosomes in a special structural unit – the nucleolus. The accuracy of all these steps is important because the functional ribosomes have a significant influence on the fidelity of translation.

Age-related studies of the synthesis of rRNA were stimulated by a report by Johnson and Strehler (1972) and Johnson et al. (1972), who found a substantial decrease of ribosomal genes (rDNA) in several tissues of the aging beagle. The loss of rDNA was tissue specific, rapid in brain, heart, and muscles, and less rapid in spleen, kidney, and liver. The authors suggested that such a decrease may reduce the synthesis of rRNA to a level insufficient to support the functions of all the ribosomes necessary for cellular functions. However, they did not compare the actual rate of synthesis of rRNA, tRNA, and mRNA to find any disproportion in the rate of synthesis. It has, therefore, remained unclear whether the loss of rDNA (estimated by the molecular hybridization) could cause some kind of "ribosomal deficiency" or whether remaining rRNA genes are still able to support the formation of ribosomes, which is apparently very slow in differentiated cells.

The possible loss of rRNA genes in aging tissues was later shown for mouse brain, spleen, and kidney tissues (Gaubatz and Cutler 1978), while loss of rDNA was shown in human myocardium and cerebral cortex (Strehler 1979; Strehler and Chang 1979). Shmookler-Reis and Goldstein (1980) found a loss of reiterated sequences during serial passage of human diploid fibroblasts. Buys et al. (1979) studied the age-dependent changes of transcription of ribosomal genes in human lymphocytes and fibroblasts. They were able to register a rather extensive loss of ribosomal RNA gene activity. However, the authors did not consider it a sign of abnormality – they expected from the results of some other tests to show that human cells may easily survive and withstand the loss of a significant part of their highly repetitive ribosomal RNA genes. A decrease of the synthesis of ribosomal RNA in hearts of aging rats was found by Yavich et al. (1978). An age-correlated loss of ribosomal RNA synthesizing capacity was shown for macronucleus in

Paramecium (Heifetz and Smith-Sonnenhorn 1981). However, in a recent study (Peterson et al. 1984) no differences in rRNA gene copy number were found during in vivo aging of mouse myocytes or in vitro aging of the W1-38 line of human fibroblasts. The authors suggest that the loss of rDNA is not a ubiquitous feature of aging of mammalian cells. In mouse heart cells the number of 28S rRNA genes per haploid genome was 90 in young, 102-107 in 15- to 25-month-old, and 93 in 39-month-old animals, with a standard deviation of about 5–6. The authors applied a different method of DNA purification and hybridization, using more extensive deproteinization procedures, and suggested that the previous reports showing a sharp decrease of rDNA were influenced by the presence of tightly DNA bound proteins in older cells which have reduced the hybridization capacity of DNA. Attempts to study age-related changes of processing of rRNAs are still absent. Indirect evidence was reported by Mori et al. (1978), who found a decrease in the cytoplasmic ratio of 28S and 18S ribosomal RNA in mouse liver and brain tissues. In polysomal RNA both 28S and 18S RNA were present in equimolar amounts. However, in cytoplasm of older tissues there was some molar excess of 18S RNA. 18S and 28S ribosomal RNAs are transcribed from the same cistron. The excess of 18S RNA can be related either to slower transportation of larger 28S RNA from nucleus to cytoplasm or a specific higher level of degradation of 28S RNA.

Transfer RNA

Strehler (Strehler et al. 1967, 1971; Strehler 1977) proposed a theory which considered some changes in the pattern of tRNAs and isoaccepting rRNAs as a cause of developmental alterations and their continuation into age-related alterations as well. The authors were able to demonstrate apparent changes of the pattern of isoaccepting tRNAs and tRNA synthetases during morphogenetic "aging" of soybean cotyledon (Bick and Strehler 1971, 1972) and plant leaves (Wright et al. 1972; Andron and Strehler 1973). However, in plants and particularly in individual plant organs the distinction between aging and genetically programmed development is difficult. Developmental aging is a special problem of gerontology and it is more relevant to plants and some short-lived animal species with a single reproduction cycle. In most animal species, and particularly in mammalian species, development and aging are well separated in time, so that the character of changes of tRNAs which are specific for development and which are relevant to real post-maturation senescence can be studied separately.

Age-related changes of the pattern of isoaccepting forms of tRNA have been reported for nematode (Reitz and Sanadi 1972) and *Drosophila* (Hosbach and Kubli 1979; Owenby et al. 1979). The appearance of some deficient, inactive molecules of tRNAs in aging *Drosophila* has also been reported (Hosbach and Kubli 1979 b). Transfer RNAs have many modified nucleotides which are necessary for their function and complex secondary structure. In aging cells some additional modifications have been observed, like the change of guanine to queuine (Singhal and Kopper 1981), or the reduction of methylation (Mays et al. 1979), which could lead to higher infidelity of translation.

There have been few attempts to study age changes of tRNA in mammalian tissues. In most cases the changes were minor and in one or two types of tRNA only (Lawrence et al. 1979). Rothstein (1982), who reviewed the literature up to 1980, suggested that for some more definite conclusions we "simply have to wait for more data to become available" (p. 187).

New data are still slow in coming. It was shown that in mouse kidney and heart the content of tRNA and the rate of tRNA synthesis decline with age (Neumeister and Webster 1981). Cook and Buetow (1982), who studied the pattern of tRNAs in the liver of the senescent female Wistar rat, did not, however, find any visible changes related to aging. No significant age-related differences were found in the extent of aminoacylation of the liver cytoplasmic tRNA population, the total tRNA synthetase activity, the rate of aminoacylation of individual tRNAs, or the overall complement of tRNA species as detected by two-dimensional gel electrophoresis. However, some undetected changes were still possible because the tRNA system (tRNAs plus aminoacyl tRNA synthetases) isolated from livers of old animals were less capable of supporting in vitro cell-free protein synthesis than were the same fractions isolated from adult (10- to 13-months-old) animals. This may indicate that some types of tRNA which show the same electrophoretic mobility are "defective," and these defects may include base modifications of a different kind. The authors have tested individual tRNAs in homologous and heterologous assays. They found that in heterologous assays adult tRNA synthetases isolated from adult animals were significantly more active than senescent synthetases when charging isoleucine, methionine, phenylalanine, proline, and glutamic acid, and less active when charging alanine, aspartic acid, and serine. There were some other differences for in vitro synthesis which were not visible in vivo.

Transfer RNA genes contain introns, but this is not the rule for all tRNA species. Only one-fifth of yeast tRNA genes contain introns (Johnson and Abelson 1983). This means that the processing pattern is different for individual tRNAs; some do have splicing, while others do not need it. It is probable that the more complex the processing of transcribed RNA, the more alteration-prone would be the functional molecules. If one could show that these tRNAs which need to be processed are also more "age-changeable," this may indicate the possibility that the error rates vary for each type of RNA macromolecule.

Messenger RNA

We discussed previously that the synthesis of rRNA declines with age. Some earlier studies (Detwiler and Draper 1962) indicated that the synthesis of messenger RNA may decline even more rapidly in aging tissues. However, if for rRNAs and for tRNAs it was possible to study some changes of individual molecular species (there are four main rRNAs and probably about 100 different species and isoforms of tRNAs), the same task was too difficult for mRNAs. Each cell has several thousand different messenger RNAs, some of them for minor protein represented by a few RNA molecules, others for major proteins represented by several million mRNAs. Despite this high heterogeneity, only about 5%–7% of cytoplasmic RNAs belong to the mRNA group; 70%–80% belong to rRNA, and 10%–15% to tRNA, both the latter groups having longer-lived molecules.

Messenger RNA is transcribed by RNA polymerase II. The structure of mRNA genes reflects the evolutionary history of different proteins. Most acient proteins, like histones or protamines, are coded for by reiterated genes assembled into special clusters. These genes normally have no introns and their transcripts have simple processing [without forming a poly(A) tail]. Genes of more recent origin, like genes for immunoglobulins, have very complex structures with many introns. Their RNA transcripts have to pass through extremely sophisticated processing before they finally form mRNAs. For most proteins the processing of their mRNAs includes the formation of precursor (initial transcript, or hnRNA), splicing, capping (from 5′ end – formation of a special structure which is necessary for later binding of mRNA to ribosome), and polyadenylation of their 3′ ends. Polyadenylation (by poly-A-polymerase) adds 50 to 250 residues of adenylic acid. (For review see Brawerman 1976; Edmonds and Winters 1976.)

If hnRNA has many introns the splicing may need to pass through several stages. Information transfer and biological reactions are never perfect and some errors are possible at every stage. *It is therefore possible to suggest that those mRNAs which have the simplest processing accumulate fewer errors, while mRNAs with complex and multistaged processing would transfer more errors into translation.* It is possible to test this hypothesis by showing, for example, that the transfer of information from DNA to histones is more accurate than the transfer of information from DNA to immunoglobulins or other proteins coded by genes with many introns. However, the actual state of the age-related studies of mRNA is still very far from the possible estimation of the accuracy of synthesis of individual messengers.

Attempts to study qualitative age changes of messenger RNA were started only recently. They became possible with the development of some methods which allow the separation of polyadenylated forms of RNA. The first to apply these methods to the study of poly(A) RNA from young and old tissues were Müller et al. (1979, 1980), who measured the synthesis of polyadenylated RNA in oviducts from adult and senescent quails and by hepatocytes isolated from rats of different ages. The authors found that in senescent animals the poly(A) stretch of mRNA is shorter than in adult animals. The rate of poly(A) RNA synthesis by hepatocytes decreased by 68% between 6 and 30 months of age. The rate of total RNA synthesis also decreased, mostly until 19 months of age. Between 19 and 30 months of age the decrease in synthesis of polyadenylated RNA continued (about 40%), while the decrease in total RNA synthesis (mainly rRNA and tRNA) was not significant. The decrease in poly(A) synthesis is most probably related to the decrease in the transcription rate. However, a decrease in the processing rate is also possible. Later Richardson et al. (1982) confirmed that the decline in the synthesis of rRNA and tRNA in aging hepatocytes was less rapid than the decrease in the synthesis of poly(A) mRNA.

The polyadenylated segment of mRNA, or poly(A), has important regulatory functions. It is relevant for the transport of mRNA through the nuclear membrane and (according to some evidence) for the regulation of the cytoplasmic functional life span of mRNA. Synthesis and degradation of poly(A) includes several enzymes, both anabolic and catabolic. Müller and collaborators were not able to analyze the individual species of mRNA which control the synthesis of specific proteins. However, they carried out a complex experiment to ascertain the effect of aging on poly(A) metabolism of mRNA in two groups of female quails: mature (250–320 days old) and older animals (3–3.5 years old) (Arendes et al. 1980; Bernd et al. 1982). They found that the average size of the poly(A) segment of mRNA decreases with age. In mature animals the average poly(A) segment was 120–180 AMP units in the oviduct and 100–110 in heart and liver. In older animals the poly(A) chains were about 70 AMP units long.

The decrease in the size of the poly(A) segment with age could be responsible for the sharp decline of mRNA synthesis. Because the methods of isolation of mRNA are now based on the binding of its polyadenylated terminus, the yields of mRNA isolated from older tissues could be lower simply because of shorter poly(A) segments. The results showing a sharp decrease in poly(A) mRNA synthesis related to aging in brain and liver cells were confirmed by several authors (Semesei et al. 1982; Dilella et al. 1982). Katsarada et al. (1982) found an age-related decline in the synthesis of specific mRNA liver malic enzyme (by measuring the substrate induction).

Chatterjee et al. (1981) were the first group who tried to find qualitative age-related changes of mRNA coding for specific hepatic proteins. Such changes could be deduced from the alterations of the pattern of synthesized proteins. However, the authors tried to approach the same problem in a more direct way, by the analysis of translational products of poly(A) mRNA isolated from liver of animals of different ages. The actual translation was carried out in vitro. Liver mRNA was mixed with the rabbit reticulocyte lysate. Newly synthesized proteins were labeled with ^{35}Smethionine and identified by autoradiography. The authors found that three proteins show evident age-related variations and they called these proteins "senescence marker proteins," or SMPs. One of these proteins was characterized as globulin (SMP-3). Aging was connected with the disappearance of mRNA for SMP-1 and SMP-23. The authors suggested that their results were consistent with the concept of genetically programmed aging.

The results of this particular work should, however, be treated with some reservations because of the very low activity of the mRNA in this in vitro system. Only four or five bands of ^{35}Smethionine-labeled proteins were visible in the areas of electrophoresis between molecular weights 12,000 and 43,000. In normal liver cytoplasm there are several dozen proteins which can be identified by in vivo synthesis with the same label and by one-dimensional SDS-gel electrophoresis. Anzai et al. (1983), who have used an improved method of in vitro synthesis and two-dimensional electrophoresis, carried out tests on poly(A) RNA translational activity with ^{35}Smethionine isolated from liver,kidney, and brain of mice of different ages. They were able to identify by autoradiography about 300 spots and most of them were highly reproducible. The authors registered an apparent tissue specificity of the pattern of spots, while the age-related variations were not significant. In kidney and brain none of these spots consistently depended on age. Only in livers did the authors observe one translation product (with a molecular weight of about 30,000) which could be associated with senescent mice. The authors concluded that most of the major genes which are expressed in the tissues of young mice (3.5–14.4 months old) and adult mice are also expressed in senescent animals (22–29 months old). The age-related protein from liver was not identified and the authors did not find this protein when they tried to analyze a liver extract of senescent mice.

This approach, like all other attempts to use to poly(A) segment for isolation of mRNA, can miss some changes of mRNA which are expressed in the reduction of poly(A) segments reported by Müller et al. (1979, 1980). It is obvious that not only the existence of mRNAs without a poly(A) segment may influence the results but also the presence of mRNAs with a short poly(A) sequence. About 30%–40% of the total mRNA in mouse liver is reported (Moffett and Doule 1981) to have poly(A) too short to bind to oligo(dT) columns which are used for isolation of poly(A) RNA. Schröder et al. (1983) have recently developed a method which is able to isolate the shorter poly(A) sequences, even oligo(A) segments down to a chain length of four nucleotide units. In nondividing mouse lymphoma cells the amount of A_{2^-6} sequence labeled by ^3H was at the level of 8% of the total amount of poly(A) sequences. This means a much higher percentage of mRNAs with short poly(A) segments. The authors applied the new method to their earlier studied experimental model of young and old female quails (Müller et al. 1979) and found that the amount of low molecular weight oligo(A) fragments also gradually decreases during aging of animals. One may assume that if the length of poly(A) segments shortens with age and the number of oligo(A) segments also decreases with age, the aging should correlate with an increase of mRNAs which are not polyadenylated.

Khasigov et al. (1983), who recently studied the rates of polyadenylation of mRNA in relation to aging, also tried to isolate poly(A) RNA and oligo(A) RNA separately. In addition they isolated nuclear precursors of mRNA from livers and brain of young and adult rats (the oldest animals were 540 days old). The rate of polyadenylation decreased with age, whereas the half-life time of precursors of mRNA increased. This means slower processing of RNA in older nuclei.

A very specific test to study the age-related changes of the pattern of mRNA was tried by Ono and Cutler (1978). They found that the amounts of endogenous leukemia virus-related and globin-related mRNA increase in the brain and liver of mice with age. The authors regard this as a possible derepression of some genes in older animals and the "leaky expression" of mRNAs which are not normally required for certain types of differentiation. These results were presented to support the theory of cellular aging as a kind of dysdifferentiation process (Cutler 1982). However, the possible appearance of "leaky mRNAs" in aging cells is only one of very many possible changes of different groups of RNA which may disturb normal function of tissues (see Table 1).

Grady and Campbell (1981) did not find changes in the RNA complexity when they studied poly(A) RNA in rat tissues. However, they have analyzed tissues of only 2- and 10-month-old animals. Yavich (1981) did not find the changes in the poly(A) mRNA pattern in myocardium from rats between 3 and 24 months of age.

If aging does correlate with the shortening of the poly(A) tail, which seems to be the case, then the changes of the mRNA population in old tissues could be selectively missed during the isolation procedure. The method selectively isolates less changed mRNA population. There are at least 10,000 different mRNA species in mouse liver (Hastie and Bishop 1976), and a method which can detect quantitative and qualitative age-related changes is still not available. It is also known that the method of in vitro synthesis only shows translation products of relatively abundant mRNA species. At the same time mRNAs of low or medium abundance are the most likely messengers for enzymes and proteins with regulatory functions – these may be the most important for age-related studies, and probably the most vulnerable to alterations. The highly abundant species of mRNA are more likely to be coded for by reiterated genes or by families of closely related genes. It has been suggested (Medvedev 1972, 1983; Cutler 1974) that gene reiteration and all the other forms of redundancy of information may act as an age-protective mechanism.

RNA Turnover

rRNA and tRNA

All forms of ribosomal RNA are quite stable; different species of tRNA have shorter half-lives, while mRNAs in most cells are very short lived. The high turnover rate of mRNAs made it possible in the late 1950s to identify this RNA as "informational" by "pulse labeling." In the 1950s and 1960s, age-related studies of turnover rates of RNA were usually carried out without fractionation of RNA into different functional groups. The first experiments in which the half-lives of RNA were measured in young and old rats for rRNA and tRNA separately were carried out by Menzies et al. (1972). The half-lives of rRNA were tissue specific and varied between 5.9 and 8.9 days in liver, spleen, kidney, and other tissues. No age-associated differences were observed. tRNA fraction was apparently very heterogeneous and had longer- and shorter-lived fractions (variations of half-lives between 1 and 11 days). The authors suggested the possible presence of abnormal tRNAs and rRNAs and their preferential degradation, but they were not able to confirm this with experimental data. In later work (Menzies and Aguilar 1973) the measurement of the decay of radioactivity of RNA was extended (up to 90 days) after a single injection of ^{14}Corotic acid. The authors found the existence of very long-lived forms of rRNA (with half-lives up to 29 days), but no clear age-related differences.

mRNA

The first study in which age-related changes of half-lives of messenger RNA were investigated was carried out by Wattiax et al. (1971). The new synthesis of mRNA was inhibited by actinomycin D, and the authors studied the functional lives of pre-existing mRNAs (by their ability to support the protein synthesis) in the thorax and ovary of *Drosophila melanogaster*. It was found that the half-lives of mRNA was shorter in older flies.

There is, as yet, no satisfactory explanation why some proteins are translated from the short-lived mRNAs and others from long-lived mRNAs. The necessity of the long-lived mRNA for terminal differentiation in reticulocytes (Gorsky et al. 1974; Nokin et al. 1976) is understandable, since this allows the reticulocytes to continue the synthesis of hemoglobin after the synthesis of most other proteins has already halted. In this case the life span of mRNA is the key mechanism of terminal differentiation.

It is possible that the newly synthesized mRNA makes fewer errors of translation than the same mRNA which is already several hours or several days old and may have accumulated diferent damages, alterations, and modifications. The repeated use of the same mRNA molecule for translation results in more chance of errors. One may suggest that in general the shorter-lived mRNAs produce fewer errors of translation than longer-lived mRNAs. This would mean that the synthesis of individual proteins may have an individual incidence of errors. Some proteins, like hemoglobin, apparently can tolerate a high proportion of altered "wrong" molecules; they are inactive and do not interfere with the main erythrocyte functions. Errors of translation of the message for enzymes could be more deleterious. It is possible that if some specific enzymes, like polymerases and enzymes of nucleotide metabolism in general, need very high accuracy of their synthesis to be functional, the mRNAs for these enzymes belong to the shorter-lived group. If the suggestion which links the length of poly(A) segment with the duration of functional life of mRNA (Sheiness and Darnell 1973; Singer and Penman 1973) is correct, the short-lived mRNAs with a short poly(A) segment should make fewer translational errors. At the same time the long-lived mRNAs, which have a shortened poly(A) that is reduced as a result of their function, may be less accurate messengers. Nokin et al. (1976) found that the newly synthesized globin mRNA with a long poly(A) stretch is very active. The reduction of this poly(A) stretch from 80 residues to 25 residues during "molecular aging" correlates with a decrease in the RNA translation efficiency [mRNA with a short poly(A) was translated 2.5–3 times slower].

We have seen form the earlier discussion that the older tissues in general have shorter poly(A) sections of their mRNA population. This is most probably due to the presence of "shortened" mRNA molecules and may explain the age-related changes of the rate of synthesis of RNA and proteins.

Enzymes of RNA Synthesis and Degradation

Most reports published in the 1960s and 1970s did not use separate measurements of activity of individual polymerases; RNA polymerase I (synthesis of rRNA), polymerase II (mRNA synthesis), and polymerase III (synthesis of tRNA). The combined RNA polymerase activity shows a modest decline with age. When the activities of individual polymerases were measured in age-related studies, it was found that RNA polymerases I and II showed a more evident decline with age than polymerase III (Rothstein 1982). However, these changes are relevant mostly for the first half of the life (Benson and Harker 1978).

There are few studies of changes of other enzymes relevant to RNA synthesis and turnover. It was reported (Bernd et al. 1982) that the activity of poly(A) polymerase is slightly increased in aging quail tissues. Activities of two catabolic enzymes – endoribonuclease IV and poly(A)-specific exoribonuclease – are markedly higher in quail senescent tissues (Müller et al. 1979, 1980). The increase of ribonuclease activity in different tissues of aging rat was also reported (Stavitskaya 1956). Goto et al. (1969) suggested that the increase of RNase in cytoplasm could be a result of a "leakage" of lysosomal enzymes in old cells.

The Problem of the Accuracy of RNA Synthesis

The problem of the accuracy of RNA synthesis is normally approached from two sides, accuracy of the pattern of transcription and the fidelity of the synthesis of each individual RNA molecule. Each of these approaches can be further fragmented. Transcription, for example, can be divided into transcription of "housekeeping" genes, common for many different types of differentiation, transcription of specialized genes, which are responsible for some differentiated functions, and transcription of inducible genes, which can be switched on a few or many cells as a result of external or internal induction. The dependence of normal life on very complex and accurate coordination of different individual acts of transcription has made it attractive to consider aging as a process of gradual accumulation of irregularities of transcription. There are several theories of aging and carcinogenesis which consider alteration of transcription as, the cause (Table 1). The analysis of finding on the pattern of transcription needs more comprehensive discussion of the age-related changes of the structure and function of chromatin; we have tried to do this in a separate review (Medvedev 1984).

Here I would like to concentrate on a much less developed area of the accuracy of transcription – the fidelity of the RNA synthesis and functions from the formation of the original transcript to the degradation of RNA molecules in cytoplasm.

Before the discovery of RNA processing it was taken for granted that the transcribed RNA repeated all mutational and other errors occurring in DNA and transferred them into proteins. Because all species of functional RNA are single-stranded polymers, it was normally assumed that no repair of previous or new errors of genetic information was possible at the RNA stage of informational transfer. In our earlier models of molecular aging (Medvedev 1962, 1964, 1966) we also considered RNA as the most error-prone stage of the transfer of information. The discovery of very sophisticated processing of RNA transcripts has made possible a very different and attractive new approach.

One may suggest that processing can and most probably does fulfil the role of a selector which eliminates errors or misinformation which has accumulated in the DNA over many previous generations or in evolution. DNA as a double helix can repair many errors and alterations. However, the same structure makes it difficult to eliminate from DNA certain types of changes and leads to the accumulation in DNA of wrong genes, pseudogenes, amplified and redundant sequences, stretches of sequences which have no useful information at all, and viral genes – a genetic load, which, if faithfully transcribed, would make well coordinated functional life impossible. This ability of DNA to preserve and accumulate useless or deleterious information is discussed in the well known concept of "selfish DNA" (Orgel and Crick 1980). Most of this junk DNA has to be avoided by the apparatus of transcription (selective transcription from initiation points to termination sequences), by repressors, or by structural changes in chromatin (condensation of chromatin in areas of domination of satellite DNA). However, many useless parts of DNA are transcribed and can be sorted out only during RNA processing (elimination of pseudogenes, introns, reiterated sequences etc.) and during transfer of functional messenger RNAs to cytoplasm (the nature of the selection process at this stage is not clear, but it may include the formation of RNP particles).

It is most probable that the RNA stage is not a simple transcription of information, but is designed to "clarify" and to "purify" the genetic message and thus acts as a filter, not a generator, of errors. RNA performs a correction function in the recreation of genes in a form which makes it possible to use these genes for synthesis of functionally sound proteins.

RNA processing can be considered as an extra repair workshop of the genetic system. At the same time, synthesis of RNA and RNA processing can generate some new simple errors of sequences, modifications which are related to the infidelity of RNA polymerases and other enzymes, errors of splicing, etc. – a kind of noise which is inevitable in any transfer of information. Direct studies of the accuracy of RNA synthesis are limited, and knowledge about the accuracy of processing is practically nonexistent. It is known that some analogues of ribonucleotides can be misincorporated into messenger RNA. Gross and Naono (1961) found synthesis of defective enzymes in many bacteria in the presence of 5-fluorouracil. Lewis and Tarrant (1971) found that the incorporation of 5-fluorouracil into RNA in *Ustilago maydis* produces altered enzymes with reduced thermostability. It was also shown (Holliday and Tarrant 1972) that the accumulation of altered proteins in the presence of this analogue increases the aging rate of human fibroblasts in culture. One could suggest that some nucleotide analogues are formed as a result of errors in the intermediate nucleotide metabolism and induce later errors in protein synthesis.

Direct studies on the fidelity of RNA synthesis were carried out only in in vitro systems (Paetkau et al. 1972; Strniste et al. 1973; Bass and Polonsky 1974) and with the use of bacterial RNA polymerase. These experiments showed a very high level of errors, but this result probably is not relevant to more perfect and specific in vivo systems. Springgate and Loeb (1975) found that the bacterial RNA polymerases are much less accurate in vitro than DNA polymerases. Eichhorn (1979) suggested that many informational errors at the stage of RNA synthesis and processing which contribute to aging could be produced by metal ions when their concentration is not optimal for their normal role, or by ions which do not play a physiological role (Hg^{2+}, Pb^{2+}, Al^{3+}). The author was able to show that RNA polymerase from *Escherichia coli,* which contains zinc as a part of its structure and requires other divalent ions (Mn^{2+}, Mg^{2+}) as activators, makes many incorporation errors (even incorporates deoxyribonucleotides into RNA) in the presence of incorrect ions or altered balance of correct ions. Some ions may produce cross-links between RNA molecules.

There are several theories which try to relate aging to alteration of the balance of metal ions. The correlation between elevation of aluminum in brain cells and Alzheimer's senile dementia is often used as an example (Eichhorn 1979). However, it is not clear that the RNA is the main or the only target for metal ion-induced errors.

RNA as an Antiaging Drug (a "Geroprotector")

RNA of different origin (from yeast and mammalian tissues) is now commercially used as a supplement for different diets and in cosmetics; this is done on the assumption that it has a rejuvenative effect or at least protects against aging. The commercial production of yeast RNA as a dietary supplement (for human consumption) started in the United States in 1977 after Frank and Miele's (1976) book on the "antiaging diet." Pearson and Shaw (1982) claim that the daily consumption of 1–5 g of pure RNA can reduce the aging rate and prolong life span. Some of these recommendations are based on experiments carried out as long ago as 1928, in which the addition of yeasts to mice diet was able to prolong their life span by 7%–12%. It is clear, however, that in 1928 the isolation of pure RNA was difficult, that there was no well balanced diet for laboratory animals and that such an effect, if reproducible, was most probably due to vitamin deficiency of the control diet. There is no RNA or nucleotide deficiency in normal diet and human tissues can synthesize nucleotides.

Cutler (1982b) suggested that the increase of dietary RNA may elevate the concentration of uric acid in tissues and blood circulation. Uric acid may have antioxidant capabilities. He tried to find a correlation in evolution between the level of uric acid and the longevity of a species. Because uric acid sediments are related to gout and some kidney problems it is hardly possible to take a simplistic approach to the usefulness of dietary consumption of pure RNA. The same is relevant for a mixture of RNA and DNA which is available on the U.S. food market under the name "Cognitex" and which is described as "a unique nutritional supplement specially designed to help prevent loss of memory associated with aging" (Life-Extension Products; Fall 1982). The sale of such products is not through the drug market, which is under strict control, but through the food market, making it clear that they were not scientifically tested.

The same can be said about so-called revitalization RNA therapy by the injection of a mixture of RNA extracted from tissues of newborn lambs (see review: Pear 1984). The mixture of RNAs prepared under the name RN-13 is used on the basis of the apparently wrong hypothesis that messenger RNAs (and other RNAs) have no species specificity, only tissue specificity, and that when injected, they can replace functional host RNAs of the same tissues of the human body.

Some more scientific approaches to RNA rejuvenation therapy – the attempts at hormonal stimulation of the synthesis of RNA or so-called hormone-replacement therapy, coupled with hypophysectomy – were carried out in rats at the age of 12 months (Denkla 1974; Bolla and Denkla 1979; Miller et al. 1980). The authors reported "a reversal of some age-associated changes," but a direct connection between this effect and RNA metabolism is not well established.

An antiaging effect was reported for centrophenoxine – a synthetic hydrochloride of dimethylaminoethyl-*p*-chlorophenoxy acetate (Nandy 1978; Rodeman and Bayreuther 1979; Zs-Nagy and K. Nagy 1980). Centrophenoxine was considered an antioxidant and "diminisher" of cross-linking react ions. However, it was also shown recently (Patro and Sharma 1984) that this drug stimulates nucleolar activity in senile Purkinje neurons in rats. This increases the synthesis of ribosomal RNA and activates protein synthesis. It is possible that the effect of centrophenoxine on the memory of old mice and on lipofuscin content (decrease) reported by Nandy (1978) is due to stimulation of protein synthesis, not an antioxidation effect of the drug.

Summary

In conclusion we would like to summarize the material discussed in this review in Table 1. This table shows the age changes of transcription and RNA which actually were found, possible age changes of RNA which have not yet been tested

Table 1. Different types of age-related changes of transcription and RNA

a) *Age changes of transcription and RNA processing*
Decrease of the total RNA content in tissues
Decrease of RNA/DNA ratio in nuclei
Decrease of rRNA content
Decrease of tRNA content
Decrease of poly(A) mRNA content
Decrease of RNA polymerase (I and II) activity
Decrease of rRNA synthesis
Decrease of tRNA synthesis
Decrease of poly(A) mRNA synthesis
Decrease of RNA turnover
Changes of RNase activity
Decrease of the nucleotide pool
Changes of life span of mRNA molecules
Reduction of the size of the poly(A) section of mRNA
Changes of the polyadenylation rate
Decrease of the rate of transport of RNA from nuclei to cyctoplasm
Post-transcriptional modifications of RNAs
Changes of the pattern of mRNAs available for translation
Changes in the pattern of transcription
Changes in the pattern of tRNAs and iso-tRNAs
b) *Possible age-related changes of RNA (suggested in some theories, but not yet tested experimentally*
Errors in the selection of hnRNA for processing
Errors of the initiation of transcription
Errors of splicing
Decrease of the accuracy of the RNA polymerases
Possible increase of the errors of RNA synthesis (incorporation of nucleotide analogues, influence of metal ions, and other factors)
Increased leakage of unprocessed RNA from nuclei
Cross-links between RNA and DNA
Leakage of RNA from mitochondria
c) *Theories of aging relating it to changes of transcription and RNA*
Synthesis of defective mRNA
General error theory (errors of DNA, RNA, and protein synthesis)
Theory of selective loss of rRNA genes
Codone restriction theory (changes of the tRNAs pattern)
Theory of dysdifferentiation
Theory of overdifferentiation (increase of repression of transciption)

experimentally, and, finally, the theories of senescence which are related mainly to changes of transcription and functions of RNA.

Acknowledgments. The author wishes to thank Robin Holliday, T.B.L. Kirkwood, and R.F. Rosenberger for helpful discussion and editorial comments, and Miss H.M. Crowne for reading the manuscript and making linguistic corrections.

References

Andron L, Strehler B (1973) Recent evidence on tRNA and tRNA acylase-mediated cellular control mechanisms: A review. Mech. Ageing Devel 2:97–116

Anzai K, Imazato Ch, Goto S (1983) mRNA population in the liver, kidney and brain of young and senescent mice: Analysis of in vitro translation products. Mech Ageing Devel 23:137–150

Arendes J, Zahn RK, Müller WEG (1980) Age-dependent gene induction in quail oviduct. XI. Alterations on the post-transcriptional level. Mech Ageing Develop 14:49–57

Bass JA, Polonsky JS (1974) On the fidelity of in vitro polynucleotide synthesis by *E. coli* RNA polymerase. FEBS Letters 48:306–309

Benson RW, Harker CW (1978) RNA polymerase activities in liver and brain tissue of ageing mice. J Gerontol 33:323–328

Berdyshev GD (1970) Transcription and its changes at the later stages of postnatal development. Usp Sovr Biol (Moscow) 70:376–396

Bernd A, Batke E, Zahn RK, Müller WEG (1982) Age-dependent gene induction in quail oviduct. XV. Alterations of the poly(A)-associated protein pattern and of the poly(A) chain length of mRNA. Mech Ageing Devel 19:361:377

Bick MD, Strehler BL (1971) Leucyl transfer RNA synthetase changes during soybean cotyledon senescence. Proc Nat Acad Sci USA 68:224–228

Bick MD, Strehler BL (1972) Leucyl tRNA synthetase activity in old cotyledons: Evidence on repressor accumulation. Mech Ageing Devel 1:33–42

Bolla R, Denckla WD (1979) Effect of hypophysectomy on liver nuclear ribonucleic acid synthesis in ageing rats. Biochem J 184:669–674

Bolla RI, Miller JK (1980) Endogenous nucleotide pools and protein incorporation into liver nuclei from young and old rats. Mech Ageing Develop 12:107–118

Brawerman G (1976) Characteristics and significance of the polyadenylate sequence in mammalian messenger RNA. Prog Nucleic Acid Res Mol Biol 17:117–148

Britton VJ, Sherman FG, Florini JR (1972) Effect of age on RNA synthesis by nuclei and soluble RNA polymerases from liver and muscle of C57BL/6J mice. J Gerontol 27:188–192

Bucher NLR, Swaffield MN (1966) Nucleic acid synthesis in relation to ageing and hepatic regeneration in rats. In: Lindop PJ, Sacher GA (eds) Radiation and ageing. Taylor and Francis, London, p 15–21

Buys CHCM, Osinga J, Anders GJPA (1979) Age-dependent variability of ribosomal RNA-gene activity in man as determined from frequencies of silver staining nucleolus organizing regions on metaphase chromosomes of lymphocytes and fibroblasts. Mech Ageing Develop 11:55–75

Castle Th, Katz A, Richardson A (1978) Comparison of RNA synthesis by liver nuclei from rats of various ages. Mech Ageing Develop 8:383–395

Chatteree B, Nath TS, Roy AK (1981) Differential regulation of the messenger RNA for three major senescence marker proteins in male rat liver. Proc Nat Acad Sci USA 256:5939–5941

Cook JR, Buetow DE (1982) The complement of cytoplasmic tRNAs, including queuosine-containing tRNAs, in adult and senescent Wistar rat liver and their levels of aminoacylation. Mech Ageing Develop 20:289:304

Cutler RG (1974) Redundancy of information content in the genome of mammalian species as a protective mechanism determining ageing rate. Mech Ageinig Develop 2:381–408

Cutler RG (1982a) Longevity is determined by specific genes: testing the hypothesis. In: Adelman RC, Roth GS (eds) Testing the theories of aging. CRC Press Inc, Boca Raton, Florida, p 26–113

Cutler RG (1982b) The dysdifferentiative hypothesis of mammalian aging and longevity. In: Giacobini E, Giacobini G, Filogamo G (eds) The aging brain. Raven Press, New York, p 1–18

Denckla WD (1974) Role of the pituitary and thyroid glands in the decline of minimal O_2 consumption with age. J Clin Invest 53:572–581

Detwiler TC, Draper HH (1962) Physiololgical aspects of aging. IV Senescent changes in the metabolism and composition of nucleic acids of the liver and muscle of the rat. J Gerontol 17:138–143

Devi A, Lindsay P, Raina PL, Sarkar NK (1966) Effect of age on some aspects of the synthesis of ribonucleic acid. Nature 212:474–475

Dilella DG, Chiang JYL, Steggles AW (1982) The quantitation of liver cytochrome P450-LM_2 mRNA in rabbits of different ages and after phenobarbital treatment. Mech Ageing Develop 19:113–125

Edmonds M, Winters MA (1976) Polyadenylate polymerases. Prog Nucleic Acid Res Mol Biol 17:149–179

Eichhorn GL (1979) Aging, genetics and the environment. Potential of errors introduced into genetic information transfer by metal ions. Mech Ageing Develop 9:291–301

Eichhorn GL (1983) Nucleic acid biochemistry and aging. Rev Biol Res Aging 1:295–303

Frank BS, Miele P (1976) Doctor Frank's no-aging diet. Dial Press, New York

Gaubatz JW, Cutler RG (1978) Age-related differences in the number of ribosomal RNA genes of mouse tissues. Gerontology 24:179–207

Gorski J, Morrison MR, Merkel CG, Lingrel JB (1974) Size heterogeneity of polyadenylate sequences in mouse globin messenger RNA. J Mol Biol 86:363–371

Goto S, Takano T, Mizuno D, Nakano T, Imaizumi K (1969) Aging and location of acid ribonuclease in liver of various animals. J Gerontol 24:305–308

Grady LJ, Campbell WP (1981) Ageing studies in rat liver1.1. Complexity of RNA from two to then months of age. Mech Ageing Develop 15:415–421

Gros F, Naono SH (1961) Bacterial synthesis of "modified" enzymes in the presence of a pyrimidine analogue. In: Harris RJC (ed) Protein biosynthesis. Academic Press, New York, p 195–205

Hastie ND, Bishop JO (1976) The expression of three abundance classes of messenger RNA in mouse tissues. Cell 9:761–774

Heifetz SR, Smith-Sonnehorn J (1981) Nucleolar changes in aging and autogamous *Paramecium tetrurelia.* Mech Ageing Develop 16:255–263

Holliday R, Tarrant GM (1972) Altered enzymes in ageing human fibroblasts. Nature 238:26–30

Hosbach HA, Kubli E (1979a) Transfer RNA in aging *Drosophila:* 1. Extent of aminoacetylation. Mech Ageing Develop 10:131–140

Hosbach HA, Kubli E (1979b) Transfer RNA in aging *Drosophila:* Isoacceptor patterns. Mech Ageing Develop 10:141–149

Johnson PF, Abelson J (1983) The yeast $tRNA^{Tyr}$ gene intron is essential for correct modification of its tRNA product. Nature 302:681–687

Johnson R, Strehler B (1972) Loss of genes coding for ribosomal RNA in aging brain cells. Nature 240:412–414

Johnson R, Chrisp C, Strehler B (1972) Selective loss of ribosomal RNA genes during the aging of post-mitotic tissues. Mech Ageing Develop 1:183–198

Kanungo MS, Koul O, Reddy KR (1970) Concomitant studies on RNA and protein synthesis in tissues of rats of various ages. Exp Gerontol 5:261–269

Katsurada A, Iritani N, Fukuda H, Noguchi T, Tanaka T (1982) Efect of aging on induction of rat liver messenger RNA activity for malic enzyme. Biochem Biphys Res Comm 109:250–255

Khasigov PZ, Glazkov VF, Delyg AA, Kuznetsov DA, Nikolaev A (1983) Age changes in metabolism of nuclear precursors of mRNA in liver and brain cortex cells of the rat. Biokhimia (Moscow) 48:179–185

Lawrence AE, Readinger JZ, Ho RW, Ackley S, Hollander M, Mays LL (1979) Age-related changes in lysine isoacceptor proportions and acylation capacity of rat liver transfer RNA's with little change in physical properties. Age 2:56–62

Lewis CM, Tarrant GM (1971) Induction of mutations by 5-fluorouracil and aminoacid analogues in *Ustilago maydis*. Mutation Res 12:349–356

Life-extention Products, Fall 1982, A Catalogue, Life Extension Foundation, Hollywood, Florida

Macieira-Coelho A, Loria E (1976) Changes in RNA synthesis during the lifespan of human fibroblasts in vitro. Gerontology 22:79:88

Mainwaring WIP (1968) Changes in ribonucleic acid metabolism of aging mouse tissue with particular reference to the prostate gland. Biochem J 110:79–86

Mays LL, Lawrence AE, Ho RW, Ackley S (1979) Age-related changes in function of transfer ribonucleic acid of rat liver. Fed Proc 38:1984–1988

Medvedev ZA (1962) Ageing at the molecular level. In: Shock NW (ed) Biological aspects of aging. Columbia Univ Press, New York, p 255–266

Medvedev ZA (1964) The nucleic acids in development and aging. Adv Gerontol Res 1:181–206

Medvedev ZA (1966) Protein biosynthesis and problems of heredity, development and ageing. Oliver & Boyd Ltd, Edinburgh

Medvedev ZA (1972) Repetition of molecular-genetic information as a possible factor in evolutionary changes of life span. Exp Gerontol 7:227–238

Medvedev ZA (1983) Developmental switches in reiterated genes may reduce the rate of age changes in DNA. Exp Gerontol 18:73–78

Medvedev ZA (1984) Age changes of chromatin. A review. Mech Ageing Develop 28:139–154

Menzies RA, Aguilar E (1973) Evidence for long-lived RNA in mammalian tissues. Mech Ageing Develop 2:349–361

Menzies RA, Mishra RK, Gold PH (1972) The turnover of ribosomal and soluble RNA in a variety of tissues of young, adult and old rats. Mech Ageing Develop 1:117:132

Miller JK, Bolla R (1980) Age-associated changes in initiation of RNA synthesis in isolated rat liver nuclei. Biochem J 188:55–60

Moffet RB, Doyle D (1981) Poly(adenylic acid)-containing and deficient messenger RNA of mouse liver. Biochem Biophys Acta 652:177–192

Mori N, Mizuno D, Goto S (1978) Increase in the ratio of 18S RNA to 28S RNA in the cytoplasm of mouse tissues during ageing. Mech Ageing Develop 8:285–297

Müller WEG, Zahn RK, Schröder CH, Arendes J (1979) Age-dependent enzymatic poly(A) metabolism in quail oviduct. Gerontology 25:61–68

Müller WEG, Zahn RK, Arendes J (1980) Age-dependent gene induction in quail oviduct X. Alterations on the post-transcriptional level (enzymic aspect). Mech Ageing Develop 14:39–48

Nandy K (1978) Centrophenoxine: Effect on aging mammalian brain. J Amer Geriatric Soc 26:74–81

Neumeister JA, Webster GC (1981) Changes in the levels and the rate of synthesis of transfer RNA in tissue of mice of different ages. Mech Ageing Develop 16:319–326

Nikitin VN, Shereshevskaya ZM (1962) Age changes of turnover of phosphorus in muscle tissues. In: Nikitin VN (ed) Proc Res Inst Biol Kharkov State Univ. Kharkov, No 33/34, p 48–55

Nokin P, Huez G, Marbaix G, Burny A, Chantrenne H (1976) Nuclear modification associated with ageing of globin messenger RNA in vivo. Eur J Biochem 62:509–517

Ono T, Cutler RG (1978) Age-dependent relaxation of gene repression: Increase of endogenous leukemia virus-related and globin-related RNA in brain and liver of mice. Proc Nat Acad Sci USA 75:4431–4435

Orgel LE, Crick FHC (1980) Selfish DNA: the ultimate parasite. Nature 284:604–607

Owenby RK, Stulberg MP, Jackobson KB (1979) Alteration of the Q family of transfer RNAs in adult *Drosophila melanogaster* as a function of age, nutrition and genotype. Mech Ageing Develop 11:91–103

Paetkau V, Coulter MB, Flintoff WF, Morgan AR (1972) Thymine-guanine base pairing during transcription of polydeoxypyrimidines in vitro. J Mol Biol 71:293–306

Pear M (1984) Revitalization therapy with live cells and RN-13. Anti-Aging News (Florida) 4:73–85

Pearson D, Shaw S (1982) Life extension. Warner Books Inc, New York

Peterson RP, Cryar JR, Gaubatz JW (1984) Constancy of ribosomal RNA genes during ageing of mouse heart cells and during serial passage of WI-38 cells. Arch Gerontol Geriatr 3:115–125

Reintz MS, Sanadi DR (1972) An aspect of translational control of protein synthesis in aging: Changes in the isoaccepting forms of tRNA in *Turbatrix aceti*. Exp Gerontol 7:119–129

Richardson A, Birchenall-Sparks MC, Staecker JL, Hardwick JP, Liu DSH (1982) The transcription of various types of ribonucleic acid by hepatocytes isolated from rats of various ages. J Gerontol 37:666–672

Rodermann von HP, Bayreuther K (1979) Verlängerung der mitotischen Lebensspanne menschlicher Glia-Zellen in einem quantitativen Zellkultursystem durch Centrophenoxin. Arzneim Forsch/Drug Res 29:124–129

Rothstein M (1982) Biochemical approaches to aging. Chapter 7. RNA. Academic Press, New York

Schneider EL, Shorr SS (1975) Alteration in cellular RNAs during the in vitro lifespan of cultured human diploid fibroblasts. Cell 6:179–184

Schröder HC, Schenk P, Baydoun H, Wagner KG, Müller WEG (1983) Occurrence of short-sized oligo(A) fragments during course of cell cycle and ageing. Arch Gerontol Geriatr 2:349–360

Semsei I, Szeszak F, Zs.-Nagy I (1982) In vivo studies on the age-dependent decrease of the rates of total and mRNA synthesis in the brain cortex of rat. Arch Gerontol Geriatr 1:29–42

Sheiness D, Puckett L, Darnell JE (1975) Possible relationship of poly(A) shortening to mRNA turnover. Proc Nat Acad Sci USA 72:1077–1081

Shereshevskaya ZM (1961) Age changes of the turnover of phosphorus-containing compounds in liver. Biochimia (Moscow) 26:708–714

Shmookler Reis RJ, Goldstein S (1980) Loss of reiterated DNA sequences during serial passage of human diploid fibroblasts. Cell 21:739–749

Singer RH, Penman S (1973) Messenger RNA in HeLa cells: kinetics of formation and decay. J Mol Biol 78:321–334

Singhal RP, Kopper RA, Nishimura S, Shindo-Okada N (1981) Modification of guanine to queuine in transfer RNAs during development and aging. Biochem Biophys Res Commun 99:120–126

Soriero AA, Talbert GB (1975) The effect of estrogen on protein and RNA concentration and on de novo synthesis of RNA in the uterus of aging ovariectomized mice. J Gerontol 30:264–268

Springgate C, Loeb LA (1975) On the fidelity of transcription by *Escherichia coli* ribonucleic acid polymerase. J Mol Biol 97:577–591

Stavitskaya LJ (1956) The age changes of ribonuclease activity in different tissues. In: Nikitin VN (ed) Proc Res Inst Biol Kharkov State Univ No 24, pp 59–63 Kharkov

Strehler BL (1977) Time, cells, aging. 2nd ed. Acad Press, New York

Strehler BL, Chang MP (1979) Loss of hybridizable ribosomal DNA from human post-mitotic tissues during aging: II. Age-dependent loss in human cerebral cortex – hippocampal and somato-sensory cortex comparison. Mech Ageing Develop 11:379–382

Strehler BL, Hendley DD, Hirsch GP (1967) Evidence on a codon restriction hypothesis of cellular differentiation. Proc Nat Acad Sci USA 57:1751–1758

Strehler BL, Hirsch GP, Gusseck D, Johnson R, Bick M (1971) Codone-restriction theory of aging and development. J Theor Biol 33:429–474

Strehler BL, Chang MP, Johnson LK (1979) Loss of hybridizable ribosomal DNA from human post-mitotic tissues during aging: I. Age-dependent loss in human myocardium. Mech Ageing Develop 11:371–378

Strniste GF, Smith DA, Hayes FN (1973) X-ray inactivation of the *Escherichia coli* deoxyribonucleic acid dependent ribonucleic acid polymerase in aqueous solution. II. Studies on initiation and fidelity of transcription. Biochemistry 12:603–608

Thakur MK (1984) Age-related changes in the structure and function of chromatin: A review. Mech Ageing Develop 27:263–286

Wattiaux JM, Mannaert L, Delcour J (1971) Protein turnover and protein synthesis following actinomycin-D injection as a function of age in *Drosophila melanogaster*. Gerontologia 17:289–299

Wright RD, Pillay DTN, Cherry J (1972/1973) Changes in leucyl tRNA species of pea leaves during senescence and after zeatin treatment. Mech Ageing Develop 1:403–412

Wulff VJ (1966) Age-associated changes in the metabolism of ribonucleic acid. In: Shock NW (ed) Perspectives in experimental gerontology. Ch. C. Thomas, Springfield, Illionois, pp 69–82

Wulff VJ, Quastler H, Sherman FG (1962) An hypothesis concerning RNA metabolism and aging. Proc Nat Acad Sci USA 48:1373–1375

Wulff V, Quastler H, Sherman FG, Samis HV (1965) The effect of specific activity of H^3-cytidine on its incorporation into tissues of young and old mice. J Gerontol 20:34–40

Wulff VJ, Samis HV, Falzone JA (1966) The metabolism of ribonucleic acid in young and old rodents. Adv Gerontol Res 2:37–76

Yavich MP (1981) Ratio of the amounts of poly A^+ and poly A^- mRNA fractions in the myocardium and the span of poly A^+ mRNA. Kardiologiia (Moscow) 21:91–94

Yavich MP, Lerman MI, Meerson FZ (1978) Rate of synthesis of RNA and proteins in the heart muscle of rat depending on age of animals. Zhur Obshchei Biol (Moscow) 39:466–473

Zs.-Nagy I, Nagy K (1980) On the role of cross-linking of cellular proteins in aging. Mech Ageing Develop 14:245–251

Aging and Drug Testing in Cultured Normal Human Cells

L. HAYFLICK [1]

Introduction

Several years ago Moorhead and I showed that cultured human cells have a finite capacity for replication in vitro (Hayflick and Moorhead 1961). We showed that embryo-derived fibroblasts which have the greatest capacity for replication in vitro undergo 50 ± 10 population doublings before division ceases in about 10–12 months. We divided these events into three phases. Phase I represents the primary culture; phase II, the active replication period; and phase III, the period when cell replication slows, ceases, and ultimately ends with complete cell degeneration and death.

After having ruled out, experimentally, trivial explanations for these events (which were historicaly invoked as the cause) we put forth the notion that the phase III phenomenon might represent aging at the cellular level (Hayflick and Moorhead 1961; Hayflick 1965). Research on this phenomenon conducted in the ensuing years by us and by many others has confirmed the finitude of normal cell replication and has substantially supported our suggestion that the phenomenon represents aging at the cellular level (Hayflick 1976, 1977, 1979, 1980 a–c).

Among the literally thousands of studies that have been done with this in vitro system, several salient observations have been made that bear on our interpretation that the phase III phenomenon represents aging at the cellular level and that its continued exploitation will enhance our understanding of biogerontology. The most important observations using this system, and made in the last 20 years, include the following:

1. There is an inverse relationship between donor age and population doubling potential, first demonstrated by us and later confirmed and greatly extended by others. This inverse relationship has now been shown to occur in normal human cells derived from lung (Hayflick 1965), skin (Martin et al. 1970; Schneider and Mitsui 1976; Goldstein et al. 1978; Vracko and McFarland 1980), liver (LeGuilly et al. 1973), arterial smooth muscle (Bierman 1978; Grunewald et al. 1983), lens cells (Tassin et al. 1979), and T-lymphocytes (Walford et al. 1981).

2. More than 60 increments and 50 decrements have been shown to occur in cultured human fibroblasts as they progress from phase II to phase III (see Hayflick, 1980 a for complete list with references). These include changes in lipid content and synthesis; carbohydrate utilization; protein content, synthesis, and

[1] Center for Gerontological Studies, University of Florida, 3357 GPA, Gainesville, Florida 32611, USA

Drugs and Aging
Ed. by D. Platt

breakdown; RNA and DNA content, synthesis, and turnover; enzyme activity and synthesis; cell cycle kinetics; morphology, ultrastructure, and cell architecture; and incorporation and stimulation.

Of great importance is the finding that many of these changes that occur in vitro before and during phase III are identical to similar changes recognized as characteristic of aging in intact humans and animals. These findings substantiate our contention that the finite capacity for replication by cultured normal cells may not, per se, be as important in understanding in vivo aging as the plethora of biochemical, physiological, and morphological changes that precede it (Hayflick 1977, 1979, 1980a–c).

It is important to note that, contrary to the misconception that fibroblast behavior may be unrelated to age changes because fibroblasts are not functional cells, is this catalogue of 110 functional properties that do change as fibroblasts age in culture. One, collagen production (Houck et al. 1971), is also a specialized physiological function.

3. The in vivo counterpart of in vitro experiments where normal cells are, respectively, transplanted or subcultivated, show identical results. That is, normal cells have a finite capacity to replicate under both conditions. These in vivo results effectively make untenable the notion that in vitro conditions are likely to be found which permit the unlimited replication of normal cells. Even when normal cells are transplanted in vivo, where ideal conditions would be expected to occur, the phase III phenomenon is expressed (Hayflick 1977, 1980a).

4. Normal human cells that are frozen at particular population doubling levels are capable of "remembering" that doubling level and, when thawed, resume doublings until the maximum number is reached (Hayflick and Moorhead 1961; Hayflick 1965). Ampules of one normal human diploid cell strain developed by us in 1962 (WI-38) have been frozen for 22 years and still accurately retain their memory of the population doubling level at which they were frozen. This is the longest period of time that living normal human cells have ever been frozen.

5. There is increasingly compelling evidence for the notion that there may be a direct relationship between species life span and population doubling potential. Published results suggest that the population doubling potential of cultured normal fibroblasts decreases as a function of life span when ten species are compared (Hayflick 1980; Rohme 1981) (Fig. 1).

6. The latent period, that is the time necessary for cell migration over a unit distance from cultured tissue explants, increases as a function of donor age (reviewed in Hayflick 1977).

7. The population doubling potential of cultured normal human fibroblasts is significantly diminished from that found with age-matched controls when cells are grown from patients with progeria, Werner's syndrome, and Cockayne's syndrome. These conditions are believed to typify accelerated aging (reviewed in Hayflick 1977).

8. One of the major theories of aging involves decreased, or less efficient, mechanisms for repair of DNA damage as a function of age. In 1974 Hart and Setlow made the important observation that cultured skin fibroblasts from long-lived species have a greater capacity to repair UV-induced damage than do cells from shorter-lived species. Later they showed that the average amount of un-

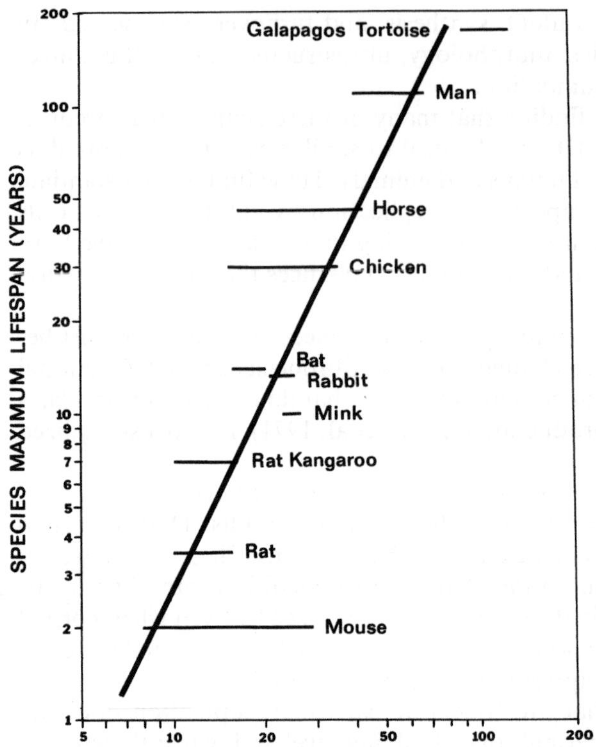

Fig. 1. Fibroblasts from the embryos of ten different species multiply in culture to a maximum number of population doublings that is roughly proportional to the life span for that species. Galapagos tortoise cells were derived from a juvenile animal

scheduled DNA synthesis decreases as cultured human cells approach phase III. (reviewed in Hayflick 1980).

Although the aforementioned classes of observations are among the more important that form the background for the field of cytogerontology, they are by no means the only ones that have been made.

Theoretical Basis for Experimental Design

The existing knowledge base in cytogerontology is now emerging from a decade or more of descriptive findings to a stage of hypothesis testing. Now that the phase III phenomenon has been established to be an intrinsic cell property and almost certainly associated with aging, this base of descriptive findings has created exciting possibilities for hypothesis testing. Thus the goal of testing theories of aging becomes possible, especially as it applies to vertebrate cells generally and to human cells specifically. These theories have been reduced in the past decade or so to six or eight nonmutually exclusive hypotheses, most of which are based on changes in the expression of information-containing molecules. These theories have been reviewed elsewhere (Hayflick 1984a).

In recent years our laboratory studies have been directed toward (a) identification of the chromosome(s) or gene loci associated with cellular senescence in the cultured normal human fibroblast strain WI-38 and (b) determination of whether these same loci are also implicated in the transformed state (immortality) of permanent cell lines.

This approach follows from previous work that led us to conclude that the chronometer(s) governing the occurrence of phase III are located in the cell nucleus.

Theories of the role of the genome in aging can be divided into two general categories. The first category considers aging as a programmed genetic event caused by (a) the active expression of specific "aging genes," (b) the active expression of "longevity genes," or (c) the passive exhaustion of accurate genetic information. Within this group of theories the fundamental cause of cellular senescence would involve mostly nuclear rather than cytoplasmic events.

The second category of theories considers senescence to be the result of progressive damage to organelles or errors in molecules not associated with the genetic apparatus. Thus, decrements that occur mostly in the cytoplasm are encompassed by these theories.

Cell Hybridization and the Location of the Chronometer

Littlefield (1973) was the first to probe cellular aging in normal human diploid fibroblasts by the use of cell hybridization techniques. He fused pairs of young and old human fibroblasts and pairs of old human fibroblasts, hoping to observe complimentation and prolongation of in vitro life span. He did not observe this and concluded that the senescent phenotype behaved as if it were dominant in all combinations of the hybrid colonies that he examined. Later Hoehn et al. (1978) fused young human fibroblasts from different sources and with slightly different total population doubling potentials. They concluded that senescence behaved codominantly. Hybrids displayed growth potentials intermediate between the parental cells.

Norwood et al. (1974) and Rabinovitch and Norwood (1980) reached essentially the same conclusion using heterokaryons composed of senescent and young human diploid fibroblasts. It should be noted, however, that one of the four cell strains that Norwood et al. examined was karyotypically 47,XXY, and therefore not normal diploid. Rather than measuring in vitro life span, they examined ^{3}H-thymidine incorporation in di- and polykaryons. Again, the senescent phenotype was observed to be dominant. Hybrid cells consisting of young and old cells behaved as if they were senescent and failed to incorporate ^{3}H-thymidine. In all of these studies, the results are consistent with both group of theories described above.

Wright and Hayflick (1975a, b) and Muggleton-Harris and Hayflick (1976) were the first to provide an answer to the question of the cytoplasmic or nuclear location of the initiating events of the phase III phenomenon. Proof of the location of the initial events would serve to distinguish between the two main categories of theories of cellular aging. We found that fusion of cytochalasin B induced anucleate cells (cytoplasts) obtained from young or old human diploid fibroblasts with young or old whole cells failed to alter the time of expected occurrence of phase III in the whole cell.

Our second study (Muggleton-Harris and Hayflick 1976) employed reconstructed cells composed of cytoplasts and karyoplasts from young and old cells. These studies confirmed the dominance of the senescent nucleus. However, cytoplasts derived from senescent cells in this study contained factors which affected the doubling potential of young nuclei. Thus, in vitro aging of human diploid fibroblasts may involve a combination of several processes.

Studies now in progress in our laboratory involve mass nuclear transplantations and biochemical selection of appropriately reconstructed cells (Wright and Hayflick 1975a, b; Muggleton-Harris and Hayflick 1976; Ringertz and Savage 1976; Lucas and Kates 1977). We anticipate that results of experiments now underway should provide an unequivocal answer to the relative contribution of nucleus and cytoplasm in the process of cellular aging. However, our studies conducted to date confirm a major role for the nucleus in cellular senescence.

The ability of immortal cell lines to rescue normal human diploid fibroblasts from cellular senescence has been the subject of many investigations (Rabinovitch and Norwood 1980; Norwood et al. 1975; Stein and Yanishevsky 1979; Muggleton-Harris and Palombo 1979; Muggleton-Harris and DeSimone 1980; Nette et al. 1982). These fully transformed cells, when fused to phase III cells, seem to possess the ability to induce DNA synthesis in the senescent genome (Rabinovitch and Norwood 1980; Norwood et al. 1975).

From cell reconstruction experiments, it was reported that either the nucleus or the cytoplasm of the transformed cell can initiate DNA synthesis in senescent human cells (Nette et al. 1982). Initiation of DNA synthesis, however, does not mean cell proliferation as exemplified by the reactivation and initiation of DNA synthesis which occurs in chick erythrocyte nuclei introduced into L cell cytoplasts (Lipisch et al. 1978). These reconstructed cells do not divide. It does seem, however, that the proliferation of fusion products between normal senescent and transformed cells, or cell parts, may occur (Muggleton-Harris and Palumbo 1979; Muggleton-Harris and DeSimone 1980) but with a low (2% or less) frequency (Muggleton-Harris and DeSimone 1980; Bunn and Tarrant 1980).

When cells that are incompletely transformed (immortal but not malignant) are fused to phase III cells, the senescent nucleus is dominant and DNA synthesis is inhibited in the immortal cell (Stein and Yanishevsky 1979).

Our current goals are twofold: First, we are attempting to determine which gene loci in human cells are responsible for governing cellular senescence (phase III). Second, we are attempting to determine which loci are associated with the ability of transformed cells to replicate indefinitely. The chromosomes in phase II normal human cells that suppress or reduce tumorigenicity in heteroploid human or rodent cell hybrids have been identified (Klinger et al. 1978).

Our studies are directed toward a determination of the location and mechanism which limits the replication of normal human cells and which, by inference, imparts unlimited replicative potential to transformed cells. The outcome of these investigations is expected to provide insights into the role of the genome in cellular aging. The role of the genome in aging may be actively expressed as a program similar to the developmental program or passively expressed as an accumulation of damage to the genome.

Drug Testing In Vitro

The use of cultured cells for the study of pharmacological and toxicological drug effects is almost as old as the field of cell culture itself. In 1895, Ringer showed that an excised frog's heart, which was known to stop beating in a 0.75% solution of NaCl, would beat for a long time if perfused with a fluid that also contained calcium and potassium chloride in concentrations known to occur in blood. Ringer also found that although each cation was toxic when present alone, toxicity could be neutralized when the correct physiological concentration of any one of the other cations was introduced. Thus was born the concept of a "balanced" salt solution where one cation is able to antagonize or neutralize the toxic effects of another. Ringer's experiments also gave birth to the concept of the in vitro testing of chemical compounds.

Despite this observation very little was done to exploit its potential because cell and tissue culturists were preoccupied in the first half of this century with refining the techniques of cell culture and the perfection of better growth media. It was not until 1949, when Enders, Weller, and Robbins discovered that the poliomyelitis virus could be grown in cultured nonneural cells, that cell culture began a period of explosive growth. That growth included exploitation of cultured cells as substrates for evaluation of the action and toxicity of drugs.

In the 35 years since the renaissance in cultured cells has taken place, considerable effort has been directed toward the use of in vitro systems in understanding drug action and toxicity. Two examples of these efforts of the many that could be given can be found in the *Collected Proceedings of the First and Second Working Conferences of Toxicity Testing In Vitro, 1975/1976,* edited by Berky and Sherrod (1977) and *Cellular Systems for Toxicity Testing,* edited by Williams et al. (1983).

In the view of Ekwall (1983) only about 50 laboratories throughout the world have been testing general toxicity using cell cultures. Some have used differentiated cells such as liver cells, neurons, blood cells, and lung cells. Most screening has been done with less differentiated cells to test for toxicity of plastics, dental materials, minerals, tobacco components, reuse water, metals, solvents, drugs, and chemicals (Ekwall 1983). In spite of the work that has been done, few validation studies have been undertaken, so that in vitro methods for general toxicity measurements cannot be considered valid, as are in vitro genetic toxicity studies.

Ekwell (1983) points out that some recent trends have developed in which the success of mutagenicity screening in vitro has created expectations that tests for general toxicity will soon be forthcoming. Also, interest in in vitro drug testing has been stimulated not only because the technique has been shown to have merit and is economical but also because drug testing in animals is drawing more fire on ethical grounds. Witness the current efforts to replace the Draize test. To these events one must add the relatively recent realization that calls into question past practices of only evaluating the efficacy and safety of drugs in young adults when most drugs are consumed by the elderly. Taken together these circumstances have provided the impetus for more serious evaluation of in vitro systems in analyzing the pharmacodynamics and pharmacokinetics of drug action and safety.

Drug Use in the Elderly

In many developed countries about 11% of the population is over the age of 65, but they account for 25–40% of all drug prescriptions (Kovar 1977; Vestal 1982; Grahnen 1985). Most of these prescriptions are for drugs with long-lasting action and, since many elderly people suffer from more than one ailment, multiple drug use is common. Bandera et al. (1983, 1984) found that in homes for the aged more than three-quarters of the residents receive some kind of pharmaceutical therapy and almost one-half receive at least three different drugs per day. The use of multiple drugs is so common that it is referred to as polypharmacy.

If one adds to this the fact that elderly persons respond to many drugs differently than do younger people for whom drugs are generally designed, then it is not surprising to learn that persons over the age of 65 have the highest incidence of adverse drug reactions. Little more needs to be said in order to justify the fact that the efficacy and safety of drugs administered to the elderly is a subject that has been neglected far too long.

Basic Biology of Cultured Cells

The study of drug reactions or, for that matter, the study of virtually anything in cell cultures presupposes an understanding of the fundamental biology of cultured cells. Despite the fact that this statement may be self-evident, my observations, especially those made over the past 10 years, persuade me to believe that the cell culture literature is virtually unintelligible because of major conceptual errors that are further compounded by the use of identical terms with multiple definitions. I will consider that my assignment here has been met if I succeed in making plain these fundamental concepts and clarifying some troublesome definitions.

It is my belief that a substantial proportion of the cancer research which is now enjoying dramatic growth because of studies on oncogenes and proto-oncogenes in cell cultures has been seriously compromised because of the failure of its practitioners to appreciate fundamental concepts in the behavior of cultured cells. I hope that my discussion of this regrettable situation in cancer biology will serve to prevent its occurrence in the emerging field of drug testing in vitro.

The fundamental phenomenon to which I refer, and upon whose understanding so much depends, was originally called an "alteration" 25 years ago (Hayflick and Moorhead 1961) but is now labelled "transformation."

How Cells are Cultured

Millions of cells can be released from virtually any piece of tissue, and from virtually any animal species, usually by use of a substance called "trypsin." The name is misleading because the substance is an aqueous extract of hog pancreas and therefore a mixture of many enzymes. The released cells are then placed in a culture vessel with growth medium, incubated at 37 °C if they are derived from homoiotherms and, after a few days, observed to have replicated.

The first vessel or vessels into which the original cells are placed is referred to as the primary culture. This definition was once important because primary cell cultures were once the only class of cultures permitted to be used for the production of human virus vaccines. The term, therefore, had not only an operational definition but a legal definition as well (United States Public Health Service Regulations, 1964). I am pleased to report that primary cultures are no longer the only cultures permitted to be used for the production of human biologicals (Hayflick 1968 a, b). Many of the world's human virus vaccines are now made in our normal human diploid cell strain WI-38 or its imitators (Hayflick 1984 b).

Once cells have divided in the primary culture to the point where the entire surface of the vessel floor is covered with cells, division stops. This condition is referred to as a confluent culture. If normal tissue is used to initiate a culture the normal cells derived from that tissue will stop dividing when the cells have replicated to the point where they are all touching neighboring cells. The cue thus received is a signal to normal cells to stop dividing. If additional cells are desired it is necessary to provide them with additional surface. The procedure by which this is accomplished is called a "subcultivation" or, in laboratory jargon, a "split."

Subcultivation

A subcultivation is accomplished first by removing the spent growth medium. The cells remain attached to the vessel floor and must then be released by the introduction of trypsin. The resulting cell suspension is then centrifuged, the trypsin discarded, and the cells resuspended in fresh growth medium. This suspension is then divided into two equal parts, placed into two new daughter culture vessels, and incubated again. After a few days the cells will once again be found to have replicated to the point of confluency, necessitating another subcultivation procedure. This process can be continued until the normal cells ultimately stop dividing, age, and die. This is the phase III phenomenon described earlier.

It is important to realize that the cell population has doubled at each subcultivation. Thus if one million cells were introduced into the primary culture, and if the vessel floor had room enough for only two million cells, the original cell population would have doubled one time. If two daughter vessels are produced from each mother vessel at every subcultivation then the cell population will be found to increase exponentially as $2^{2 \cdots n}$ each time confluency is reached. For normal human fibroblasts the number of population doublings that will occur before phase III is reached is 50 ± 10 (Hayflick and Moorhead 1961).

The Finite Replicative Capacity of Cultured Normal Cells

When we derived cells from human embryonic tissue and cultivated them in this way some 25 years ago we were surprised to find that the cells underwent about 50 population doublings over a period of about 10 months and then slowly stopped dividing. After an additional period of several weeks or months the cultures died (Hayflick and Moorhead 1961).

Our surprise arose because the dogma of that time insisted that once cultured cells were grown successfully for a few doublings, any ultimate cell death could only be blamed on errors in culture technique. The dogma further maintained that because any failure of cultured cells to replicate was due to human error, all cultured cells were intrinsically immortal. Indeed, a number of authentic immortal populations were then known and this lent support for the belief. There was, for example, the HeLa cell and the L cell which were truly immortal cell populations. We were surprised that our cultures had failed after about 50 population doublings because the identical culture conditions consistently permitted the luxurious growth of the identical cells at population doublings less than 50.

We suggested that the reason why our cultured cells consistently failed to replicate indefinitely was because they were normal cells. We further suggested that the immortal cell populations like HeLa and L cells were immortal because they were abnormal in one or more important properties (Hayflick and Moorhead 1961; Hayflick 1965).

The Transformation of "Transformation"

We called those cell populations that had properties identical to the cells composing the tissue of origin "cell strains" and the immortal cell populations having abnormal properties, "cell lines" (Hayflick and Moorhead 1961). The phenomenon by which a cell strain becomes a cell line we called an "alteration." Not only are these terms not used by others to describe these phenomena but an understanding of the phenomena has become hopelessly blurred in the scientific literature. The names, of course, are unimportant, but the phenomena that they describe are. I had hoped that other terms might be used to distinguish these classes of cells and the phenomenon of alteration but that has not happened. The phenomenon of alteration did come to be known as "transformation," but in the last 20 years this term has become so abused that despite its original clear definition and common usage, few now agree on what it means. The term is so abused that unless it is defined upon use it is impossible to assume safely what is meant by its user.

We proposed that the term "alteration" be used instead of "transformation" because the latter term had a precise definition in the field of bacteriology from which most cell culturists then came (Hayflick and Moorhead 1961; Hayflick 1965). We wanted the term "transformation" to be reserved in the likely event that transformation identical to pneumococcal transformation would be discovered to occur some day in eukaryotic cells. But our proposal was ignored and "transformation" became the term used allegedly to describe the event for the next 20 years. A few years ago transformation identical to pneumococcal transformation was reported to occur in mammalian cells. Of course, a new term had to be invented for a phenomenon that already exists in microbiology (Murray et al. 1981). The new term chosen was "transfection," which allegedly means in cell biology what transformation means in bacteriology!

The original meaning given by us to the term "alteration," and now subsumed by its synonym "transformation," is an in vitro phenomenon in which a normal cell population that we call a cell strain acquires abnormal properties such as immortality, aneuploidy, ability to grow in suspension culture (anchorage independence), and, frequently, ability to grow as a tumor in inbred or immunologically compromised animals (Hayflick and Moorhead 1961; Hayflick 1965). The transformed population we called a "cell line." Although not always demonstrable, a transformation implies the acquisition of cancer cell properties by a cell population previously shown to be normal. These fundamental concepts and definitions of terms are not generally used in the current scientific literature. They will be used here because the clarity of understanding of these essential concepts and definitions is paramount in appreciating how cell cultures can best be used in the assessment of drug activity in vitro.

It is important to stress that the transformation phenomenon does not result in the sudden acquisition by normal cells of the full complement of abnormal properties. Major features such as immortality, aneuploidy, anchorage independence, and growth in proper host animals occur in different sequences in different transformations.

I will give here one example of literally hundreds that could be given to illustrate the misleading way in which the transformation phenomenon is currently abused in the literature.

Transformation is, of course, at the core of all fundamental research into the cause of cancer. That is, how is a normal cell converted into a cancer cell? This question obviously presupposes that all cancer researchers who study why or how normal cells become cancer cells begin their work with normal cells. Yet that is simply not true. The *alleged* normal cells most frequently used today internationally for transformation studies are not *normal* cells at all. They are already transformed. In fact, they are cancer cells or abnormal cells even before the army of investigators who use them try to transform them to what they already are – cancer cells. These notorious rodent cell lines are BHK-21, Balb 3T3, and C3H10T1/2.

In my view more than 75% of all transformation studies reported in the literature today are conducted using these cell lines, which are already proven to be abnormal or cancer cells. The most surprising fact is that in the case of Balb 3T3 proof that these cells form vasoformative sarcomas or malignant hemangioendotheliomas was published almost 10 years ago. Did these papers appear in obscure journals? Not unless you call *Science* and *Research Cancer* obscure journals (Boone 1975; Boone et al. 1976). In spite of this 3T3, BHK-21, and C3H10T1/2 are referred to frequently in literally hundreds of published papers as normal cells. They are not. No self-respecting mouse or hamster has in its anatomy a cell that has the characteristics of 3T3, BHK-21, or C3H10T1/2. These cell lines are, therefore, the archtypical artifact. To work with them is to abandon terrestrial biology in favor of Martian biology. Publication of work using such cell populations for transformation and other studies should be restricted to exobiology journals.

This fundamental misconception, or self-delusion, is one of the most serious impediments to the conduct of proper cancer research today. It has compromised virtually all results and made the interpretation of experiments almost impossible. The rectification of this intellectual folly would be equivalent to a major breakthrough in cancer research without the necessity for the expenditure of more money or the exertion of greater effort. The situation is even more disheartening when one realizes that *normal* cultured rodent cell strain populations *do* exist. In fact they have been grown for decades even before the first transformed rodent cell line was discovered in the 1940s. Why, then, are normal cell strains rarely used for transformation studies when they are the obvious cell of choice? Frankly, I do not know. I can only guess that there is a mistaken belief on the part of newcomers to the field that normal cells do not exist or that they are difficult to culture. Neither is true.

Nevertheless, there is hope that the aforementioned considerations finally are coming to be appreciated. The National Institute of Environmental Health Sciences, National Institutes of Health in the USA has very recently asked for research to be done on the development and utilization of a human cell-mediated system where primary human liver cells are to be used for the metabolic activation of chemicals and cocultivated with human target cells to be used to detect genetic damage caused by metabolic intermediates. They also seek research on the development and utilization of a human cell system for the detection of genotoxic chemicals in which metabolic activation of the chemicals and measurement of genetic endpoints can be accomplished in the same cells.

Cultured Normal Cells do Exist

My purpose in coming down as hard as I have on the use of transformed cells is to persuade the pharmacological community not to follow the poor example set by the cancer biologists. The testing of drugs in vitro is on the threshold of increasing dramatically. I would assume that pharmacologists are interested in understanding the effect of drugs on normal cells and not on cells that lack any in vivo counterpart. It requires no great leap of intellect to argue that if cell cultures are to be used for drug testing, logic dictates that those cultures consist of normal cells.

As indicated earlier, normal cells can be grown easily in cell culture. Not only can normal rodent and other animal cells be cultured but normal human cells can be cultured as well. Indeed, normal human cells have been cultured in hundreds of laboratories for almost 25 years (Hayflick and Moorhead 1961). We know more about the biology of one normal human cell strain, WI-38, developed by us in 1962, than we know about any other cultured cell population. WI-38 is the most highly characterized cell population in the world. It is a fibroblast population but other kinds of normal human cells can also be grown in culture. In spite of this the use of normal human cells for transformation studies is virtually nonexistent. The reason for this cannot be satisfactorily explained. It is almost as though cancer biologists are much more interested in studying and eliminating cancer in rodents than they are in studying and eliminating cancer in humans.

It is often argued that rodent cell populations are studied because human cells are very difficult to transform. Rodent cell lines are easy to transform, of course, because they are already transformed! It is a bit like the drunkard who was found by a policeman to be crawling on his hands and knees one night under a lamppost. When asked by the officer what he was doing, the drunkard answered, "I'm looking for my wallet." "Where did you lose it?" asked the policeman. "Oh, I lost it down the road about fifty meters" said the drunk. "Then why are you looking for it here?", the policeman asked. "Because the light is better" replied the drunk.

The major advantages of using normal human cells for drug evaluation is that they are normal and they are human, two important facts that have not been appreciated by cancer biologists and others who continue to use abnormal cell lines. Nor is the use of normal-cell lines limited to monolayer cultures. The technology for maintaining organ cultures and true tissue cultures is now sufficiently well advanced to make these systems attractive possibilities for the study of drug action on organized tissues. Normal human cell populations either derived from old donors or in the senescent phase from young donors represent likely opportunities for drug testing at a time when increasing pressure is being applied by national control authorities to evaluate drugs on the population that uses them the most – the elderly.

There are, of course, circumstances in which abnormal human cell populations should be used for drug evaluation. These would be cell populations derived from individuals with heritable disorders whose flawed metabolic expression is displayed in individual cultured cells. There are hundreds of these anomalies from which cell populations can be obtained either directly from the afflicted individuals or from several cell banks located throughout the world.

Another example of opportunities for drug testing in vitro bears on the search for anticancer drugs. In recent years an assay called the clonogenic assay has come into favor. This assay is based on the reasonable argument that stem cells are responsible for tumor repopulation after therapy and metastatic growth (Buick and Pollak 1984). When human tumor cells are cloned they frequently give rise to colonies with substantial proliferative capacity compared with other cells in the population. It is these cells that are considered to be the most important target cells for the assessment of anticancer compounds. This view is predicated on the supposition that the cells that are capable of the largest proliferative capacity in vitro may be the most important cells in determining growth properties of the tumor in vivo. Note that the cell populations are not human cell lines but primary human tumor tissue removed from patients and tested in the clonogenic assay as described.

Special Considerations of Drug Testing In Vitro

General toxicity, that is acute lethality, organ-specific toxicity, and toxicity relative to other drugs must be distinguished from long-term toxicity or mutagenesis, carcinogenesis, and teratogenesis (Berky and Sherrod 1977). The efficiency of a drug may depend on the administration of a very high dose for a short period of time, as in the case of broad spectrum antibiotics, or a high dose for years, as in the case of tranquilizers. Compounds may be given by different routes. All of these variables must be considered when designing and assessing the performance of drugs in in vitro tests.

Participants at the First and Second Working Conference of Toxicity Testing In Vitro (Berky and Sherrod 1977) have summarized their findings as follows: *With respect to general toxicity testing of drugs, current in vivo systems are relatively low in cost, simple, and efficient. They offer a wide variety of proven endpoints. Cell culture methods appear to have no advantages.* This statement was made before the current pressure by antivivisectionists resulted in serious efforts to replace animals in tests similar to the Draize test. Valid and feasible in vitro test systems exist for testing the potential mutagenicity of chemical agents. The validity of these tests have been demonstrated in *Salmonella, E. coli,* repair mutants, yeast, and to a lesser degree mammalian cells. A feasible system does not yet exist for rapid in vitro carcinogenicity testing. However, a reasonable correlation exists between carcinogenicity and mutagenicity.

In order to give credibility to the use of in vitro systems as valid tools for the in vivo assessment of drugs and chemicals, it must be shown that known compounds toxic to humans correlate with in vitro tests.

Conclusions

The phenomenon of aging has been shown to occur in cultured normal human cells. Among the many age-correlated changes that occur in these cells are (a) an inverse relationship between donor age and the number of population doublings that normal cultured cells will undergo, (b) over 125 incremental and decremental changes that occur in many areas of cell biochemistry and cell behavior as normal human cells age in vitro, (c) inverse correlation of cell migration from cultured tissue explants with donor age, (d) reduction of the population doubling potential of cell cultures derived from patients with syndromes mimicking age acceleration, such as progeria, as compared with age-matched controls (e) a direct correlation between species life span and population doubling potential of their cultured fibroblasts, and (f) greater capacity of the cultured cells of long-lived species to repair UV irradiation-induced DNA damage, as compared with cells of less long-lived species.

Current research is directed toward a determination of the gene loci in cultured normal human cells (WI-38) that are responsible for governing cell senescence and those loci that govern immortality in transformed cells.

Drug testing in vitro must avoid the use of transformed or abnormal cells whose in vivo counterparts do not exist. Highly characterized normal human cells are available and are ideal candidates for developing in vitro drug assay systems.

References

Bandera R, Bollini P, Garattini S (1984) Long and short acting benzodiazepines in the elderly: kinetic differences and clinical relevance. Curr Med Res Opin, 8 Suppl 4:94–107

Berky J, Sherrod PC (eds) (1977) Short term in vitro testing for carcinogenesis, mutagenesis, and toxicity. Collected Proceedings of the First and Second Working Conferences of Toxicity Testing In Vitro, 1975–1976. Franklin Institute, Philadelphia

Bierman EL (1978) The effect of donor age on the in vitro lifespan of cultured human arterial smooth-muscle cells. In Vitro 14:951–955

Boone CW (1975) Malignant hemangioendotheliomas produced by subcutaneous inoculation of Balb/3T3 cells attached to glass beads. Science 188:68–70

Boone CW, Takeichi N, Paranjpe M (1976) Vasoformative sarcomas arising from Balb/3T3 cells attached to solid substrates. Cancer Res 36:1626–1633

Buick RN, Pollak MN (1984) Perspectives on clonogenic tumor cells, stem cells, and oncogenes. Cancer Res 44:4909–4918

Bunn CL, Tarrant GM (1980) Limited lifespan in somatic cell hybrids and cybrids. Exp Cell Res 127:385–396

Ekwall B (1983) Screening of toxic compounds in mammalian cell cultures. Ann NY Acad Sci 407:64–77

Goldstein S, Moerman EJ, Soeldner JS, Gleason RE, Barnett DM (1978) Chronologic and physiological age affect replicative lifespan of fibroblasts from diabetics, prediabetics, and normal donors. Science 199:781–782

Grahnen A (1985) Drug metabolism and actions in the aged. In: Hartz S (ed) Nutrients, medicines, and aging. (in press)

Grunewald J, Mey J, Schonleben W, Hauss J, Hauss WH (1983) Cultivated human arterial smooth muscle cells. The effect of donor age, blood pressure, diabetes and smoking on in vitro growth. Path Biol 31:819–823

Hart RW, Setlow RB (1974) Correlation between deoxyribonucleic acid excision-repair and lifespan in a number of mammalian species. Proc Natl Acad Sci USA 71:2169–2173

Hayflick L (1965) The limited in vitro lifetime of human diploid cell strains. Exp Cell Res 37:614–636

Hayflick L (1968 a) Cell substrates for human virus vaccine preparation – general comments. Natl Canc Inst, Monograph No. 29:83–91

Hayflick L (1968 b) An analysis of the potential oncogenicity of human virus vaccine cell substrates. Proc Symp on Oncogenicity of Virus Vaccines. Yugoslav Acad Sci and Arts, p 39–46

Hayflick L (1976) The cell biology of human aging. New Eng J Med 295:1302–1308

Hayflick L (1977) The cellular basis for biological aging. In: Finch C, Hayflick L (eds) Handbook of the biology of aging. Van Nostrand Reinhold, New York, p 159–186

Hayflick L (1979) Progress in cytogerontology. Mech Ageing Dev, Special volume on Research Frontiers in Biological Ageing Research 9:393–408

Hayflick L (1980 a) Cell aging. In: Eisdorfer C (ed) Annual review of gerontology and geriatrics. Springer, New York, p 26–68

Hayflick L (1980 b) The cell biology of human aging. Scientific American 242 no. 1:58–65

Hayflick L (1980 c) Recent advances in the cell biology of aging. Mech Ageing Dev 14:59–79

Hayflick L (1984 a) Theories of biological aging. In: Andres R, Bierman E, Hazzard W (eds) Principles of geriatric medicine. McGraw Hill, New York, p 9–21

Hayflick L (1984 b) The coming of age of WI-38. In: Maramorosch K (ed) Advances in cell culture, vol 3. Academic, New York, p 303–316

Hayflick L, Moorhead PS (1961) The serial cultivation of human diploid cell strains. Exp Cell Res 25:585–621

Hoehn H, Bryant EM, Martin GM (1978) The replicative lifespans of euploid hybrids derived from short-lived and long-lived human skin fibroblast cultures. Cytogenet Cell Genet 21:282–295

Houck JC, Sharma VK, Hayflick L (1971) Functional failures of cultured human diploid fibroblasts after continued population doublings. Proc Soc Exptl Biol and Med 137:331–333

Klinger HP, Baim AS, Eun CK, Shows TB, Ruddle FH (1978) Human chromosomes which affect tumorigenicity in hybrids of diploid human with heteroploid human or rodent cells. Cytogenet Cell Genet 22:245–249

Kovar M (1977) Health of the elderly and use of health services. Public Health Res 92:9–19

LeGuilly Y, Simon M, Lenoir P, Bourel M (1973) Long-term culture of human adult liver cells: Morphological changes related to in vitro senescence and effect of donor's age on growth potential. Gerontologia 19:303–313

Lipsich LA, Lucas JJ, Kates JR (1978) Cell cycle dependence of the reactivation of chick erythrocyte nuclei after transplantation into mouse L 929 cell cytoplasts. J Cell Physiol 97:199–208

Littlefield JW (1973) Attempted hybridizations with senescent human fibroblasts. J Cell Physiol 82:129–132

Lucas J, Kates J (1977) Nuclear transplantation with mammalian cells. In: Prescott DM (ed) Methods in cell biology, vol 15. Academic, New York, p 359–370

Martin GM, Sprague CA, Epstein CJ (1970) Replicative lifespan of cultivated human cells. Effect of donor's age, tissue, and genotype. Lab Invest 23:86–92

Muggleton-Harris AL, DeSimone DW (1980) Replicative potentials of various fusion products between WI-38 and SV_{40} transformed WI-38 cells and their components. Somat Cell Genet 6:689–698

Muggleton-Harris AL, Hayflick L (1976) Cellular aging studied by the reconstruction of replicating cells from nuclei and cytoplasms isolated from normal human diploid cells. Exp Cell Res 103:321–330

Muggleton-Harris AL, Palumbo M (1979) Nucleo-cytoplasmic interactions in experimental binucleates formed from normal and transformed components. Somat Cell Genet 5:397–407

Murray MJ, Shilo B-Z, Shih C, Weinberg RA (1981) Three different human tumor cell lines contain different oncogenes. Cell 25:355–361

Nette EG, Sit HL, King DW (1982) Reactivation of DNA synthesis of aging diploid human skin fibroblasts by fusion with mouse L karyoplasts, cytoplasts and whole L cells. Mech Ageing Dev 18:75–87

Norwood TH, Pendergrass WR, Sprague CA, Martin GM (1974) Dominance of the senescent phenotype in heterokaryons between replicative and post-replicative human fibroblast-like cells. Proc Natl Acad Sci USA 71:2231–2235

Norwood TH, Pendergrass WE, Martin GM (1975) Reinitiation of DNA synthesis in senescent human fibroblasts upon fusion with cells of unlimited growth potential. J Cell Biol 64:551–556

Rabinovitch PS, Norwood TH (1980) Comparative heterokaryon study of cellular senescence and the serum-deprived state. Exp Cell Res 130:101–109

Ringer S (1895) Further observations regarding the antagonism between calcium salts and sodium, potassium and ammonium salts. J Physiol 18:425–429

Ringertz NR, Savage RE (1976) Cell hybrids. Academic, New York

Rohme D (1981) Evidence for a relationship between longevity of mammalian species and life spans of normal fibroblasts in vitro and erythrocytes in vivo. Proc Nat Acad Sci USA 78:5009–5013

Schneider EL, Mitsui Y (1976) The relationship between in vitro cellular aging and in vivo human aging. Proc Nat Acad Sci USA 73:3584–3588

Stein G, Yanishevsky RM (1979) Entry into S phase is inhibited in two immortal cell lines fused to senescent human diploid cells. Exp Cell Res 120:155–165

Tassin J, Malaise E, Courtois Y (1979) Human lens cells have an in vitro proliferative capacity inversely proportional to the donor age. Exp Cell Res 123:388–392

United States Public Health Regulations: Biological Products, Title 42, Part 73, Publication No. 437, United States Department of Health Education and Welfare, Revised 1964

Vestal RB (1982) Pharmacology and aging. J Am Geriatrics Soc 32:144–149

Vracko R, McFarland BM (1980) Lifespan of diabetic and non-diabetic fibroblasts in vitro. Exp Cell Res 129:345–350

Walford RL, Jawaid SQ, Naeim F (1981) Evidence for in vitro senescence of T-lymphocytes cultured from normal human peripheral blood. Age 4:67–70

Williams GM, Dunkel VC, Ray VA (eds) (1983) Cellular systems for toxicity testing, vol 407. Ann NY Acad Sci

Wright WE, Hayflick L (1975a) Use of biochemical lesions for selection of human cells with hybrid cytoplasms. Proc Natl Acad Sci USA 72:1812–1816

Wright WE, Hayflick L (1975b) Contributions of cytoplasmic factors to in vitro cellular senescence. Fed Proc 34:76–79

Aging, Cancer, and the Life Span of Cells in Vitro

A. Macieira-Coelho and B. Azzarone [1]

Relationship Between Growth Potential in Vitro and Aging

Several experiments support the idea that there is a relationship between the limited life span of human fibroblasts and aging of the donor. The first claim was published by Hayflick (1965), who found that human fibroblasts originated from adult donors have a shorter doubling potential than those originated from human embryos. These results were rapidly followed by other attempts to test the relationship of the doubling potential in vitro with the age of the donor of the post-natal cells. Thus it was ascertained that cells obtained from human adults early during their life span in vitro have proliferation kinetics similar to those of embryonic cells during the last stages of their in vitro life span (Macieira-Coelho and Pontén 1969; Schneider and Mitsui 1976); that the potential number of doublings in vitro is inversely proportional to the age of the donor (Martin et al. 1970); and that cells originating from individuals with premature aging have a reduced division potential (Salk et al. 1981).

An inverse relationship between age of the donor and the doubling potential in vitro was also found with cells from other human tissues besides fibroblasts (for review see Macieira-Coelho 1981 a). Moreover, a relationship between the limited life span of cultivated cells and the age of the donor was reported with tortoise fibroblasts (Goldstein 1974).

One obvious question is whether there is a direct relationship between the life spans of the different species and the doubling potential of the respective cells in vitro. According to some investigators there is none (Stanley 1975); others, however, claim to have found such a relationship (Röhme 1981). Unfortunately the latter author compared embryonic with adult cells from the different species and in the case of embryonic cells the whole embryo was used, which gives origin to highly heterogeneous cell populations. Hence as long as the same type of cell is not used for comparison, the question will remain unsettled.

Relationship Between Growth Potential In Vitro and Cancer

Another pitfall when making interspecies comparisons arises from the tendency of fibroblasts from some species to acquire the capacity to replicate indefinitely in vitro. Indeed, the investigator comparing life spans of fibroblast-like cells may

[1] Laboratoire de Pathologie Cellulaire, F-94804 Villejuif Cédex, France

Drugs and Aging
Ed. by D. Platt

have the feeling of going "through a looking glass" and penetrating a nonsense world. Chicken embryonic fibroblasts, for instance, like those from human donors, will invariably die after a certain number of doublings (Lima and Macieira-Coelho 1972). On the other hand, mouse cells behave in exactly the opposite way and invariably become spontaneously permanent cell lines (Todaro and Green 1963). Cells from other rodents can spontaneously develop permanent lines with a variable frequency: the probability of obtaining a permanent cell line from Syrian hamster fibroblasts is higher than that for rabbit but less than for Chinese hamster or mouse (Terzi and Hawkins 1975).

This difference in the probability of yielding a permanent cell line seems to be a crucial property of cells since it is related to the response of these cells to viral, chemical, and physical carcinogens. Thus chicken fibroblasts infected with Rous sarcoma virus (RSV), although transformed in the sense that they lose contact inhibition of growth, have a shorter life span than identical populations of noninfected cells (Pontén 1970), and the probability of obtaining permanent cell lines is low. Furthermore, the sarcomas induced by these transformed cells are not transplantable and seem to propagate by infection of new cells which die after a few divisions (Bergs and Groupé 1963; Pontén 1970). Mouse sarcomas obtained by the in vitro infection of cells with oncogenic viruses, however, are transplantable and present the type of clonal growth where all cells in the tumor are derived from the first transformed cells.

Human cells seem to have an intermediate behavior in regard to the response to oncogenic viruses when compared with chicken and mouse, since they can be transformed, for instance by SV40 virus, and yield with an intermediate frequency immortal cell populations (Pereira-Smith and Smith 1981).

The relative position of these cell types in regard to the response to oncogenes is identical. Thus oncogenes can facilitate the immortalization of rat cells (Land et al. 1983) (a phenomenon which in any case occurs spontaneously with these cells), they cannot immortalize human fibroblasts (Sager et al. 1983), and they transform without immortalization chicken cells (Stehelin et al. 1976).

The same type of response is found with chemical carcinogens and with ionizing radiation. Indeed, radiation accelerates the immortalization of mouse cells, it may have no effect or only prolong the life span of human cells, and it shortens the division potential of chicken fibroblasts (Macieira-Coelho et al. 1976).

The same response occurs with chemical carcinogens. One can thus produce a scale (Fig. 1), with at the one end cells like chicken fibroblasts which very rarely give origin to permanent cell lines in response to carcinogens, and at the other end cells which spontaneously produce immortal populations and where carcinogens and oncogenes only accelerate a natural phenomenon. Finally in between are cells in which carcinogens can prolong the life span but rarely give rise to immortal populations.

Pertinent to this subject is the fact that within the human species there seems to be a relationship between the growth potential in vitro of postnatal fibroblasts and the presence of a tumor in the donor or the proneness of the donor to develop a tumor. Indeed, the life span of skin fibroblasts from some cancer patients seems to be more unstable than that of those obtained from normal donors (Azzarone et al. 1976). Moreover it was found that the growth potential in vitro of normal

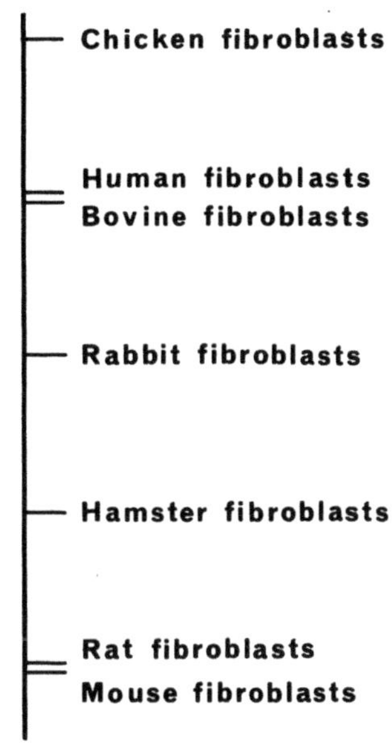

Fig. 1. Scale representing from top to bottom the increasing probability of obtaining immortal cell lines with fibroblasts from different species either spontaneously or with oncogenes and viral, chemical, and physical carcinogens

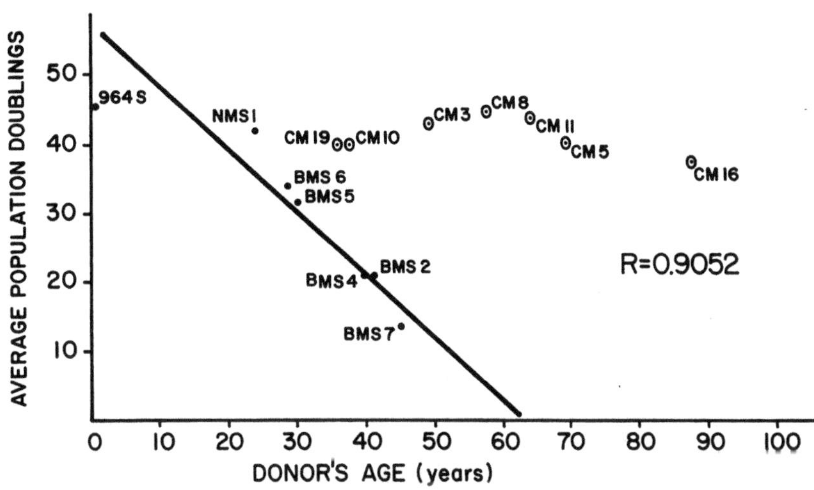

Fig. 2. Age of the donor versus average population doublings of the skin fibroblast strains derived from a human embryo (964 S) and from patients with benign mammary lesions (●) or breast cancers (⊙). The *straight line* is the regression fitting the plot corresponding to the fibroblasts originating from donors with benign lesions. The correlation coefficient is indicated on the chart. (Azzarone et al. 1984)

skin fibroblasts from mammary cancer patients had no correlation with the age of the donor (Azzarone et al. 1984), as is the case with fibroblasts from normal donors (Fig. 2). The fibroblasts from the cancer patients also responded in an abnormal way to three biological parameters: anchorage dependence, colony formation on monolayers of normal epithelial cells, and saturation densities in overcrowded cultures (Azzarone et al. 1984). In addition, the fibroblasts obtained from the cancer patients had a cell subset with a greater growth potential, which could invade foreign tissues in vitro and which had proliferation kinetics different from those of the control cells.

A prolongation of the life span of fibroblasts from donors at high risk of cancer, through variations in the culture conditions, has also been described (Diatloff-Zito and Macieira-Coelho 1982).

Another analogy between interspecies differences in fibroblast behavior and differences between human fibroblasts from different donors concerns the response to viral, chemical, and physical carcinogens. Indeed, skin fibroblasts from human donors with cancer or at high risk of cancer seem more susceptible to transformation by carcinogens than those obtained from normal donors. Thus although immortalization of normal human cells is a rare event, the doubling potential from donors with cancer (Rhim et al. 1980; Azzarone et al. 1980) or at high risk of cancer (Diatloff and Macieira-Coelho 1979) can be prolonged by carcinogens.

Putative Mechanisms of the Correlation Between Aging, Cancer, and the Growth Potential of Somatic Cells

The study of the response of the different types of cell to ionizing radiation gave some clues to the intriguing relationship described above.

Cells with a lower division potential are more sensitive to radiation (Bourgeois et al. 1981); however, the doubling potential of cells more prone to transformation can be increased by radiation (Macieira-Coelho et al. 1976). These data suggest that ionizing radiation under the experimental conditions utilized (low dose rate) accentuates the intrinsic growth potential of fibroblasts and only accelerates changes in the cell genome which anyway take place during cell replication.

These changes could be the chromosome rearrangements that inevitably occur during cell division and which are known to be increased by ionizing radiation (Macieira-Coelho 1980). Thus it was attempted to establish whether there is any correlation between genome rearrangements and the response of the different fibroblast populations to radiation. Results showed that ionizing radiation did not increase the number of chromosome rearrangements, but that the response to radiation seemed to be correlated with the potential for rearrangements of the nonirradiated target cells. The findings are illustrated in Fig. 3. No chromosome rearrangements were observed in cells whose life span was shortened by radiation. By contrast, a high level of rearrangements was observed in the cell population (nonirradiated) whose doubling potential was increased by radiation. Finally, the cells whose life span was not affected by radiation had an intermediate number of chromosome rearrangements. These results suggest that the effect of radiation depends upon the potential of the populations for chromosome rearrangements; in other words, that the survival in vitro and the sensitivity to radiation depend upon the plasticity of the cell genome.

Another pertinent observation was the finding that in the irradiated cells most of the breaks involved in exchanges (53 out of 62) concerned the centromeric and telomeric regions (Fig. 4). Thus the intrachromosomal break distribution was

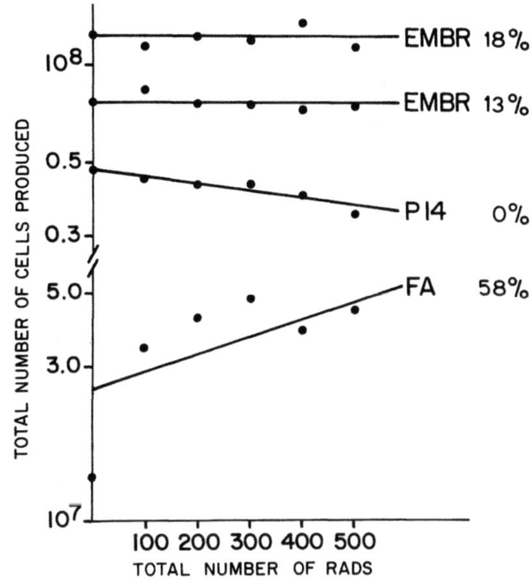

Fig. 3. Regression lines fitting the plot of the total number of cells produced by fibroblast populations from different donors either nonirradiated or irradiated with different doses of low dose rate radiation. The % indicates the frequency of chromosome rearrangements observed in the respective nonirradiated cells through their in vitro life span

preferentially located at regions rich in repetitive DNA, which has been implicated in recombinational events (Bourgeois et al. 1981).

On the other hand when one compares cells from different species it seems that those in which radiation increases the probability of immortalization also have a higher frequency of recombinational events in the genome. This is the case for mouse cells, where bridges between chromosomes and radial figures can be easily found before immortalization (Fig. 5). Further evidence of the plasticity of the mouse genome is the rapidity with which the genome can change from the diploid to the tetraploid state (Fig. 6) and the higher frequency of sister chromatid exchanges as compared with human cells (Table 1).

These results led to a new paradigm for the explanation of the relative probability of cells to have limited or unlimited growth potential (Macieira-Coelho 1979, 1980, 1981 b, 1984). According to this paradigm, the trigger for a progressive shift in cell behavior could be the DNA strand switching, sister chromatid exchanges, and displacement of transposable elements occurring during cell division. Transcription from the reorganized DNA strands could depend inter alia on the efficiency of repair enzymes, the presence of a reparable matrix, the conformation of chromatin, gene amplification, the presence of palindromes, and the switching on and off of transposable elements. In some cells this genome reorganization during cell division leads to aging. In other cells there is a higher probability of the turning on of chromatin regions, creation of independently replicating units, maintenance of transcription, and immortalization. Carcinogens and oncogenes would just have the role of activators of this latent potential.

Since the somatic cells of cancer patients and of donors at high risk of cancer can express in vitro this potentiality, the results imply that at least in some situations, cancer is a generalized disease which eventually becomes expressed predominantly in a localized area.

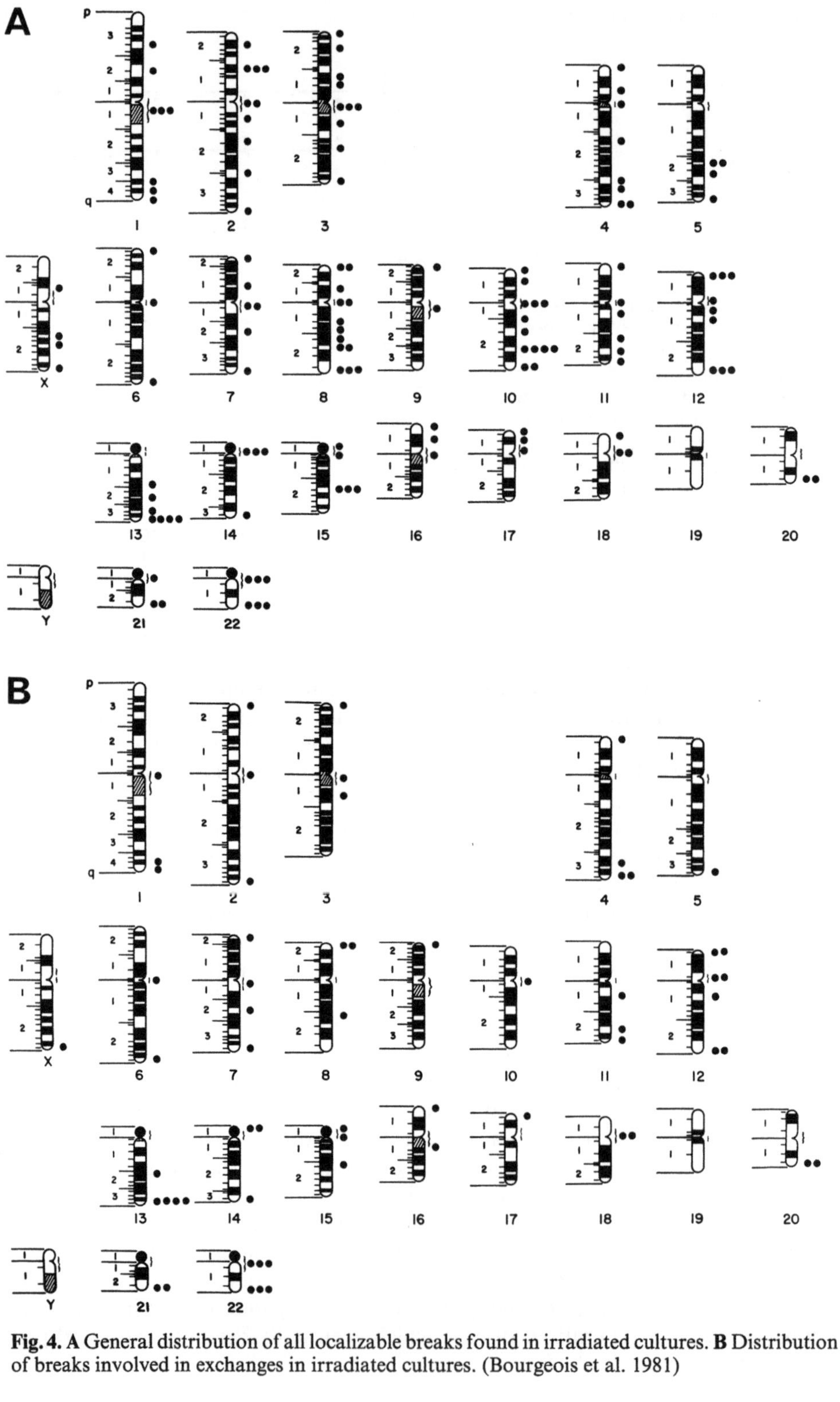

Fig. 4. A General distribution of all localizable breaks found in irradiated cultures. **B** Distribution of breaks involved in exchanges in irradiated cultures. (Bourgeois et al. 1981)

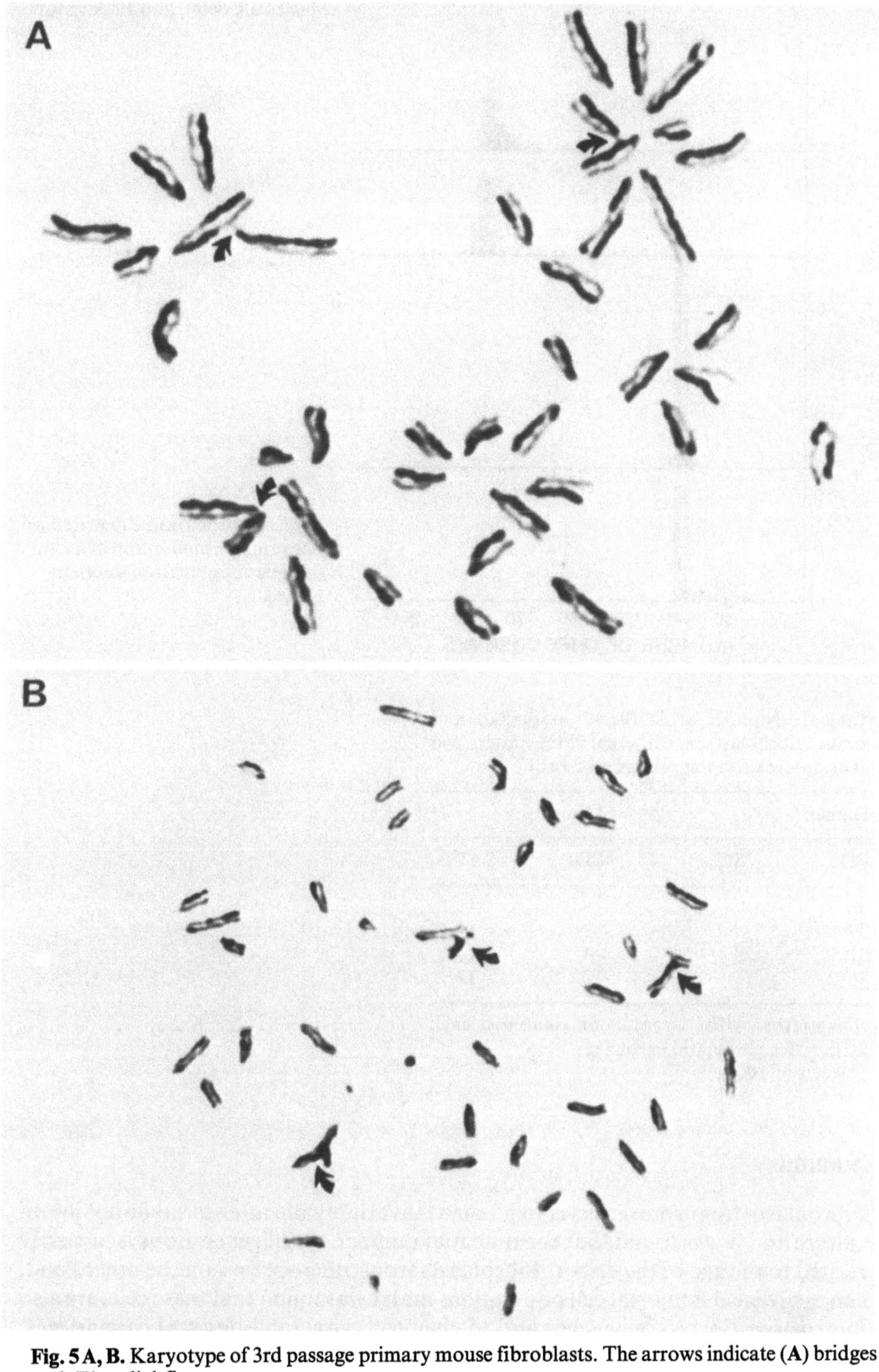

Fig. 5 A, B. Karyotype of 3rd passage primary mouse fibroblasts. The arrows indicate **(A)** bridges and **(B)** radial figures

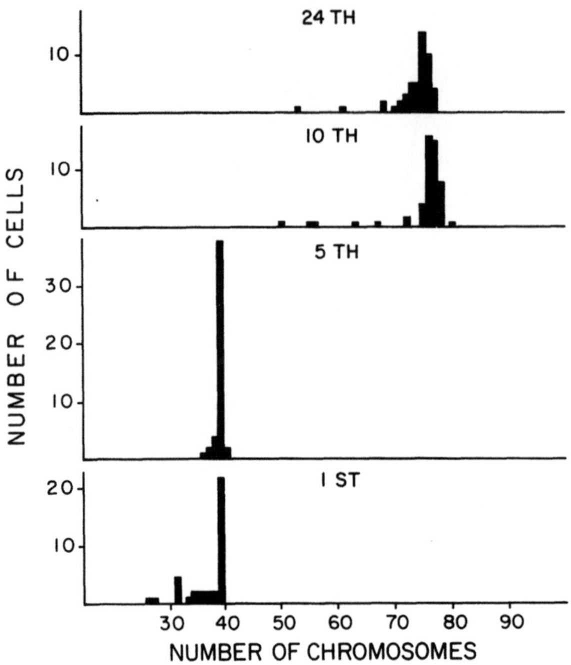

Fig. 6. Chromosome distribution of primary mouse fibroblasts at different population doubling levels

Table 1. Number of SCE/cell[a] in human and mouse fibroblasts at different PDL after two division cycles in the presence of BrdU

Human		Mouse	
PDL	SCE	PDL	SCE
33	7	1	11
37	5	3	11
41	8	4	17
46	6	12	12

Abbreviations: PDL, population doubling level; SCE, sister chromatid exchanges
[a] Mean of 100 cells

Summary

Fibroblasts from some species (e.g., man) invariably die after serial doublings in culture and it was found that the potential number of cell generations is inversely related to the age of the donor. Fibroblasts from other species, on the other hand, can easily yield immortal cell populations and it was found that these cells are also more susceptible to oncogenes and to chemical, viral, and physical carcinogens. The results suggest that these agents just accentuate an intrinsic potential for transformation.

Within the human species fibroblasts from some donors with cancer or at high risk of cancer have a tendency for an increased growth potential so that the number of population doublings does not correlate with the donor's age. The data seem to show that at least in some cases neoplasia is a generalized disease with repercussions for all somatic cells.

Acknowledgements. This work was supported by a contract from EURATOM.

References

Azzarone B, Pedullá D, Romanzi CA (1976) Spontaneous transformation of human skin fibroblasts derived from neoplastic patients. Nature 262:74–75

Azzarone B, Diatloff-Zito C, Billard C, Macieira-Coelho A (1980) Effect of low dose rate radiation on the division potential of cells in vitro. VII. Human fibroblasts from young and adult donors. In Vitro 16:634–638

Azzarone B, Mareel M, Billard C, Scemama P, Chaponnier C, Macieira-Coelho A (1984) Abnormal properties of skin fibroblasts from patients with breast cancer. Int J Cancer 33:759–764

Bergs VV, Groupé V (1963) Low malignancy of Rous sarcoma cells as evidenced by poor transplantability in turkeys. Science 139:922–923

Bourgeois CA, Raynaud N, Diatloff-Zito C, Macieira-Coelho A (1981) Effect of low dose rate ionizing radiation on the division potential of cells in vitro. VIII. Cytogenetic analysis of human fibroblasts. Mech Ag Dev 17:225–235

Diatloff C, Macieira-Coelho A (1979) Effect of low dose rate ionizing radiation on the division potential of cells in vitro. V. Human skin fibroblasts from donors with a high risk of cancer. J Natl Cancer Inst 63:55–59

Diatloff-Zito C, Macieira-Coelho A (1982) Effect of growth arrest on the doubling potential of human fibroblasts in vitro: a possible influence of the donor. In Vitro 18:606–610

Goldstein S (1974) Aging in vitro: growth of cultured cells from the Galapagos tortoise. Exp Cell Res 83:297–301

Hayflick L (1965) The limited in vitro lifetime of human diploid cell strains. Exp Cell Res 37:614–636

Land H, Parada LF, Weinberg RA (1983) Tumorigenic conversion of primary embryo fibroblasts requires at least two cooperating oncogenes. Nature 304:596–602

Lima L, Macieira-Coelho A (1972) Parameters of aging in chicken embryo fibroblasts cultivated in vitro. Exp Cell Res 70:279–284

Macieira-Coelho A (1979) Reorganization of the cell genome as the basis of aging in dividing cells. In: Orimo H, Shimada K, Iriki M, Maeda D (eds) Recent Advances in Gerontology. Excerpta Medica, Amsterdam, p 11

Macieira-Coelho A (1980) Implications of the reorganization of the cell genome for aging or immortalization of dividing cells in vitro. Gerontology 26:276–282

Macieira-Coelho A (1981 a) Tissue culture in aging research: present status and prospects. Experientia 37:1050–1053

Macieira-Coelho A (1981 b) Possible implications of the reorganization of the cell genome for the transfer of information in dividing cells. In: Danon D, Schock NW, Marois M (eds) Aging: a challenge to science and society, vol I. Oxford University Press, Oxford, p 136–145

Macieira-Coelho A (1984) Genome reorganization during cellular senescence. Mech Ag Dev 27:257–262

Macieira-Coelho A, Pontén J (1969) Analogy in growth between late passage human embryonic and early passage human adult fibroblasts. J Cell Biol 43:374–377

Macieira-Coelho A, Diatloff C, Malaise E (1976) Doubling potential of fibroblasts from different species after ionizing radiation. Nature 261:586–588

Martin GM, Sprague CA, Epstein CJ (1970) Replicative life span of cultivated human cells. Effects of donor's age, tissue and genotype. Lab Invest 23:86–92

Pereira-Smith O, Smith JR (1981) Expression of SV40 T antigen in finite life-span hybrids of normal and SV40-transformed fibroblasts. Som Cell Gen 7:411–421

Pontén J (1970) The growth capacity of normal and Rous virus transformed chicken fibroblasts in vitro. Int J Cancer 6:323–332

Rhim JS, Huebner RJ, Arnstein P, Kopelovitch L (1980) Chemical transformation of cultured human skin fibroblasts derived from individuals with hereditary adenomatosis of the colon and rectum. Int J Cancer 26:565–569

Röhme D (1981) Evidence for a relationship between longevity of mammalian species and life spans of normal fibroblasts in vitro and erythrocytes in vivo. Proc Natl Acad Sc USA 78:5009–5013

Sager R, Tanaka K, Lan CC, Ebina Y, Anisowicz A (1983) Resistance of human cells to tumorigenesis induced by cloned transforming genes. Proc Natl Acad Sc USA 80:7601–7605

Salk D, Bryant E, Au K, Hoehn H, Martin G (1981) Systematic growth studies, cocultivation, and cell hybridization studies of Werner syndrome cultured skin fibroblasts. Hum Genet 58:310–316

Schneider EL, Mitsui Y (1976) The relationship between in vitro cellular aging and in vivo human age. Proc Natl Acad Sc USA 73:3584–3588

Stanley JF, Pye D, MacGregor A (1975) Comparison of doubling numbers attained by cultured animal cells with life span of species. Nature 255:158–159

Stehelin D, Guntaka RV, Varmus HE, Bishop JM (1976) Purification of DNA complementary to nucleotide sequences required for neoplastic transformation of fibroblasts by avian sarcoma viruses. J Mol Biol 101:349–365

Terzi M, Hawkins TSC (1975) Chromosomal variation and the establisment of somatic cell lines in vitro. Nature 253:361–362

Todaro GJ, Green H (1963) Quantitative studies of the growth of mouse embryo cells in culture and their development into established lines. J Cell Biol 17:299–313

The Effect of Age on Rat Liver Drug Metabolism

C. F. A. van Bezooijen, G. J. M. J. Horbach, and C. F. Hollander [1]

Introduction

The elderly use drugs more often than do young persons. In the Netherlands, about 80% of people older than 80 years regularly use drugs, which is high in comparison with the 20% of the 20- to 30-year olds. In addition, the elderly use more drugs simultaneously (Smith 1979). Furthermore, the incidence of adverse drug reactions in the elderly is about 2–3 times higher than in young people (Seidl et al. 1966; Hurwitz et al. 1969; Smidt and McQueen 1972). This high incidence of adverse drug reactions in old age may be due to age-related changes in drug interactions, compliance, pharmacodynamics, and pharmacokinetics. Changes in the pharmacokinetics of drug handling with age might be due to changes in absorption, volume of distribution, metabolism, and excretion. Our attention here will be concentrated on the effect of age on the drug metabolizing capacity of the liver. Many studies on this subject have been performed in rats during the past several years. These studies will be reviewed. Age-related changes in many anatomical, histopathological, biochemical, and physiological factors which may be relevant to changes in the drug metabolizing activity of the rat liver with age will also be considered.

Age-Related Changes in Rat Liver: Anatomical and Histopathological Features in Relation to Drug Metabolism

Since the hepatocytes are the cells in which drug metabolism mainly takes place, changes in liver weight with age due to changes in hepatocyte mass may play an important role in drug metabolism. Literature data as given in Table 1 reveal that liver weight increases in female and male rats with age for all strains investigated. Next to changes in liver weight, changes in the liver weight/body weight ratio are of importance, especially if the dose administered is based on body weight. A literature review on the liver weight/body weight ratio revealed a decrease or no change in this ratio with age (van Bezooijen 1984). The observed increase in liver weight might be due to a shift to a higher polyploidy of the hepatocyte with age (van Bezooijen et al. 1984a). However, these changes appear to occur in early life (Table 2) and are therefore not really aging phenomena.

[1] TNO Institute for Experimental Gerontology, P.O. Box 5815, 2280 HV Rijswijk, The Netherlands

Drugs and Aging
Ed. by D. Platt

Table 1. Changes in rat liver weight with age

Strain	Sex	Age (months)	Liver weight (g)	Reference
Wistar	Female	3 vs 24	8.3→12.9	Uchida et al. (1982)
Wistar	Female	3 vs 24	7.1→12.0	Devasagayam et al. (1983)
Wistar	Male	3 vs 24	9.1→12.9	Kitani et al. (1978b)
Wistar	Male	4 vs 36	11.1→15.1	McMartin et al. (1980)
Wistar	Male	3 vs 23	11.7→16.0	Uchida et al. (1982)
RU	Female	3 vs 27	6.1→ 9.2	De Leeuw-Israel (1971)
WAG/Rij	Female	3 vs 30	4.6→ 5.6	Kitani et al. (1981)
WAG/Rij	Female	3 vs 36	4.7→ 6.7	Horbach et al. (1984)
WAG/Rij	Male	3 vs 30	7.6→ 8.9	Kitani et al. (1981)
BN/Bi	Female	3 vs 30	4.4→ 5.8	Kitani et al. (1981)
Fischer 344	Male	6 vs 16	10.9→16.5	Rikans and Notley (1981)
Fischer 344	Male	3 vs 27	5.9→10.0	Schmucker et al. (1982)
Sprague-Dawley	Male	2 vs 20	8.3→14.7	Varga and Fischer (1978)
Sprague-Dawley	Male	2.5 vs 16	10.5→19.1	Weigand et al. (1980)
Sprague-Dawley	Male	3 vs 16	16.4→25.9	Uchida et al. (1982)

Table 2. Proportions of diploid and polyploid hepatocytes in livers of female WAG/Rij rats of different ages

Age (months)	MD 2n (%)	BD 2×2n (%)	MT 4n (%)	BT 2×4n (%)	MO 8n (%)	BO 2×8n (%)	MDH 16n (%)
0.5	97	2	1				
1	36	48	9	4	3		
1.5	2	22	56	12	8		
3	5	14	60	17	3	1	
12		4	72	21	3		
24	3	4	59	26	6	2	
30	11	3	46	19	18	4	
36	11	3	37	30	10	7	4

Abbreviations: MD, mononuclear diploid; BD, binuclear diploid; MT, mononuclear tetraploid; BT, binuclear tetraploid; MO, mononuclear octaploid; BO, binuclear octaploid; MDH, mononuclear decahexoid

Cytochrome P-450, which is an important enzyme in liver drug metabolism, is localized in the smooth endoplasmic reticulum (SER). Therefore, morphological changes in the SER may be indicative for changes in drug metabolism. An increase in the cytoplasmic volume occupied by SER was observed in female Wistar rats at between 12 and 27 months of age (Pieri et al. 1975). These data were reproduced by Meihuizen and Blansjaar (1980) for female WAG/Rij rats at between 3 and 35 months. However, a study performed by Schmucker et al. (1977) revealed a decrease in the amount of SER in male Fischer rats at between 10 and 30 months. These data indicate that changes in the amount of SER with age may be strain and/or sex dependent.

Other factors which could influence liver drug metabolism are changes in liver structure due to spontaneous lesions. This hypothesis is supported by the finding of Zurcher et al. (1982) that the bromsulfophthalein retention in rats was increased due to bile duct hyperplasia. In old age, many spontaneous nonneoplastic age-related liver lesions are observed in various rat strains. Especially, foci or areas of cellular alterations have been found in male Wistar rats (McMartin et al. 1980) and in female WAG/Rij rats (Burek 1978). Bile duct hyperplasia in male Fischer rats (Coleman et al. 1977), bile duct cysts in female BN/BiRij rats (Burek 1978), hepatic telangiectasis in female and male WI rats (Gellatly 1967), and periportal inflammation in male Sprague-Dawley rats (Anver et al. 1982) occur at frequencies higher than 50%. However, no data exist correlating these changes with altered drug metabolism. One should be aware that these changes, like the mentioned bile duct hyperplasia, may influence the outcome of metabolizing processes in the liver.

Age-Related Changes in Rat Liver: Biochemical and Physiological Factors Related to Drug Metabolism

After fractionation of the hepatocytes, the smooth endoplasmic reticulum is found in the microsomal fraction. Stier et al. (1982) hypothesized that age-related changes in the lipid composition of rat liver microsomal membranes could be of importance for the functioning of the drug metabolizing enzymes present in these membranes. The cholesterol/phospholipid ratio increases with age (Grinna 1977; Schmucker et al. 1982). An increase in this ratio may result in a decrease in the fluidity of the membranes and consequently in a decrease in the activity of the monooxygenases (Stier et al. 1982).

Besides possible age-related changes in the capacity of the individual hepatocyte to metabolize drugs, changes in liver blood flow and in hepatic uptake of the drug with age may influence the biotransformation activity of the total liver. Age-related changes in hepatic blood flow are of especial importance for drugs with a high extraction ratio (for details, see below). Liver blood flow in rats decreases with age, especially during the first 12 months (Varga and Fischer 1978). To study the effect of age on hepatic uptake, Kroker et al. (1980) used the system of the perfused rat liver. They observed that in old rats the hepatic uptake of a bile acid was decreased to a lesser extent than was its secretion. Therefore, for bile acids, the hepatic uptake is not a rate-limiting step in their removal from the blood by the liver.

Changes in the Rat Liver Excretory Functions with Age

The effect of age on excretory functions of the rat liver has been studied with exogenous dyes such as bromsulfophthalein and indocyanin green. The plasma retention of these substances or the half-life ($t\frac{1}{2}$) of disappearance, when the substance is supplied at suboptimal doses, depends on liver blood flow and the excretion capacity of the liver. To differentiate between these two possibilities, the maximal excretion capacity (T_m) has to be determined by measuring the concentration of the dye in the bile during a continuous dye infusion. A decrease in the maximal excretion capacity was observed for bromsulfophthalein (Kitani et al. 1978 a and 1981). Kitani (1977) also observed a decrease in the maximal removal rate of indocyanin green with age. Ouabain, a cardiac glycoside which is not metabolized by the liver, clearly shows an age-dependent decrease in its biliary excretion (Kitani 1978 b). These data reveal an age-related decrease in biliary excretion in rats.

Aging and Rat Liver Drug Metabolism

Drugs handled by the liver can be subdivided into those with a high and those with a low extraction ratio. The extraction ratio is an important characteristic of the hepatic clearance: the hepatic clearance is the product of liver blood flow and the extraction ratio.

a) Drugs with a high extraction ratio are those of which 70% or more is removed during the first passage through the liver. Examples of drugs with a high extraction ratio are chlormethiazole, labetol, lignocaine, morphine, nortryptiline, pentazocine, pethidine, propoxyphene, and propranolol. The normal hepatic blood flow is about 10 ml·min^{-1} for 2-month-old rats (Varga and Fischer 1978). A drug with an extraction ratio of 0.70 would have a clearance of 7 ml·min^{-1}. The hepatic clearance of such a drug is primarily determined by liver blood flow. As mentioned above, a decrease in liver blood flow with age is observed, especially during the first year of life.

b) Drugs with a low extraction ratio are those of which 20% or less is removed during the first passage through the liver.

These drugs can be subdivided into those which bind to a low or to a high extent to serum proteins. Since only the unbound drug is probably available for hepatic uptake, the clearance of drugs which are poorly bound to serum proteins depends mainly on the hepatic drug metabolizing system. Examples of such drugs are antipyrine, acetaminophen, chloramphenicol, and theophylline. On the other hand, the hepatic clearance of drugs which are highly bound to serum proteins depends not only on the liver drug metabolizing system but also on the extent of protein binding. Such drugs are diazepam, warfarin, and phenytoin. It is known that the albumin concentration in plasma is unchanged in old rats (de Leeuw-Israel 1971; Horbach et al. 1983). However, indications for structural changes in the albumin molecule have been observed (Horbach et al. 1983). Consequently, age-related changes in the hepatic clearance of drugs with a low extraction ratio and which are highly bound to serum proteins are not due to quantitative changes in serum albumin concentrations but might be influenced by structural changes in the albumin molecule.

The drug metabolizing system of the liver comprises two phases. Phase I involves oxidation, reduction, dealkylation, and hydrolysis reactions. Parent drugs or their phase I metabolites can be conjugated in the phase II reaction with glucuronic acid, sulfuric acid, or glutathione. Important phase I enzymes are the monooxygenases, which insert one oxygen atom into the drug. In addition to this oxidation reaction, these enzymes are also able to reduce drugs. Therefore, they are also called the mixed-function oxidase system. A trivial name is cytochrome P-450. For its drug metabolizing activities, cytochrome P-450 requires cytochrome *b5* and NADPH-cytochrome *c* reductase.

Age-related changes in cytochrome P-450 and cytochrome *b5* content and NADPH-cytochrome *c* reductase activity have been reviewed (van Bezooijen 1984). No change with age in the cytochrome *b5* concentration was reported in male rats. Except for some where no age-related differences were reported, most studies show a decrease in the cytochrome P-450 concentration and in the NADPH-cytochrome *c* reductase activity. In addition, the specific activity of NADPH-cytochrome *c* reductase appeared to be two times higher in young rats than in old ones (Schmucker et al. 1982). Furthermore, an increased thermostability of this enzyme was observed in old rats as compared with young rats. So, along with a decrease in the concentration of NADPH-cytochrome *c* reductase, a decrease in the specific activity with age occurred. A kinetic analysis of NADPH-cytochrome *c* reductase revealed that the K_m for NADPH as substrate did not change, while the V_{max} decreased with age (Schmucker and Wang 1983).

The effect of age on specific drug-metabolizing enzymes in rat liver microsomes has been studied by many investigators (see the review of van Bezooijen 1984). In male rats, most enzyme activities decreased with age; exceptions were the activity of epoxide hydrase and nitroanisole-*O*-demethylase, which increased. In female rats, most enzyme activities did not change with age, except for an increase and a decrease in amino *N*-demethylase and a decrease in 7-ethoxycoumarin-*O*-deethylase.

With respect to phase II reactions, many studies on the effect of age on different forms of glutathione and glutathione-related enzymes have been performed. A decrease, an increase, and no change with age have been observed (Birnbaum and Baird 1979; Kitahara et al. 1982; Spearman and Leibman 1984). Contradictory results for changes with age were also observed for the glucuronidation capacity (Ali et al. 1979; Fujita et al. 1982; Kitahara et al. 1982). These discrepancies are probably due to sex and strain differences but may also be attributed to the possibility that age has a different effect on the several molecular forms of glutathione-*S*-transferase and UDP-glucuronyltransferase.

The Effect of Age on the Liver Drug Metabolizing Capacity In Vivo

Only a few studies have been performed on the influence of age on the metabolism of drugs in intact rats. Studies by Kato and Takanaka (1968), Kitani et al. (1982a, b), and Fiume et al. (1983) indicated a decreased metabolizing capacity for carisoprodol and pentobarbital, for digitoxin, and for anthracene and chrysene, respectively.

In studying the effect of age on the in vivo metabolism of drugs, it should be taken into consideration that besides the capacity of the liver to metabolize drugs, extrahepatic factors such as neurological and endocrinological as well as circulatory aspects may be of importance.

In addition, changes in drug absorption, drug distribution, and kidney elimination with age should be taken into account when drawing conclusions concerning age-related changes in the liver metabolizing capacity in rodents. Changes in drug absorption or volume of distribution would result in changes in blood levels and consequently in a changed drug supply to the liver. The well-known decreased kidney elimination would result in prolonged presence of the hydrophilic metabolites at higher blood levels in the body.

The use of isolated intact hepatocytes has the advantage that extrahepatic influences are excluded. In addition, the hepatocytes contain all cytoplasmic and mitochondrial factors which influence rates of drug metabolism and are lacking in the in vitro system of isolated microsomes. Therefore, data obtained on the drug-metabolizing capacity of hepatocytes isolated from rats of different ages can be expected to provide useful information on the role of the liver in age-related changes in the kinetics of drug metabolism of rats in vivo.

The Drug Metabolizing Capacity of Hepatocytes Isolated from Rats of Different Ages

Up to now, the metabolism of digitoxin and aflatoxin B1 has been studied with hepatocytes isolated from rats of different ages.

Digitoxin (DT_3) is metabolized via different metabolic pathways, viz., degraded by hydrolysis and hydroxylation reactions. The resulting active metabolites and DT_3 itself can be inactivated by conjugation with glucuronic or sulfuric acid. Therefore, by studying the influence of age on the metabolic patterns of DT_3, information on the effect of age on hydrolysis, hydroxylation, and conjugation reactions can be obtained.

In a recent study (van Bezooijen et al. 1984b), hepatocytes were isolated from 3-, 18-, 30-, and 36-month-old male BN/Bi rats. It was observed that the relative distribution pattern of the digitoxin metabolites did not change with age. This result does not agree with the observations of Ohta et al. (1984), who used male Wistar rats and observed a more pronounced decrease for the hydrolyzed metabolites. Probably, changes in the metabolite pattern with age might be strain dependent.

A decrease in apparent V_{max} (see Fig. 1) and no change in apparent K_m was found with age (van Bezooijen et al. 1984b). Consequently, the intrinsic hepatic clearance ($Cli = V_{max}/K_m$) decreased linearly with age (Fig. 2), which was significant at the age of 36 months as compared with the values for 3 and 18 months. Ohta et al. (1984) observed a sharper decrease in V_{max} and also a decrease in K_m. When they compared their data with our previously published data obtained with hepatocytes isolated only from 3- and 30-month-old rats (van Bezooijen et al. 1982), they explained these discrepancies by referring to differences in plasma testosterone levels. These differences might be the result of a high incidence of testicular tumors in the Wistar-derived rat strains used by Ohta et al. (1984). This condition is rarely found in our male BN/BiRij rats (Burek 1978).

The observations that there was no change with age in the relative distribution pattern and that the intrinsic hepatic clearance decreased with age indicate that the hydroxylation, hydrolysis, and conjugation reactions decreased equally with age. Especially, the observation that the contributions of the metabolites digitoxi-

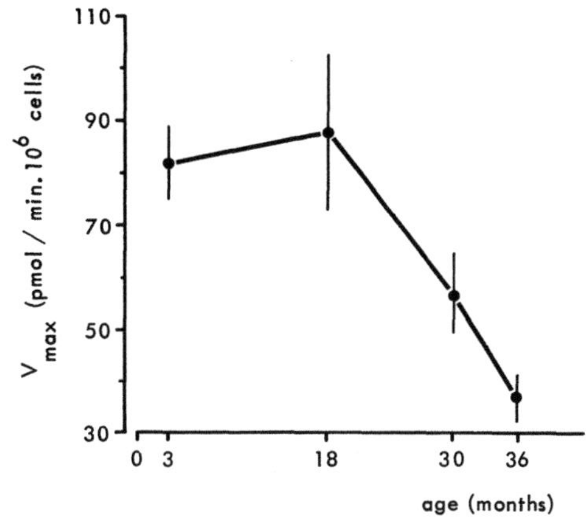

Fig. 1. The effect of age on the apparent V_{max} of DT_3 biotransformation by hepatocytes isolated from male BN/BiRij rats of different ages. $\pm 1.0 \times 10^6$ cells·ml^{-1} were incubated for 1 h with DT_3 concentrations of 20, 25, 30, 40, 60, and 100 μM. Values for V_{max}, are expressed as mean ±SD. The number of rats used per age group was 4, 5, 4, and 6 for 3-, 18-, 30-, and 36-month-old rats, respectively

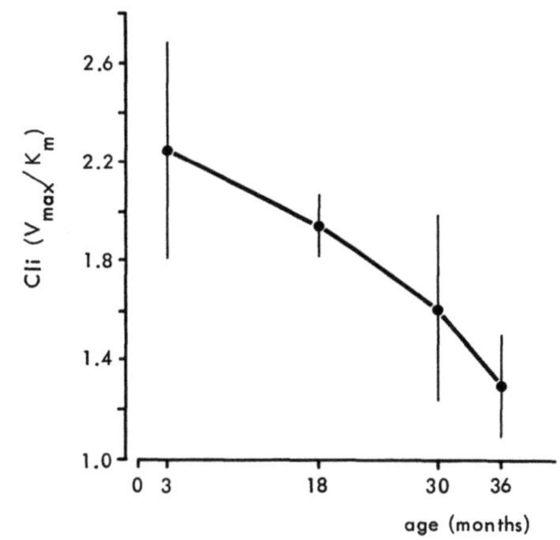

Fig. 2. The effect of age on the intrinsic hepatic clearance (*Cli*) of DT_3 biotransformation by hepatocytes isolated from male BN/BiRij rats of different ages. For technical details, see Fig. 1

genin-bis-digitoxoside (which is only formed by the hydrolysis reaction) and digoxin (which is the result of a hydroxylation reaction) to the pattern of metabolites did not change with age supports this conclusion. Kitani et al. (1982a, b), however, observed that in vivo the conjugation reaction itself did not decrease with age, but as a consequence of a decrease in hydrolysis and/or hydroxylation, less digitoxigenin-mono-digitoxoside, the preferred substrate for glucuronidation (Castle 1979 and Schmoldt and Promies 1982), may be available for conjugation. The observed age-related decrease in the conjugation capacity of the isolated hepatocytes may be explained in the same way.

Richardson et al. (1982) observed that the rate of aflatoxin B1 metabolism by hepatocytes isolated from 30-month-old male Fischer 344 rats was approximately one-half that observed with hepatocytes isolated from 6-month-old rats.

Those three studies prove that the metabolizing capacity of hepatocytes decreases with age. So, the observed decrease in the drug metabolizing activity of the liver in vivo is at least partly attributable to the decrease in the drug metabolizing capacity of the individual hepatocytes.

Discussion

Age-related changes in the in vivo rat liver drug metabolizing capacity can be due to changes in many factors, including the liver weight, the shift in ploidy status of the hepatocytes, the amount of smooth endoplasmic reticulum, the occurrence of spontaneous nonneoplastic liver lesions, the lipid composition of the liver microsomes, liver blood flow, hepatic uptake and excretion, the mixed function oxygenases, and specific liver microsomal drug metabolizing enzymes.

In contrast to the observed increase in rat liver weight with age, a decrease was found in humans. This discrepancy complicates the interpolation of data obtained in vivo in rats to the human situation. The occurrence of spontaneous nonneoplastic liver lesions varies greatly from strain to strain. These lesions may influence the drug metabolizing capacity of the liver, as was observed for bromsulfophthalein retention in rats with bile duct hyperplasia (Zurcher et al. 1982). Even tumors or lesions outside the liver may play a role in liver drug metabolism, as was proposed by Ohta et al. (1984). They speculated that the high incidence of testicular tumors which was observed in Wistar rats and not in BN/BiRij rats explained the differences in the digitoxin metabolism with age for these different rat strains (cf. above).

Phase I metabolism represents a complex system. The components cytochrome P-450 and NADPH-cytochrome *c* reductase are multienzymatic in nature and are dependent on a continuous supply of NADPH, which itself is generated by other multienzyme systems. It would be interesting to determine the effect of age on the various forms of cytochrome P-450. Possibly, the different effects of age on the liver drug metabolizing capacity might be attributable to different effects of age on the different isozymes of cytochrome P-450. The use of isolated microsomes, intact rats, or isolated hepatocytes, systems used to study the effect of age on liver drug metabolism, has some drawbacks. Isolated microsomes are lacking in cytoplasmic and mitochondrial substrate and cofactor supply. In in vivo studies, complicating extrahepatic factors such as neurological, endocrinological, and circulatory aspects may influence conclusions on the drug metabolizing activity of the liver. Changes in drug absorption, distribution, or kidney excretion may also complicate these conclusions. Isolated hepatocytes possess the cytoplasmic and mitochondrial cofactors and the extrahepatic influences are excluded. However, it is difficult to transpose quantitative data obtained in vitro with isolated hepatocytes to the in vivo situation, since no data on the effect of age on the number of hepatocytes per liver are available. In addition, hepatocytes are a heterogeneous population. Also with respect to the drug metabolizing system, the intralobular localization of the hepatocytes is important for their functioning (Moody et al. 1983). This localization is lost in the in vitro situation. In conclusion, all systems have serious drawbacks but in connection with each other they can provide useful information on the influence of age on rat liver drug metabolism.

Acknowledgments. The authors wish to thank Dr. A. C. Ford for editing the English text and Miss Marion Roggenkamp for carefully typing the manuscript.

References

Ali M (1979) The influence of old age and of renal failure on hepatic glucuronidation in the rat. Br J Pharmacol 66:498–499

Anver MR, Cohen BJ, Luttuada CP, Foster SJ (1982) Age-associated lesions in barrier-reared male Spraque-Dawley rats: a comparison between HAP:(SD) and Crl:COBS$^{(r)}$CD$^{(r)}$SD stocks. Exp Aging Res 8:3–24

Birnbaum LS, Baird MB (1979) Senescent changes in rodent hepatic epoxide metabolism. Chem Biol Interact 26:254–256

Burek JD (1978) Pathology of aging rats. In: Burek JD (ed). CRC Press, West Palm Beach, Florida

Castle MC (1979) Digitoxin metabolism by rat liver homogenates, subcellular fractions and isolated hepatocytes: stimulation by spironolactone and pregnenolone-16α-carbonitrile. J Pharmacol Exp Therapeutics 211:120–126

Coleman GL, Barthold SW, Osbaldiston GW, Foster SJ, Jonas AM (1977) Pathological changes during aging in barrier reared Fischer 344 male rats. J Gerontol 32:258–278

De Leeuw-Israel FR (1971) Aging changes in the rat liver. Thesis, Leiden

Devasagayam ThPA, Pushpendran ChK, Eapen J (1983) Changes in enzymes of hepatic rough and smooth microsomes during postnatal development and ageing of rats. Mech Age Dev 21:365–375

Fiume M, Guaitani A, Modica R, Bartosek I (1983) Effect of fasting, induction, sex and age on clearance of benz(a)anthracene and chrysene by isolated perfused rat liver. Toxicol Lett 19:73–79

Fujita S, Uesugi T, Kitagawa H, Suzuki T, Kitani K (1982) Hepatic microsomal monooxygenase and azoreductase activities in aging Fischer-344 rats. Importance of sex difference for aging studies. In: Kitani K (ed) Liver and aging – liver and drugs. Elsevier Biomedical Press, Amsterdam, p 55–72

Gellatly JBM (1967) In: Cotchin E, Roe FJC (eds) Pathology of laboratory rats and mice. Blackwell Scientific Publications, Oxford, p 22

Grinna LS (1977) Age-related changes in the lipids of the microsomal and the mitochondrial membranes of the rat liver and kidney. Mech Ageing Dev 6:197–205

Horbach GJMJ, Yap SH, van Bezooijen CFA (1983) Age-related changes in albumin elimination in female WAG/Rij rats. Biochem J 216:211–221

Horbach GJMJ, Princen HMG, Van der Kroef M, Van Bezooijen CFA, Yap SH (1984) Changes in the sequence content of albumin mRNA and in its translational activity in the rat liver with age. Biochem Biophys Acta 783:60–66

Hurwitz N, Wade OL (1969) Intensive hospital monitoring of adverse reactions to drugs. Brit Med J 1:531–536

Kato R, Takanaka A (1968) Metabolism of drugs in old rats (II). Metabolism in vivo and effect of drugs in old rats. Jpn J Pharmacol 18:389–396

Kitahara A, Ebina T, Ishikawa T, Soma Y, Sata K, Kanai S (1982) Changes in activities and molecular forms of rat hepatic drug metabolizing enzymes during aging. In: Kitani K (ed) Liver and aging – liver and drugs. Elsevier Biomedical Press, Amsterdam, p 135–142

Kitani K (1977) Functional aspects of the ageing liver. In: Platt D (ed) Liver and ageing. FK Schattauer Verlag, Stuttgart New York, p 5–17

Kitani K, Kanai S, Miura R (1978 a) Hepatic metabolism of sulfobromophthalein (BSP) and indocyanine green (ICG) in aging rats. In: Kitani K (ed) Liver and aging. Elsevier/North-Holland Biomedical Press, Amsterdam, p 145–156

Kitani K, Kanai S, Miura R, Morita Y, Kasahara M (1978 b) The effect of ageing on the biliary excretion of ouabain in the rat. Exp Gerontol 13:9–17

Kitani K, Zurcher Ch, van Bezooijen CFA (1981) The effect of aging on the hepatic metabolism of sulfobromophthalein in BN/Bi female and WAG/Rij male and female rats. Mech Age Dev 7:381–393

Kitani K, Sato Y, van Bezooijen CFA (1982 a) The effect of age on the biliary excretion of digitoxin and its metabolites in female BN/Bi rats. Arch Gerontol Geriatr 1:43–54

Kitani K, Sato Y, Nokubo M (1982 b) Biliary elimination of cardiac glycosides in aging rats. Sex and strain differences. In: Kitani K (ed) Liver and aging – liver and drugs. Elsevier Biomedical Press, Amsterdam, p 179–191

Kroker R, Hegner D, Anwer MS (1980) Altered hepatobiliary transport of taurocholic acid in aged rats. Mech Ageing Dev 12:367–373

McMartin DN, O'Connor JA, Fasco MJ, Kaminsky LS (1980) Influence of aging and induction of rat liver and kidney microsomal mixed function oxidase systems. Toxicol Appl Pharmacol 54:411–419

Meihuizen SP, Blansjaar N (1980) Stereological analysis of liver parenchymal cells from young and old rats. Mech Ageing Dev 13:111–118

Moody D, Taylor LA, Smuckler EA, Levin W, Thomas PE (1983) Immunohistochemical localization of cytochrome P-450a in liver sections from untreated rats and rats treated with phenobarbital or 3-methylcholanthrene. Drug Metab Dispos 11:339–343

Ohta M, Sato Y, Kanai S, Kitani K (1984) The digitoxin metabolism in isolated hepatocytes from young and old male rats. Arch Gerontol Geriatr 3:249–258

Pieri C, Nagy IZs, Mazzufferi G, Giuli C (1975) The aging of rat liver as revealed by electron microscopic morphometry – I. Basic parameters. Exp Gerontol 10:291–304

Richardson A, Sutter MA, Jayaraj A, Webb JW (1982) Age-related changes in the ability of hepatocytes to metabolize aflotoxin b1. In: Kitani K (ed) Liver and aging – liver and drugs. Elsevier Biomedical Press, Amsterdam, p 119–132

Rikans LE, Notley BA (1981) Decline in hepatic microsomal monooxygenase components in middle-aged Fischer 344 rats. Exp Geront 16:253–259

Schmoldt A, Promies J (1982) On the substrate specificity of the digitoxigenin monodigitoxoside conjugating UPD-glucuronyltransferase in rat liver. Biochem Pharmacol 31:2285–2289

Schmucker DL, Wang RK (1982) Qualitative changes in rat liver microsomal NADPH cytochrome c (P-450) reductase during aging. Age 5:105–110

Schmucker DL, Wang RK (1983) Age-dependent changes in rat liver microsomal NADPH cytochrome c (P-450) reductase: a kinetic analysis. Exp Geront 18:313–321

Schmucker DL, Mooney JS, Jones AL (1977) Age-related changes in the hepatic endoplasmic reticulum: a quantitative analysis. Science 197:1005–1007

Schmucker DL, Wang RK, Kwong P (1982) Age-dependent alterations in rat liver microsomal NADPH cytochrome c (P-450) reductase. In: Kitani K (ed) Liver and aging – liver and drugs. Elsevier Biomedical Press, Amsterdam, p 75–96

Seidl LG, Thornton GF, Smith JW, Cluff LE (1966) Studies on the epidemiology of adverse drug reactions. III. Reactions in patients on a general medical service. John Hopkins Med J 199:299–315

Smidt NA, McQueen EG (1972) Adverse reactions to drugs: A comprehensive hospital inpatient survey. New Zealand Med J 76:397–401

Smith CR (1979) Use of drugs in the aged. John Hopkins Med J 145:61–64

Spearman ME, Leibman K (1984) Effects of aging on the hepatic and pulmonary glutathione s-transferase activities in male and female Fischer 344 rats. Biomed Pharmacol 33:1309–1313

Stier A, Finch SAE, Greinert R, Höhne M, Müller R (1982) Membrane structure and function of the hepatic microsomal cytochrome P-450 system. In: Kitani K (ed) Liver and aging – liver and drugs. Elsevier Biomedical Press, Amsterdam, p 3–17

Uchida K, Matsubara T, Ishikawa Y, Itoh N (1982) Age-related changes in cholesterol-bile acid metabolism and hepatic mixed function oxidase activities in rats. In: Kitani K (ed) Liver and aging – liver and drugs. Elsevier Biomedical Press, Amsterdam, p 195–211

Van Bezooijen CFA (1984) Influence of age-related changes in rodent liver morphology and physiology on drug metabolism – a review. Mech Ageing Dev 25:1–22

Van Bezooijen CFA, Sakkee AN, Boonstra-Nieveld IHJ, Bégue JM, Guillouzo A, Knook DL (1982) The effect of age on digitoxin biotransformation by isolated hepatocytes. In: Kitani K (ed) Liver and aging – liver and drugs. Elsevier Biomedical Press, Amsterdam, p 167–176

Van Bezooijen CFA, Bukvic SJ, Sleyster ECh, Knook DL (1984 a) Bromsulfophthalein storage capacity of rat hepatocytes separated into ploidy classes by centrifugal elutriation. In: Van Bezooijen CFA (ed) Pharmacological, morphological, and physiological aspects of liver aging. EURAGE, Rijswijk, p 115–120

Van Bezooijen CFA, Sakkee AN, Boonstra-Nieveld IHJ, Knook DL (1984b) A decrease in the capacity of hepatocytes isolated from aged male BN/BiRij rats to metabolize digitoxin. Biochem Pharmacol 33:3709–3711

Varga F, Fischer E (1978) Age-dependent changes in blood supply of the liver and the biliary excretion of eosine in rats. In: Kitani K (ed) Liver and aging. Elsevier/North-Holland Biomedical Press, Amsterdam, p 327–339

Weigand W, Hannappel E, Brand K (1980) Effect of starvation and refeeding a high-protein or high-carbohydrate diet on lipid composition and glycogen content of rat liver in relation to age. J Nutr 110:669–674

Zurcher Ch, van Zwieten MJ, Solleveld HA, van Bezooijen CFA, Hollander CF (1982) Possible influence of multiple pathological changes in aging rats on studies of organ aging, with emphasis on the liver. In: Kitani K (ed) Liver and aging – liver and drugs. Elsevier Biomedical Press, Amsterdam, p 19–36

Effects of Hydrocortisone and Heparin on Growth and Glycosaminoglycan Synthesis of Cultured Human Fibroblasts (WI-38)

D. O. Schachtschabel, G. Sluke, and J. Wever [1]

Introduction

In contrast to "nonaging" tumor cells with unlimited proliferation potential in vitro (cell culture), normal diploid fibroblasts and epithelial cells undergo a limited number of divisions in culture, and are finally mortal (for review see Hayflick 1977; Cristofalo and Stanulis-Praeger 1982). According to Hayflick and Moorhead (1961), the growth behavior of normal fibroblasts in culture can be differentiated into three phases: the primary culture of freshly isolated (from the in vivo tissue) normal cells is termed phase I. Following subcultivation, these subcultures (phase II) are mainly composed of dividing cells. However, with increasing subcultivations and population doublings, there is a relative increase of slowly or nondividing cells in the total population, resulting in a deceleration of the average population doubling rate (phase III). Finally, after a finite number of population doublings the whole population primarily consists of nonproliferating ("phase out") cells. Such "division-arrested" cells (phase III phenomenon according to Hayflick and Morrhead 1961) die off in the course of several weeks or months. This phase III phenomenon was interpreted as an expression of aging at the cellular level (Hayflick and Moorhead 1961), and the limited life span of normal human and animal cells is regarded as a genetically programmed event (for review see Hayflick 1977; Cristofalo and Stanulis-Praeger 1982). Phase III ("senescent") cultures exhibit several characteristics which are similar to properties arising during in vivo aging, such as increases in lysosomal activities or residual bodies and lipid content (for review see Hayflick 1977; Reff and Schneider 1981; Cristofalo and Stanulis-Praeger 1982). And it is supposed that the two processes (the phase III phenomenon and in vivo aging) are regulated by similar mechanisms. Phase III fibroblasts – in comparison with phase II cells – are also characterized by a decreased responsiveness to growth factors (Plisko and Gilchrest 1983; Phillips et al. 1984; Schachtschabel et al. 1983; Tsuji et al. 1984). A distinctive feature of fibroblasts is their relatively high rate of glycosaminoglycan (synonymous with mucopolysaccharide) synthesis and excretion, especially of hyaluronic acid. Decreased synthesis rates of cell-bound and cell-released (medium) glycosaminoglycans (GAGs) were observed with "senescent" human fibroblasts in culture (Schachtschabel and Wever 1978; Schachtschabel et al. 1979; Wever et al. 1980; Sluke et al. 1981; Vogel et al. 1981), accompanied by a relative decrease in hya-

[1] Institut für Physiologische Chemie, Philipps-Universität, Lahnberge, D-3550 Marburg/F.R.G.

Drugs and Aging
Ed. by D. Platt

luronic acid and increase in heparan sulfate (Wever et al. 1980; Sluke et al. 1981; Matuoka and Mitsui 1981). Such changes in GAG synthesis were also found with cultured, "senescent" trabecular meshwork cells, derived from human eyes (Schachtschabel et al. 1982a, b). In this connection, we have discussed heparan sulfate as a "signal" or regulation factor for cell proliferation (Wever et al. 1980). Because of the structural similarity between heparan sulfate and heparin, we have tested the influence of addition of heparin to the culture medium of fibroblasts (WI-38), which resulted in growth inhibition and changes in GAG synthesis (Schachtschabel et al. 1979; Wever et al. 1980). The results of the second part of the present paper extend these former findings.

It is well established from in vivo investigations that glucocorticoids [e.g., hydrocortisone (=cortisol); or the synthetic derivative dexamethasone] have distinct influences on connective tissue metabolism, as on GAG (and proteoglycan) or collagen synthesis. We have recently described an inhibitory action of hydrocortisone on the synthesis of cell-released (medium) GAGs (Schachtschabel and Sluke 1984). In contrast to the medium GAGs, the pattern of cell-bound GAGs was changed by hydrocortisone, with an increase in hyaluronic acid synthesis and a decrease in sulfated GAGs. On the other hand, addition of hydrocortisone or other glucocorticoids to the culture medium of normal (diploid) fibroblasts results in an increase (by ca. 20%) of the number of population doublings, with a delay of the onset of phase III (Macieira-Coelho 1966; Cristofalo 1970; Grove and Cristofalo 1977; Nichols et al. 1977; Ban et al. 1980; Kondo et al. 1983). The mechanism of this "senescence-delaying" effect of hydrocortisone is unknown.

Material and Methods

Cultivation of the utilized embryonic lung fibroblasts (WI-38) in plastic culture flasks (Falcon or Nunc) with a growth surface of 25 cm^2, subculturing by trypsinization, the incubation with radioactive precursors, determination of cell number (of the fixed and with "Kernechtrot"-stained monolayer cells) or protein and ^{14}C-glucosamine-labeled cellular or medium GAGs have been described in former publications (Schachtschabel et al. 1977, 1979; Schachtschabel and Sluke 1984; Wever et al. 1980; Sluke et al. 1981).

The last possible subcultures of phase III ("phase out" cultures) were regarded as those which did not reach confluence within 4 weeks after the last subcultivation (1:2 split). Figure 1 shows typical cells from a proliferating phase II culture, and Fig. 2 cells from a phase out culture. Phase III cultures were defined as those comprising the last five population doublings before phase out.

The utilized *medium* was basal medium Eagle (BME diploid) with Earle's salts (Gibco) supplemented with nonessential amino acids (Sluke et al. 1981), antibiotics (135 µg/ml streptomycin sulfate, 100 IU/ml penicillin-G-sodium), and 10% fetal calf serum (Gibco). The dialyzed fetal calf serum was also obtained from Gibco.

Heparin (from beef lung, 152 U/mg) and heparan sulfate were gifts from Upjohn Co. The GAGs and hydrocortisone were obtained from Sigma Chemical Co. Stock solutions of GAGs were prepared by dissolving in regular culture medium

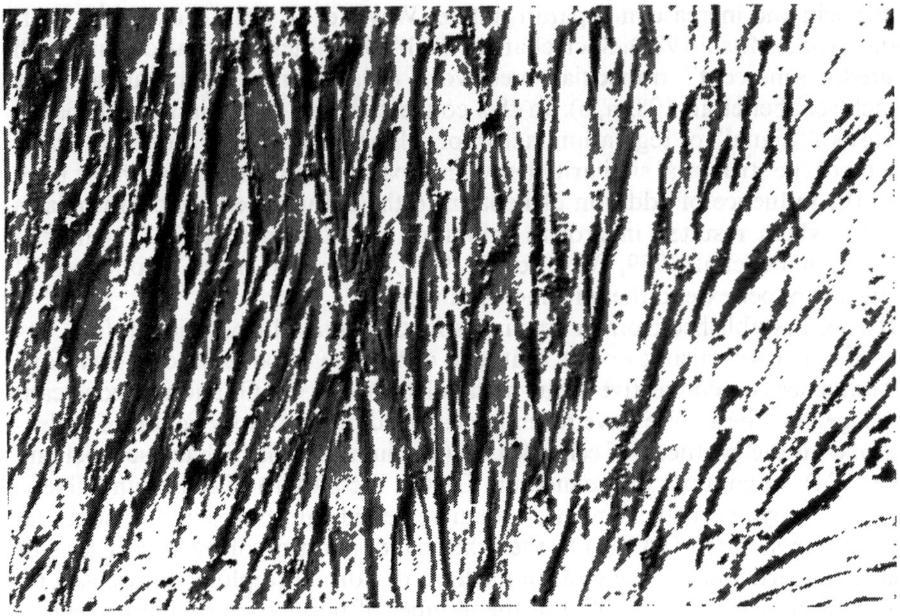

Fig. 1. Monolayer culture of human diploid fibroblasts (WI-38) in growth phase II. Photographed in living state, X 160

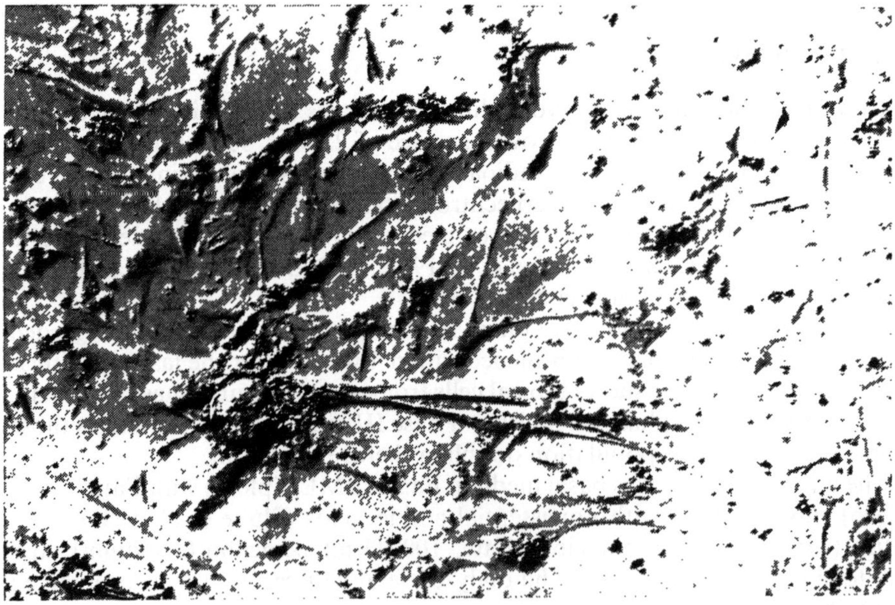

Fig. 2. "Phase out" monolayer culture of human diploid fibroblasts (WI-38) in growth phase III. Phase out culture is the last possible, "senescent" phase III subculture and consists of degenerating, irregularly shaped cells. The granula derive from disintegrated cells. Photographed in living state, X 160

(usually at 10 times the final experimental concentration). Hydrocortisone was dissolved in ethanol (9 mg/ml) and diluted thereafter with culture medium (5 μg/ml is equivalent to ca. 1.4×10^{-5} M). All stock solutions and media were sterilized by filtration (pore size: 0.2 μm).

Results and Discussion

Influence of Hydrocortisone on Growth

Addition of hydrocortisone (1.4×10^{-7} M) to the culture medium of phase II cultures results in a small though significant increase in proliferative activity. The results of a typical experiment are shown in Fig. 3. This stimulatory effect can also be shown by measuring DNA synthesis by ^{3}H-thymidine incorporation (Table 1). Following addition of dialyzed serum DNA synthesis of control cultures is reduced by about 65% (from 24380 to 8246 cpm) (Table 1); however, addition of hydrocortisone to cultures with dialyzed serum leads to a relatively stronger stimulation of DNA synthesis (by 52% instead of 14% with undialyzed serum). Thus, dialysis causes a loss of serum "growth factors" (insulin, platelet-derived growth factor? – and perhaps also of hydrocortisone, which might explain the stronger hydrocortisone effect in the presence of dialyzed serum). On the other hand, complete removal of serum (Table 1) leads to a very strong reduction in DNA synthesis in controls (2807 instead of 24380 cpm). Addition of hydrocortisone to such serum-free cultures has no effect on ^{3}H-thymidine incorporation into DNA, indicating that hydrocortisone only acts "in concert" with other serum factors.

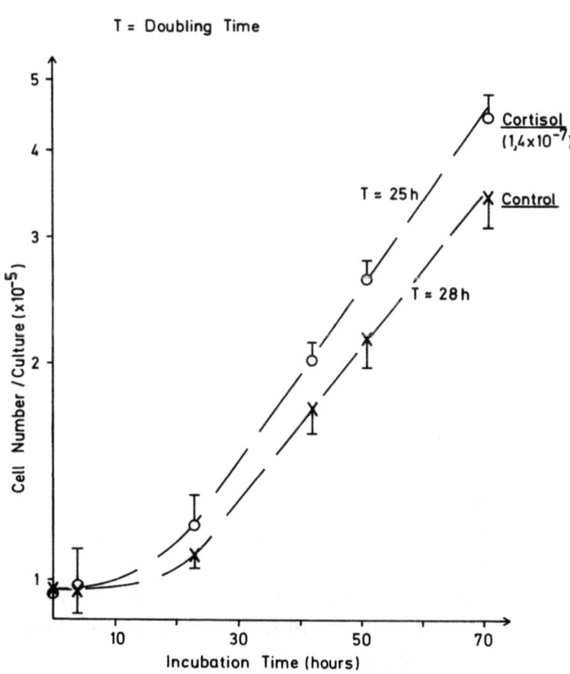

Fig. 3. Influence of cortisol treatment (1.4×10^{-7} M) on the proliferation of human embryonic lung fibroblasts (WI-38) in culture. A batch of cultures, each receiving the same cell number, was seeded at 0-time (with addition of hydrocortisone in the case of treatment) following trypsinization of parent cultures. Each value reflects the mean of two cultures

Table 1. Influence of hydrocortisone treatment (1.4×10^{-7}, 20 h) on incorporation of ^{3}H-thymidine into the DNA of WI-38 cells cultured in Eagle's medium (see Materials and Methods) without or supplemented with 10% fetal calf serum (FCS) (regular or dialyzed). Duplicate cultures were preincubated for 3 days in the respective media, before the media were renewed with addition of hydrocortisone (none in controls) and ^{3}H-thymidine (during the last 20 h)

Addition	^{3}H-thymidine incorporation (cpm/10^6 cells/20 h)	
	Control	Hydrocortisone
10% FCS	24,380 ± 1,110 (100%)	27,246 ± 413 (114%)
10% dialyzed FCS	8,246 ± 538 (100%)	12,549 ± 654 (152%)
No serum	2,807 ± 224 (100%)	2,863 ± 232 (102%)

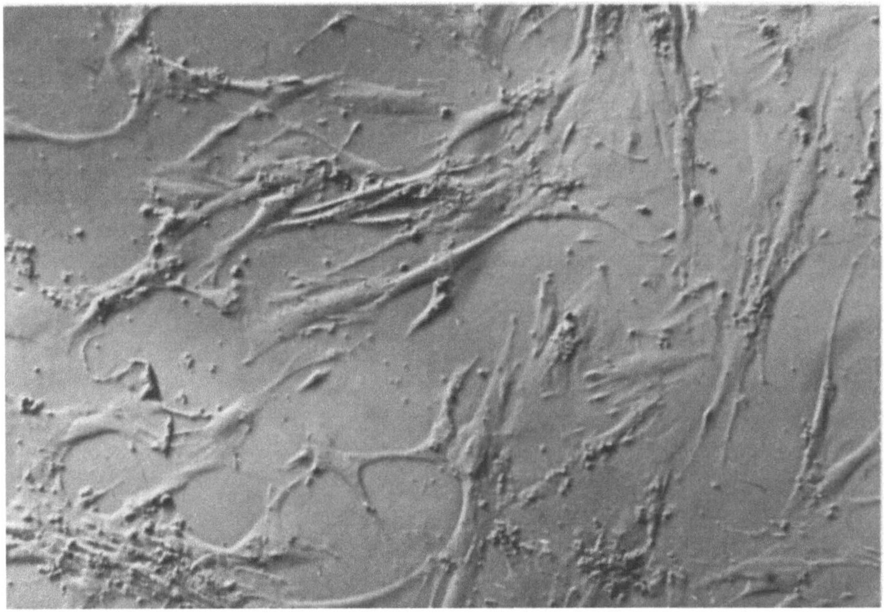

Fig. 4. Monolayer culture of WI-38 fibroblasts, derived from a phase II culture in the exponential growth phase, but cultivated for 6 weeks in BME medium supplemented with 10% *dialyzed* fetal calf serum (for details, see "Results"), with medium changes every 4 days. The cultures underwent ca. two population doublings during this period and finally appeared like "senescent" phase III cultures (compare with Fig. 2). Photographed in living state, X 160

In the presence of *dialyzed serum,* phase II cultures still undergo about two population doublings. Thereafter, the cells start to degenerate and they have the appearance of phase III cells (granulation, larger surface area, etc.) (Fig. 4). In the presence of hydrocortisone (1.4×10^{-7} M) such cultures with dialyzed serum pass through four population doublings. Thus, hydrocortisone exerts a significant multiplication-stimulating effect in the presence of dialyzed serum.

Influence of Hydrocortisone on GAG Synthesis

Incorporation of ^{14}C-glucosamine or ^{35}S-sulfate into medium GAGs occurs in a near-linear mode during an incubation period of at least 44 h, while the incorporation of both precursors into cellular GAGs levels off after a nearly linear incorporation rate for the first 20 h (Sluke et al. 1981). The same kinetics were found in the presence of hydrocortisone (Schachtschabel and Sluke 1984). However, as can be seen in Table 2, hydrocortisone treatment resulted in a significant, inhibitory effect on the incorporation of both precursors into medium GAGs: by 22%–24% in the case of phase II cultures, and by ca. 50% in the case of phase III cultures. Thus, "senescent" phase III cells appear to be more sensitive toward inhibition by hydrocortisone (Schachtschabel and Sluke 1984). The same holds true for cellular GAGs (Table 2). However, there was also a slight but significant difference between ^{35}S-sulfate and ^{14}C-glucosamine cell labeling, namely the latter is not or is somewhat less inhibited than ^{35}S-sulfate incorporation into cellular GAGs (Table 2).

An analysis of the GAG pattern offers an explanation for this difference: while the relative amount of hyaluronic acid and sulfated GAGs in the medium was not affected by hydrocortisone, the same treatment resulted in a relative (and absolute) increase in cell-bound hyaluronic acid and a decrease in cellular sulfated GAGs (Table 3). The distribution pattern of sulfated GAGs (chondroitin sulfate, dermatan sulfate, heparan sulfate) was not significantly changed by hydrocortisone treatment (Schachtschabel and Sluke 1984). Thus, the question arises of a possible functional significance of this cell-bound hyaluronic acid, especially since there is a continuous decrease in ^{14}C-glucosamine labeled cellular hyaluronic acid with increasing in vitro aging (Sluke et al. 1981; Schachtschabel et al. 1982b, Table 3). Most of this cell-bound hyaluronic acid appears to be localized at the cell surface and/or in the extracellular matrix, since it is removable from the monolayer cells by trypsin treatment (unpublished results). Hyaluronic acid has been implicated in cell-to-cell and cell-to-substratum adhesion (Culp 1974; Underhill and Dorfman 1978; Kraemer and Barnhart 1978; Forrester and Lackie

Table 2. Influence of short-term treatment (40 h) with hydrocortisone (1.4×10^{-7} M) on ^{14}C-glucosamine or ^{35}S-sulfate incorporation into cellular or medium glycosaminoglycans (GAGs) of WI 38 cultures at middle and late ("senescent") population doubling level

Radioactive precursor	Population doublings until phase out[a]	n	% Incorporation of hydrocortisone-treated cultures (cpm/mg cell protein/40 h of controls = 100%)	
			Cellular GAGs	Medium GAGs
^{14}C-glucosamine	20–8	20	101±5	76±3
^{35}S-sulfate	20–8	22	79±3	78±6
^{14}C-glucosamine	2–1	8	88±6	51±7
^{35}S-sulfate	2–1	8	64±4	50±2

[a] Phase out cultures are the last possible cultures of phase III, which do not reach confluence within 4 weeks (see also "Material and Methods")

Table 3. Influence of short-term treatment (40 h) with hydrocortisone (1.4×10^{-7} M) on the distribution of incorporated ^{14}C-glucosamine between hyaluronic acid (Hyal.) and sulfated glycosaminoglycans (sulfat. GAGs) in the cells and medium of WI-38 cultures at middle and late ("senescent") population doubling level

Treatment	Population doublings until phase out[a]	*n*	Relative incorporation of ^{14}C-glucosamine			
			Cells		Medium	
			Hyal. (%)	Sulfat. GAGs (%)	Hyal. (%)	Sulfat. GAGs (%)
–	20–8	22	19±6	81±6	58± 5	42± 5
Hydro-cortisone	20–8	10	32±3	68±3	59± 8	41± 8
–	2–1	10	8±4	92±4	38±11	62±11
Hydro-cortisone	2–1	6	22±5	78±5	33± 4	67± 4

[a] For definition of phase out, see footnote to Table 2 and "Material and methods"

1981; Underhill and Toole 1981, 1982). At least in the case of 3T3 and BHK cell cultures transformation with tumor viruses (simian virus 40; polyoma virus) resulted in a strongly reduced amount of cell coat hyaluronic acid (Underhill and Toole 1982). Furthermore, hyaluronic acid appears to be accumulated at those cell adhesion sites of the substratum at which cell movements start (Rollins and Culp 1979). Whether the reduced migratory activity of in vivo or in vitro aged cells (for review see Cristofalo and Stanulis-Praeger 1982; Macieira-Coelho 1983) is related to such a change in the cell surface composition is unknown. Cell-derived fibronectin in aggregated form but not plasma fibronectin displayed appreciable binding affinity for hyaluronic acid, and it is conceivable that such interactions might interfere with potential heparan proteoglycan binding to fibronectin, resulting in a destabilization of attachment sites (for review see Laterra and Culp 1982; Hynes and Yamada 1982).

The increased rate of synthesis of cell-associated hyaluronic acid following hydrocortisone treatment might provide at least a partial explanation in molecular terms for changes in cell surface properties ("decreased adhesion") which might account for, for example, the known increased saturation density of cultured fibroblasts caused by hydrocortisone (for review see Cristofalo and Stanulis-Praeger 1982; Schachtschabel and Sluke 1984). In this connection it would be of interest to determine whether the migratory activity of cultured fibroblasts changes in the presence of hydrocortisone. However, an effect of hyaluronic acid on the interaction with constituents of the cells or culture medium other than fibronectins (e.g., growth factors) has to be taken into consideration, too (Turley and Moore 1984). Furthermore, growth-influencing effects of glucocorticoids (such as hydrocortisone) might be mediated by changes in cellular growth factor receptors (e.g., Fanger et al. 1984).

Influence of Heparin on Cell Proliferation

Exposure of WI-38 cultures in the exponential growth phase to heparin (100 μg/ml) resulted in a striking growth retardation (Schachtschabel et al. 1979; Wever et al. 1980, Fig. 5). The extent of inhibition was about the same in the case of both short-term (up to 5 days) and long-term (ca. 4 weeks) treatment with heparin (Fig. 5). Thus, heparin causes a change in the proliferation rate. This is reversible, if one removes heparin from the medium (results not shown in a figure). The inhibitory effect of heparin was already seen at 20 μg/ml (Wever et al. 1980). Heparan sulfate was also inhibitory (though about five fold less so than heparin), while no growth inhibition was observed with chondroitin 4- or chondroitin 6-sulfate, dermatan sulfate, or hyaluronic acid at concentrations up to 500 μg/ml (Schachtschabel et al. 1979). It should be stressed that exposure to heparin did not result in cell death, as evidenced by the ability of these cells to grow for extended periods (months) in the presence of heparin (100 μg/ml). There was no significant difference in viability between control and heparin-treated cells as judged by the degree of trypan blue staining. However, the heparin-treated cells appeared to adhere more tightly to the substratum and to one another, since longer trypsinization periods in comparison with controls were required for detachment and disaggregation of cells. This was especially pronounced with "senescent" phase III cells. These observations suggest changes in cell surface properties following heparin treatment, as will be outlined in more detail below. In regard to growth-

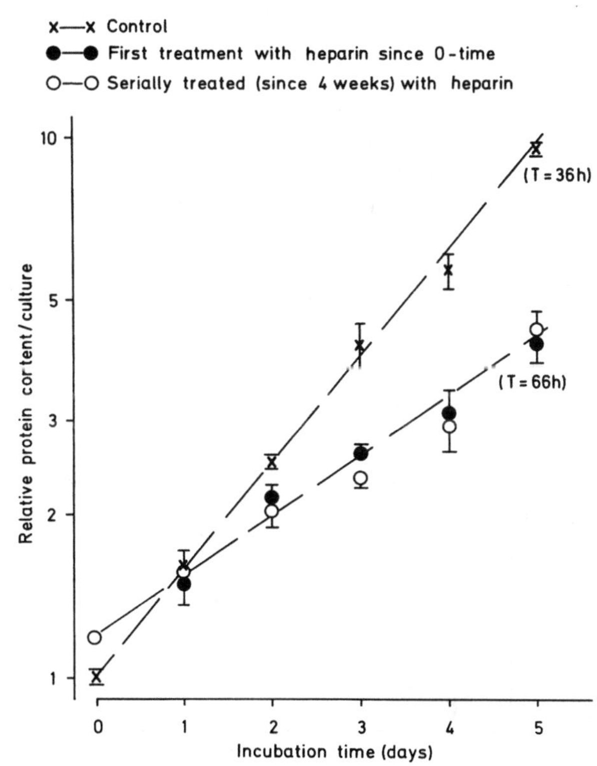

Fig. 5. Influence of heparin (100 μg/ml) on growth of WI-38 cultures in logarithmic phase. The cultures were seeded 2 days before 0-time (with heparin addition in serially treated cultures). In the case of first treatment, heparin was added at 0-time. Medium changes occurred at 0-time and after 3 days (with addition of heparin in the case of treatment)

inhibitory effects, the suppression of smooth muscle cell proliferation and the prevention of scarring by heparin should also be mentioned (Clowes and Karnowsky 1977; Castellot et al. 1982).

Influence of Heparin on GAG Synthesis

Treatment of phase II WI-38 cultures with heparin (100 μg/ml) resulted in significantly increased rates of cellular GAG synthesis, as measured by the incorporation of ^{14}C-glucosamine (Fig. 6; Wever et al. 1980). This increase occurred after a lag period of ca. 16 h. The synthesis of cell-released (medium) GAGs was less affected by heparin than that of cell-bound GAGs (Wever et al. 1980). Chondroitin 4- or 6-sulfate and hyaluronic acid in concentrations between 2.5 and 2500 μg/ml did not stimulate the synthesis of ^{14}C-glucosamine-labeled GAGs. Actually, slightly inhibitory effects were observed with hyaluronic acid (Wever et al. 1980). Stimulation of GAG synthesis occurred at heparin concentrations of 20, 100, 200, and 500 μg/ml and with heparan sulfate at between 100 and 500 μg/ml (results not shown in a figure). Also, ^{35}S-sulfate incorporation into cell-bound GAGs was elevated by heparin, though to a lesser degree than ^{14}C-glucosamine (Wever et al. 1980). The increased GAG synthesis rate was also observed after long-term (several weeks) treatment with heparin – in fact it was still more pronounced. Characterization of the individual GAG types labeled with ^{14}C-glucosamine or ^{35}S-sulfate of control and heparin (100 μg/ml, short- and long-term)-treated cells revealed stimulatory effects of heparin, especially on the synthesis of cell-bound hyaluronic acid and heparan sulfate (Table 4; similar but somewhat less pronounced effects were already observed after 40 h treatment with heparin). The altered cellular GAG pattern is reversible following heparin removal from cultures in the exponential growth phase. Thus, already 40 h later, incorporation of ^{14}C-glucosamine or ^{35}S-sulfate into cell-bound heparan sulfate was significantly reduced, and control values for hyaluronic acid and heparan sulfate were reached after about 4–7 days (results not shown in a figure).

In order to find out whether heparin interacts with the cells and perhaps has a "competitive" effect on cell-bound GAGs, these GAGs were prelabeled with ^{35}S-sulfate (for 40 h), and after three washes with "cold" medium the cultures

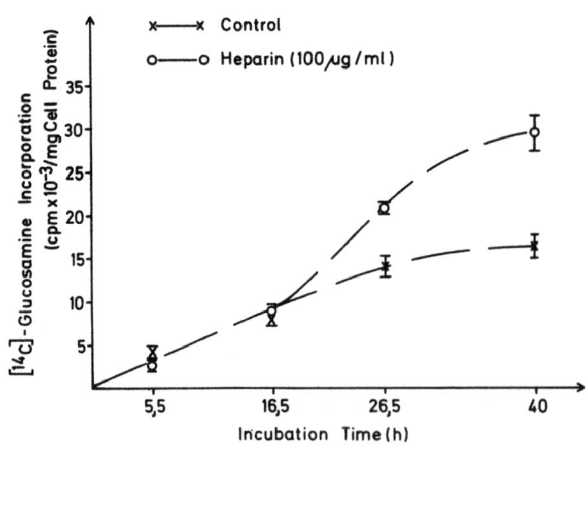

Fig. 6. Influence of heparin (100 μg/ml) on incorporation of [^{14}C]-glucosamine into cellular GAGs of WI-38 cultures as a function of incubation time. Heparin treatment started at 0-time. Each value reflects the mean of two cultures. The *ordinate* represents the incorporation of ^{14}C-glucosamine into total cell-bound GAGs

Table 4. Influence of long-term (6 weeks) treatment with heparin (100 µg/ml) on the synthesis of cell-bound glycosaminoglycans by phase II cultures in the exponential growth phase. Subcultivations (1:4 splits) were performed every 1–2 weeks. For the present experiments, subcultures (ca. 150 µg cell protein per culture) of control and long-term heparin (100 µg/ml)-treated cells were seeded at 0-time. Following incubation for 2 days, the medium of all cultures was renewed (with readdition of heparin in the case of treatment) and the cultures were incubated for further 40 h in the presence of ^{14}C-glucosamine or ^{35}S-sulfate. For determination of individual GAGs, see "Material and Methods". Results (cmp/mg cell protein; for each condition two cultures) of the individual GAGs of treated cultures expressed as % of the individual control GAGs, which add up to 100%. For example, in the case of ^{14}C-glucosamine incorporation, 110% hyaluronic acid in heparin-treated cells means about a six fold increase in ^{14}C-glucosamine incorporation in comparison with hyaluronic acid labeling of control cells (18%)

Culture n	Radioactive precursor	Relative incorporation (cpm/mg cell protein) of ^{14}C-glucosamine or ^{35}S-sulfate into cell-bound GAGs (Related to the respective control values, which add up to 100%)			
		Hyaluronic acid	Chondroitin sulfate	Dermatan sulfate	Heparan sulfate
Control	^{14}C-glucosamine	18 ± 0	15 ± 2	19 ± 4	48 ± 1
Heparin (100 µg/ml)	^{14}C-glucosamine	110 ± 7	11 ± 2	11 ± 3	88 ± 7
Control	^{35}S-sulfate	–	23 ± 1	25 ± 3	52 ± 2
Heparin (100 µg/ml)	^{35}S-sulfate	–	22 ± 4	9 ± 5	117 ± 6

were incubated in "cold" medium without ("controls") or with heparin (100 µg/ml) for further 31 h (Fig. 7). Thereafter, cell-bound and medium-released ^{35}S-labeled GAGs were determined. Incubation in the presence of heparin resulted in a significantly increased removal of ^{35}S-labeled GAGs. Results regarding the characterization of these GAGs indicate that this increase is predominantly caused by liberation of heparan sulfate. Therefore, we assume that exogenous heparin is able to compete with structurally similar heparan sulfate (probably located at the cell surface and/or pericellularly) and to replace it, at least in part.

As reported earlier (Wever et al. 1980; Sluke et al. 1981), senescent WI-38 cells (phase III) exhibited a change in the pattern of synthesized GAGs, with a relative increase in heparan sulfate and a decrease in hyaluronic acid. This raises speculation as to whether heparan sulfate might act – at least in the case of these normal (nontumorigenic) fibroblasts – as a growth-inhibitory regulation factor, and whether heparin might – because of structural similarities – mimic the effect of endogenous heparan sulfate. The molecular mechanism for the described effects of heparin (or heparan sulfate) is unknown. The effects could be due to an interaction with cell surface sites (as indicated by Fig. 7), which might interfere with membrane-associated processes for GAG synthesis (e.g., enzymes) or/and cell growth (e.g., receptor sites for growth factors; interaction with fibronectin). In this connection we feel it necessary to mention reports about a role of heparan

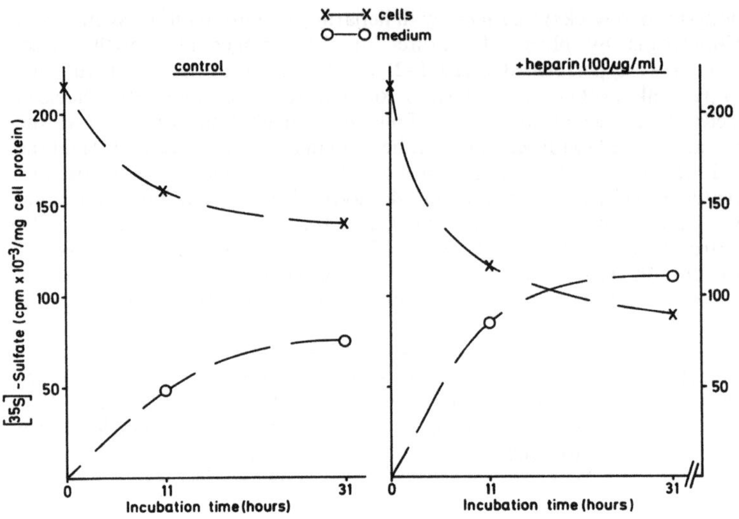

Fig. 7. Release of [^{35}S]-prelabeled cellular GAGs in controls and following treatment with heparin. The cultures (all with the same cell number) were prelabeled with ^{35}S-sulfate for 40 h. Following three washes with medium at 0-time, the cultures were "postincubated" in ^{35}S-sulfate-free medium in the presence or absence of heparin. After 11 or 31 h, the incorporation of ^{35}S-sulfate into cell-bound or cell-released ("medium") GAGs was determined. Each time point reflects the mean result of two cultures (deviation from the mean less than $\pm 5\%$). The *ordinate* represents the incorporation of ^{35}S-sulfate into total cellular or medium GAGs

sulfate (or heparan sulfate proteoglycan) and heparin in membrane-associated processes, such as binding to fibronectin (a mediator between cells and the extracellular matrix), to actin (interaction with the cytoskeleton of the cells!), or to platelet factor 4 (for review see Hynes and Yamada 1982; Hörmann 1982; Lark and Culp 1984; Woods et al. 1984). Actually, the latter observations indicate a transmembranous linkage of cell surface heparan sulfate proteoglycan(s) to the microfilament bundles of the cytoplasm and to the extracellular matrix. Such interactions might be important for mediating regulatory influences on cell growth, adhesion, locomotion, or the synthetic and secretory activity in regard to GAGs or proteoglycans (Schachtschabel et al. 1979; Wever et al. 1980). In this connection, an inductive effect of heparin and related GAGs on the secretion of specific smooth muscle cell proteins is of interest (Majack and Bornstein 1984). However, it cannot be ruled out that the effects of heparin result – at least in part – from intracellular action following fluid-phase or receptor-mediated endocytosis (Castellot et al. 1983) or from an interaction with specific serum constituents (e.g., platelet factor 4) influencing growth ("growth factors") and GAG synthesis. *In conclusion,* while both hydrocortisone and heparin increased the synthesis of cell-bound hyaluronic acid, heparin also stimulated the synthesis of cellular heparan sulfate. On the other hand, hydrocortisone treatment resulted in a significant inhibition of cellular and medium sulfated GAGs (including heparan sulfate; Schachtschabel and Sluke 1984). The proliferation rate (and the number of population doublings) was increased by hydrocortisone, while heparin (or heparan sulfate; Schachtschabel et al. 1979) exposure resulted in a decline in the proliferation rate of WI-38 fibroblasts, without affecting cell viability. It is assumed that exogenous heparin mimics – because of its structural similarity – the effects of "endogenous" heparan sulfate, possibly by interaction with specific cell surface sites.

Summary

Addition of *hydrocortisone* (=cortisol, 1.4×10^{-7} M) to the culture medium of normal (diploid) human fibroblasts (WI-38) with a finite number of population doublings resulted in increased proliferative activity. Following addition of dialyzed fetal calf serum (instead of regular FCS) to the culture medium, the proliferation rate was strongly reduced. After several weeks in this medium, the cells started to degenerate and took on the appearance of "senescent" phase III cells (granulation, larger surface area, etc.). Addition of hydrocortisone to cultures with dialyzed serum increased the number of population doublings (four instead of two). The synthesis of "secreted" medium glycosaminoglycans (GAGs: hyaluronic acid, heparan sulfate, chondroitin sulfate, dermatan sulfate), as followed by ^{14}C-glucosamine or ^{35}S-sulfate incorporation, was evenly reduced by hydrocortisone, with stronger inhibitory effects in the case of "senescent" phase III than with "younger" phase II cells. On the other hand, the pattern of cell-bound GAGs was changed by hydrocortisone treatment, leading to an increase in hyaluronic acid and a decrease in sulfated GAGs. Possible functions of cell-bound hyaluronic acid were suggested in regard to cell surface properties (cell adhesion, interaction with pericellular matrix).

Short- (several days) or long-term (several weeks) treatment with *heparin* resulted in a concentration-dependent retardation of the proliferation rate of WI-38 fibroblasts, without affecting cell viability. The average population doubling time increased nearly twofold (from 36 to 66 h) in the presence of 100 µg/ml heparin. Heparin treatment caused increased synthesis and deposition of cell-bound heparan sulfate and hyaluronic acid. Incubation of ^{35}S-sulfate prelabeled cells in the presence of heparin resulted in an increased liberation – compared with controls – of ^{35}S-labeled GAGs (predominantly heparan sulfate). It is assumed that exogenous heparin competes with structurally related heparan sulfate (probably located at the cell surface) and mimics the effects of "endogenous" heparan sulfate. This interaction with cell surface sites might interfere with membrane-associated processes in regard to GAG synthesis and cell growth (e.g., receptor sites for growth factors; interaction with fibronectin or platelet factor 4; effects on membrane-localized enzymes). The role of heparan sulfate as an inhibitory regulation factor for cell growth of these fibroblasts was discussed. It appears that an increase in cellular hyaluronic acid, as caused by hydrocortisone treatment, is "growth favorable" (as also indicated by the relative decrease during in vitro aging of these fibroblasts: Sluke et al. 1981), while an elevation in cellular heparan sulfate correlates with growth inhibition.

References

Ban S, Nikaido O, Sugawara T (1980) Modifications of doubling potential of cultured human diploid cells by ionizing radiation and hydrocortisone. Exp Gerontol 15:539–549

Castellot JJ Jr, Favreau LV, Karnovsky MJ, Rosenberg RD (1982) Inhibition of vascular smooth muscle cell growth by endothelial cell-derived heparin. J Biol Chem 257:11256–11260

Castellot JJ, Wong K, Herman B, Albertini DF, Wright TC, Hoover RL, Karnovsky MJ (1983) Binding and internalization of heparin by vascular smooth muscle cells. J Cell Biol 97 (5, Pt 2):430a (Abstr)

Clowes AW, Karnowsky MJ (1977) Suppression by heparin of smooth muscle cell proliferation in injured arteries. Nature 265:625–626

Cristofalo VJ (1970) Metabolic aspects of aging in diploid human cells. In: Holeckova E, Cristofalo VJ (eds) Aging in cell and tissue culture. Plenum Press, New York, p 83–119

Cristofalo VJ, Stanulis-Praeger BM (1982) Cellular senescence in vitro. In: Maramorosch K (ed) Advances in cell culture, vol 2. Academic Press, New York, pp 1–68

Culp LA (1974) Substrate-attached glycoproteins mediating adhesion of normal and virus transformed mouse fibroblasts. J Cell Biol 63:71–83

Fanger BO, Viceps-Madore D, Cidlowski JA (1984) Regulation of high- and low-affinity epidermal growth factor receptors by glucocorticoids. Arch Biochem Biophys 235:141–149

Forrester JV, Lackie JM (1981) Effect of hyaluronic acid on neutrophil adhesion. J Cell Sci 50:329–344

Grove GL, Cristofalo VJ (1977) Characterization of the cell cycle of cultured human diploid cells: effects of aging and hydrocortisone. J Cell Physiol 90:415–422

Hayflick L (1977) The cellular basis for biological aging. In: Finch CE, Hayflick L (eds) Handbook of the biology of aging. Van Nostrand-Reinhold Comp, New York, p 159–186

Hayflick L, Moorhead PS (1961) The serial cultivation of human diploid cell strains. Exp Cell Res 25:585–621

Hynes RO, Yamada KM (1982) Fibronectins: multifunctional modular glycoproteins. J Cell Biol 95:369–377

Hörmann H (1982) Fibronectin-mediator between cells and connective tissue. Klin Wochenschr 60:1265–1277

Kondo H, Kasuga H, Noumura T (1983) Effects of various steroids on in vitro lifespan and cell growth of human fetal lung fibroblasts (WI-38). Mech Ageing Develop 21:335–344

Kraemer PM, Barnhart BJ (1978) Elevated cell-surface hyaluronate in substrate-attached cells. Exp Cell Res 114:153–157

Lark MW, Culp LA (1984) Multiple classes of heparan sulfate proteoglycans from fibroblast substratum adhesion sites. Affinity fractionation on columns of platelet factor 4, plasma fibronectin, and octyl-sepharose. J Biol Chem 259:6773–6782

Laterra J, Culp LA (1982) Differences in hyaluronate binding to plasma and cell surface fibronectins. Requirement for aggregation. J Biol Chem 257:719–726

Macieira-Coelho A (1966) Action of cortisone on human fibroblasts in vitro. Experentia 22:390–391

Macieira-Coelho A (1983) Changes in membrane properties associated with cellular aging. In: Bourne GH, Danielli JF (eds) International review of cytology, vol 83. Academic Press, Orlando, p 183–220

Majack RA, Bornstein P (1984) Heparin and related glycosaminoglycans modulate the secretory phenotype of vascular smooth muscle cells. J Cell Biol 99:1688–1695

Matuoka K, Mitsui Y (1981) Changes in cell-surface glycosaminoglycans in human diploid fibroblasts during in vitro aging. Mech Ageing Develop 15:153–163

Nichols WW, Murphy DG, Cristofalo VJ, Toji LH, Greene AE, Dwight SA (1977) Characterization of a new human diploid cell strain, IMR 90. Science 196:60–63

Phillips PD, Kaji K, Cristofalo VJ (1984) Progressive loss of the proliferative response of senescing WI-38 cells to platelet-derived growth factor, epidermal growth factor, insulin, transferrin, and dexamethasone. J Gerontol 39:11–17

Plisko A, Gilchrest BA (1983) Growth factor responsiveness of cultured human fibroblasts declines with age. J Gerontol 38:513–518

Reff M, Schneider EL (1981) Cell culture aging. Molecul and Cellul Biochem 36:169–176
Rollins BJ, Culp LA (1979) Glycosaminoglycans in the substrate adhesion sites of normal and virus-transformed murine cells. Biochem 18:141–148
Schachtschabel DO, Sluke G (1984) Einfluß von Cortisol auf Glykosaminoglykansynthese und Wachstum von diploiden, menschlichen Fibroblasten (WI-38) in Abhängigkeit von der In-vitro-Alterung. Z Gerontol 17:141–149
Schachtschabel DO, Wever J (1978) Age-related decline in the synthesis of glycosaminoglycans by cultured human fibroblasts (WI-38). Mech Ageing Develop 8:257–264
Schachtschabel DO, Bigalke B, Rohen JW (1977) Production of glycosaminoglycans by cell cultures of the trabecular meshwork of the primate eye. Exp Eye Res 24:71–80
Schachtschabel DO, Wever J, Sluke G, Wever G (1979) Influence of exogenous glycosaminoglycans on growth and glycosaminoglycan synthesis of cultured human diploid fibroblasts (WI-38). Z Gerontol 12:19–26
Schachtschabel DO, Wilke K, Wehrmann R (1982a) In vitro cultures of human and monkey trabecular meshwork. In: Lütjen-Drecoll E (ed) Basic aspects of glaucoma research. Schattauer Verlag, Stuttgart, p 211–220
Schachtschabel DO, Rohen JW, Wever J, Sames K (1982b) Synthesis and composition of glycosaminoglycans by cultured human trabecular meshwork cells. Graefe's Arch Clin Exp Ophthalmol 218:113–117
Schachtschabel DO, Weyel G, Koch D (1983) Altered responsiveness of DNA synthesis and cell growth to serum or growth factors during in vitro ageing of cultured human diploid fibroblasts (WI-38). In: Abstracts 7th European Symposium on Basic Research in Gerontology, Budapest, p 47
Sluke G, Schachtschabel DO, Wever J (1981) Age-related changes in the distribution pattern of glycosaminoglycans synthesized by culture human diploid fibroblasts (WI-38). Mech Ageing Develop 16:19–27
Tsuji Y, Ide T, Ishibashi S, Nishikawa K (1984) Loss of responsiveness in senescent human TIG-1 cells to the DNA synthesis-inducing effect of various growth factors. Mech Ageing Develop 27:219–232
Turley E, Moore D (1984) Hyaluronate binding proteins also bind to fibronectin, laminin, and collagen. Biochem Biophys Res Commun 121:808–814
Underhill C, Dorfmann A (1978) The role of hyaluronic acid in intercellular adhesion of cultured mouse cells. Exp Cell Res 117:155–164
Underhill CB, Toole BP (1981) Receptors for hyaluronate on the surface of parent and virus-transformed cell lines. Binding and aggregation studies. Exp Cell Res 131:419–423
Underhill CB, Toole BP (1982) Transformation-dependent loss of the hyaluronate-containing coats of cultured cells. J Cellul Physiol 110:123–128
Vogel KG, Kendall VF, Sapien RE (1981) Glycosaminoglycan synthesis and composition in human fibroblasts during in vitro cellular aging (IMR-90). J Cell Physiol 107:271–281
Wever J, Schachtschabel DO, Sluke G, Wever G (1980) Effect of short- or long-term treatment with exogenous glycosaminoglycans on growth and glycosaminoglycan synthesis of human fibroblasts (WI-38) in culture. Mech Ageing Develop 14:89–99
Woods A, Höök M, Kjellen L, Smith CG, Rees DA (1984) Relationship of heparan sulfate proteoglycans to the cytoskeleton and extracellular matrix of cultured fibroblasts. J Cell Biol 99:1743–1753

The Influence of Esberitox on the Phagocytic Activity of Young and Old Isolated Perfused Rat Livers

T. VÖMEL [2] and D. PLATT [1,2]

Macrophages play an important role in the immunological system: They function as primary antigen acceptors and present them to the lymphocytes. They also phagocytose antigen–antibody complexes, thus removing the litter from the bloodstream (Katz 1980). So, the macrophages play the first and the last role in the immunological process. They determine which particles are to be eliminated, and also form the last indispensable effector organ in the immunological network. The increase of infections and tumorous diseases with age coincides with decreasing activity of especially the T-lymphocytes (Makinodan et al. 1976). Possibly to compensate for the decrease in the activity of the T- and consequently the B-lymphocyte system, the activity of the macrophages increases with age (Kay 1980; Price and Makinodan 1972). Therefore, the macrophages are more important than ever in the old organism. In spite of this importance, there have been only a few studies on the age-dependent reactions of the reticulohistiocytic system (RHS) to drugs, possibly because the RHS forms a disseminated organ which makes it hard to investigate in the intact organism. There are multiple interactions with other cell systems which make it necessary to use models for studying the macrophage system, but up to now few investigators have used these models to study the influence of drugs. Two experimental set-ups have been investigated sufficiently: The isolated perfused liver on the one hand, and isolated macrophage populations in cell cultures on the other. The isolated perfused liver offers several advantages over macrophage cell cultures: Firstly, the liver presents a less artificial model; secondly, the macrophages remain in their physiological cell context, which promotes their function (Price and Makinodan 1972); and thirdly, phagocytosis can be standardized and quantified. The liver contains approximately 85% of the phagocytic capacity of the RHS (Hopf and Ramadori 1980; Vömel and Platt 1982), which makes the isolated perfused rat liver a fairly quantitative model for the investigation of the RHS. The negative influence of corticoids (Miller and Meinykovych 1982), heparin (Bentley-Phillips et al. 1982), and colchicine (Sanui et al. 1982) on the macrophage system is widely known. Different substances seem to block different phases of phagocytosis. A positive effect on the phagocytic activity of polymorphonuclear granulocytes is claimed for an extract from the roots of *Echinacea,* known as Esberitox on the German market (Quadripur 1976). The age-related influence of Esberitox on the phagocytic capacity of rat livers is the subject of this paper.

[1] Institut für Gerontologie der Universität Erlangen-Nürnberg und [2] 2. Medizinische Klinik, Klinikum Nürnberg, D-8500 Nürnberg/F.R.G.

Drugs and Aging
Ed. by D. Platt

The experiments were carried out with animals of our own extraction. The young but mature animals were 10–12 months old and weighed 250 g; the old animals were 24–26 months old and weighed 380 g. They were anesthetized by intraperitoneal injection of 32 μg thiopental and anticoagulated with 1500 IU heparin. After removing the livers from the bodies (Vömel and Platt 1983), they were perfused for 2 h, as shown in Table 1. The perfusion fluid in the cyclic perfusion system was 150 ml of a hemoglobin- and protein-free medium which was replenished with oxygen in one part of the cycle. Samples to determine the rate of phagocytosis and the liver function parameters were taken at 0, 20, 40, 60, 80, 100, and 120 min. Different kinds of particles were offered to differentiate between the nonspecific and the specific recognition of material for phagocytosis: 120 mg ink with a particle diameter of 4 μm in 150 ml perfusion fluid was used to test the nonspecific recognition mechanism, and 10^6 red blood cells/ml were applied to test the specific recognition mechanism. Table 2 shows the 16 differing groups, each containing ten rats. 0.32 mg Esberitox/g body weight was administered to some groups in the perfusion fluid; other groups received the same amount for 7 days by intraperitoneal injection as pretreatment. After the last sample had been taken, the livers were fixed by perfusion with yellow fix for 10 min and prepared for electron microscopy (Ito and Karnovsky 1968). The results were checked statistically for significance by variance analysis and comparison of multiple mean values by Scheffe.

Figure 1 shows the results of the experiments with colloidal ink in the perfusion fluid. There were no significant differences between the control group and the Esberitox-treated animals, but a significant difference could be established between young and old animals ($P \leqq 0.05$).

Whereas the young livers reduced the ink concentration to 32%–36% of the original concentration after 120 min of perfusion, the old livers only achieved

Table 1. Perfusion of the isolated rat liver

Buffer medium:
free of Hb and proteins
with oxygen
Total volume: 150 ml in cyclic perfusion 120 min
Samples: 0, 20, 40, 60, 80, 100, 120 min

Table 2. Design of the study

Animals	Control	Phagocytosis	
		RBC	Colloidal carbon
10–12 months	×	×	×
24–26 months	×	×	×
10–12 months + Esberitox perfusion	×	×	×
10–12 months pretreated with Esberitox	×	×	×
24–26 months + Esberitox perfusion	×	×	×
24–26 months pretreated with Esberitox	×		

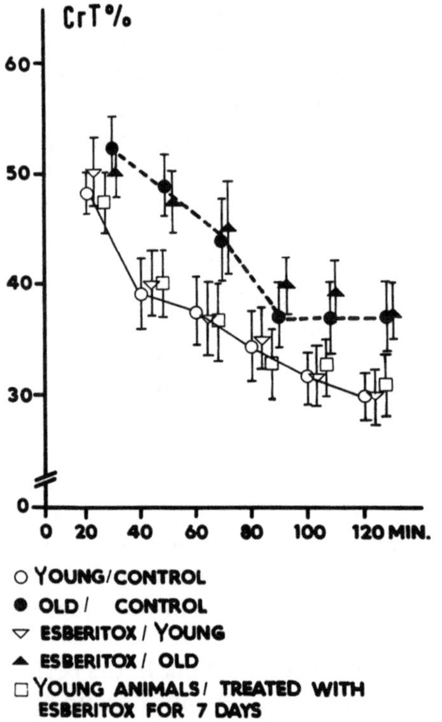

Fig. 1. Relative concentration of India ink in the perfusion medium

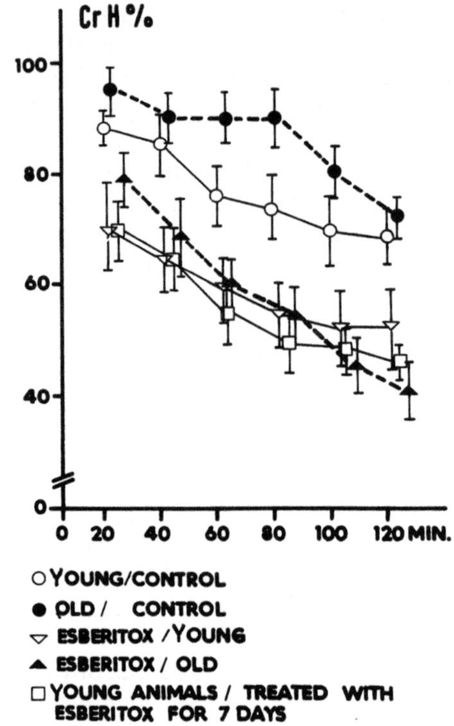

Fig. 2. Relative concentration of hemoglobin in the perfusion medium

39%–41%. A significant difference ($P \leqq 0.01$) emerged between the Esberitox-treated groups and the controls when red blood cells were used as colloidal particles. There was a small, nonsignificant difference between the Esberitox pretreatment groups and the those in which Esberitox was added to the perfusion liquid. The control group showed a significant difference between young and old animals, which disappeared under the influence of Esberitox. Figure 2 shows the old animals to have had a greater increase in the rate of phagocytosis. After 120 min of perfusion the young livers had reduced the original erythrocyte concentration to 76%. When Esberitox was added to the perfusion medium, the erythrocyte concentration sank to 54% and even went down to 47% in the case of pretreated animals. The old rat livers of the control group reduced the erythrocyte concentration to 80%. The other values also were above those of the young animals. With Esberitox in the perfusion fluid the old livers could lower the erythrocyte concentration to 42%. Glutamic oxalo-acetic transaminase (Gor) is a parameter of liver function and correlates especially with phagocytosis and the stability of the cell membrane. The activity of this enzyme remained significantly lower under the influence of Esberitox. Those groups that were offered colloidal ink for phagocytosis showed no change in the phagocytic capacity but an increased cell membrane stability with Esberitox. Those livers that were perfused

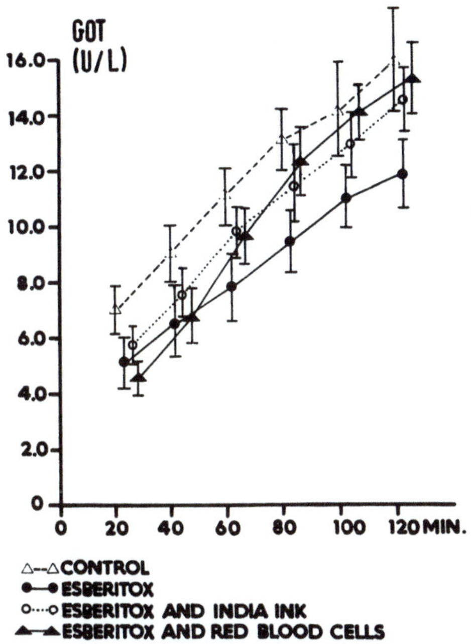

Fig. 3. Activities of glutamic oxalo-acetic transaminase

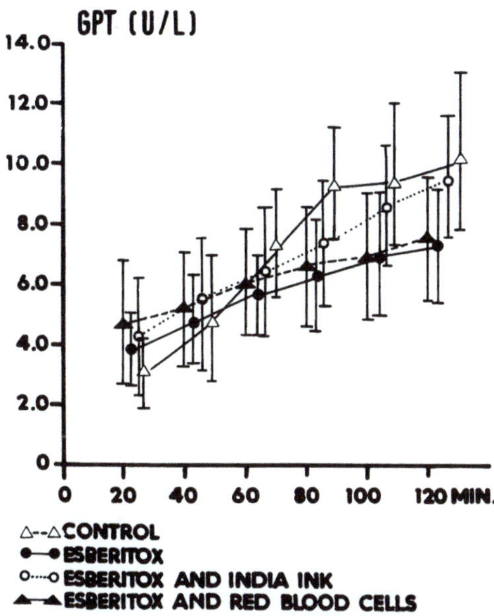

Fig. 4. Activities of glutamic pyruvic transaminase

with red blood cells performed a distinctly higher rate of phagocytosis as well as a greater cell membrane stability under the influence of Esberitox in both young (Fig. 3) and old animals.

Glutamic pyruvic transaminase is a parameter of the mitochondrial and the cell membrane stability and, to a lesser degree, the phagocytic activity. It generally showed the same tendency in young (Fig. 4) and old animals as GOT.

The potassium level showed no significant difference between any of the groups of either young (Fig. 5) or old animals. The cytoplasmic quotient of lactate of pyruvate rose 4 times higher than the control level during the perfusion of young livers with Esberitox, while the pretreated animals' quotient rose to not quite twice the control level (Fig. 6). With Esberitox treatment the aged animal livers reached only 30% more than the controls did. After 60–80 min perfusion, the lactate pyruvate quotient reached its higher level and remained constant.

The reaction of β-hydroxybutyrate indicates the mitochondrial redox situation; no significant differences were evident in respect of it for either young or old rat livers (Fig. 7). There was a high variability in the liver function parameters of young and old animals, though no statistically significant differences. These data are not presented in an extra table, as this would complicate matters unnecessarily.

No difference between the control group and the Esberitox-treated group could be established when ink was used as the colloidal particles in the perfusion fluid. Neither the morphological aspect of the liver parenchyma cells nor the in-

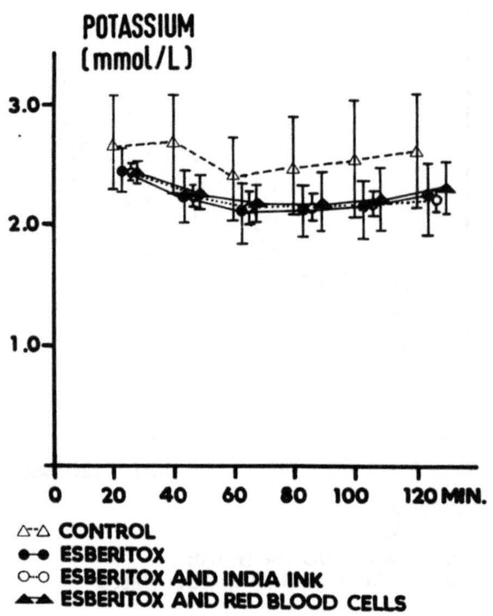

Fig. 5. Potassium content in the perfusion medium

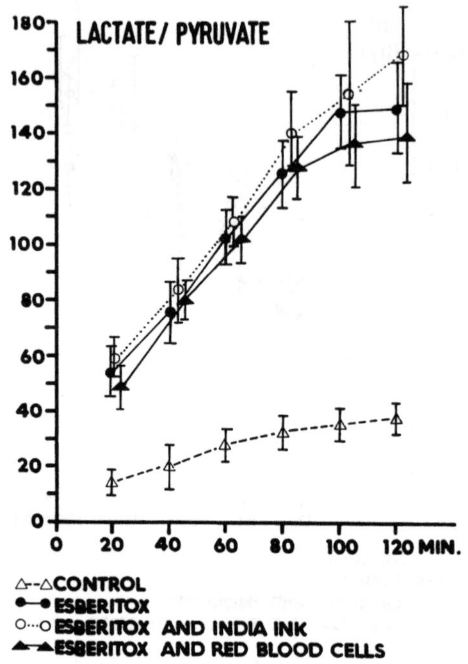

Fig. 6. Quotient of lactate/pyruvate

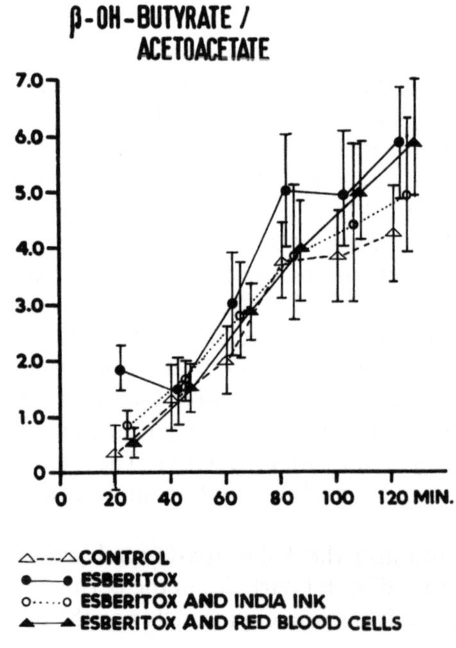

Fig. 7. Quotient of β-OH-butyrate/acetoacetate

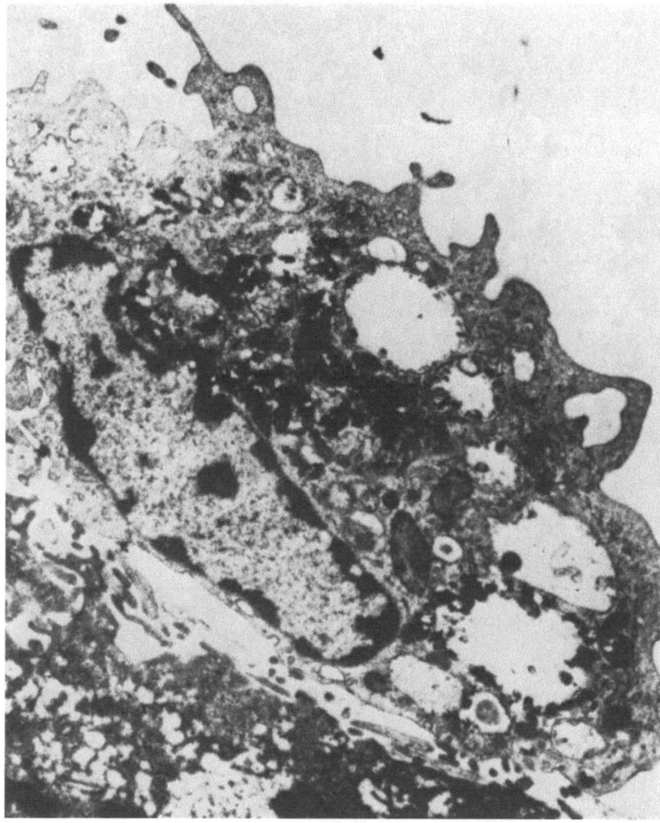

Fig. 8. Young rat liver cells under the influence of Esberitox (× 11 200); phagocytosis of colloidal carbon

gestion of ink by the Kupffer cells was altered by Esberitox (Figs. 8, 9). In the erythrocyte perfusions there were no morphological differences between the Esberitox-treated group and the control group. The number of adhered cells also gave no significant differences, which was to be expected. The main difference lay in the incorporation of a few erythrocytes by Kupffer cells. This demonstrates the influence of Esberitox on the second step of specific phagocytosis, i.e., the ingestion of the adhered material (Figs. 10, 11).

The number and the metabolic activity of polymorphonuclear granulocytes are significantly higher under the influence of Esberitox (Gerhardt 1972). The metamorphosis of monocytes to Kupffer cells takes 3–5 days (Whitelaw and Batho 1975), which made a 7 days' pretreatment sufficient. Cell reduplication is probably of little importance for our results, since pretreated animals showed the same phagocytic activity as those that only received Esberitox during the perfusion itself. Nonspecific absorption, the first phase of phagocytosis, is obviously independent of Esberitox: Ink as an inert substance is absorbed by a nonspecific mechanism and is not phagocytized differently under drug influence (Sauer et al.

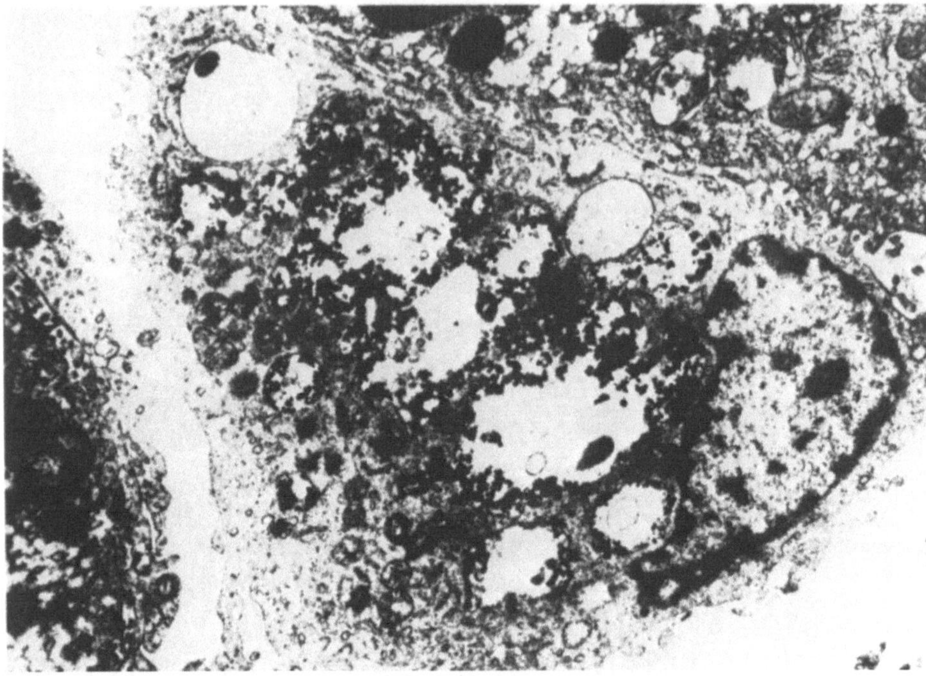

Fig. 9. Old rat liver cells under the influence of Esberitox (× 12000); phagocytosis of colloidal carbon

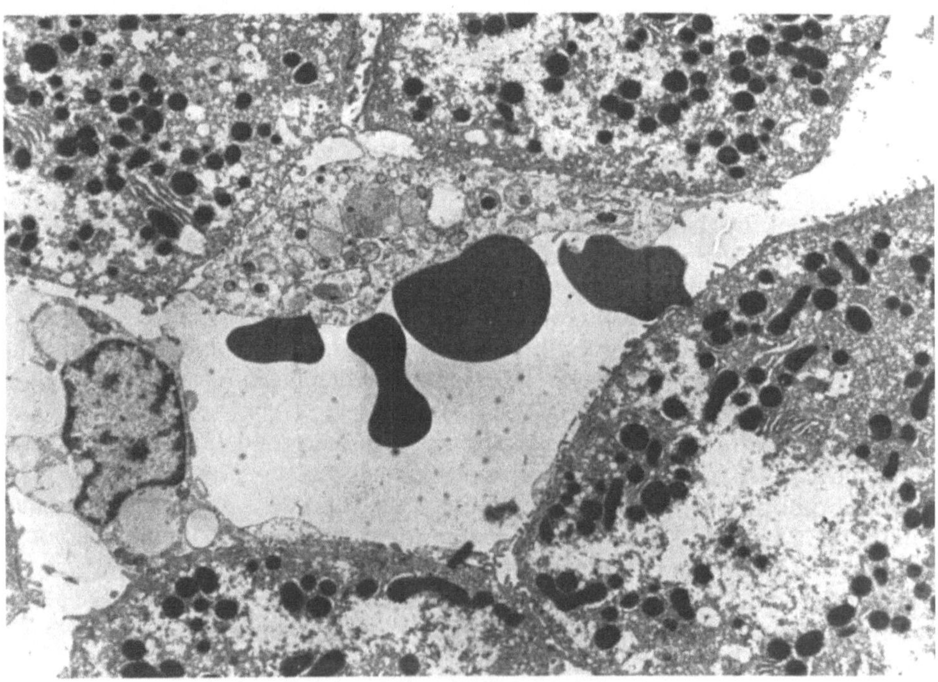

Fig. 10. Young rat liver cells under the influence of Esberitox (× 11000) with adhered erythrocytes

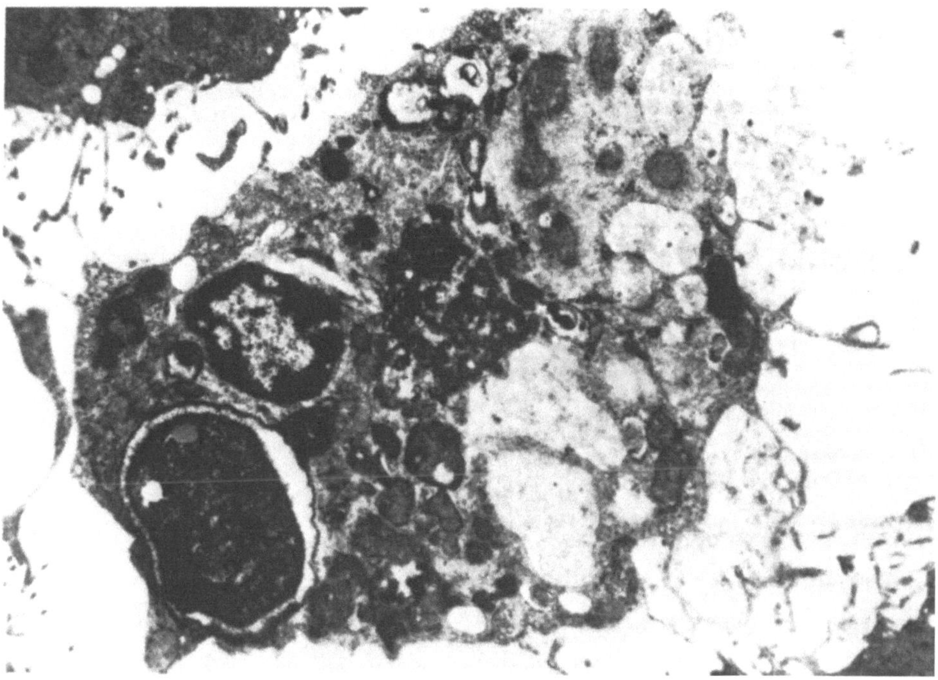

Fig. 11. Old rat liver cells under the influence of Esberitox (× 15 000) with complete phagocytosis of 1 RBC

1982). The specific absorption of erythrocytes is due either to complement and immunoglobulins or to a direct receptor mechanism. Up to now it has not been possible to discriminate between these two forms of binding. Our results indicate a significant positive influence of Esberitox on the first specific phase of phagocytosis (Fig. 12). Ingestion forms the second phase of phagocytosis and depends on the available cell energy (Weisdorf et al. 1982; Horwitz 1982). This energy limits the phagocytic capacity during liver perfusion (Vömel and Platt 1983; Schauer et al. 1982). Phagocytosis of red blood cells takes a half-life of 100–110 min (Hunt et al. 1981). The model of the isolated perfused liver shows the same kinetics with a half-life of 10–100 min depending on the phagocytosed cells (Hager 1983), but only for the first step of phagocytosis, the absorption of particles. The second step of ingestion takes much more time in vitro than in vivo, which may be explained by the limited cell energy supply. Esberitox obviously has a positive influence on the second step also, since the redox quotients stabilize on a new level in spite of an initial significant rise. The membrane function is characterized by the activity of the glutamic oxalo-acetic transaminase and the glutamic pyruvic (Scholz 1968; Lehninger 1972). The membrane appeared more stable under the influence of Esberitox. The significant differences between young and old animals during the control perfusion with red blood cells disappear in the drug-treated groups. A similar phenomenon occurs with piracetam (Vömel 1984), which also induces a significant increase of phagocytic activity in old animals, to the level of young animals.

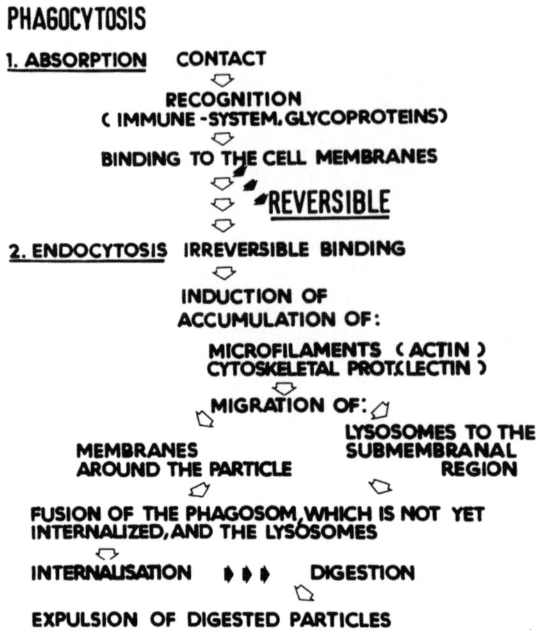

Fig. 12. Mechanism of phagocytosis

Conflicting results have been reported on the effect of antibiotics on the MPS: The same substance has been found to hinder or enhance phagocytosis, and to spur or to slow down leukotaxis by different investigators (Milatovic 1983).

Summary

The influence of *Echinacea* extracts (Esberitox) on the phagocytic activity of Kupffer cells was tested by the perfusion of isolated rat livers. The nonspecific phagocytosis of colloidal ink was not altered. The specific phagocytosis of red blood cells was significantly enhanced by Esberitox in young and old animals, both when the substance was added to the perfusion fluid and when the animals received 7 days' pretreatment. The combination of these data with the liver function parameters indicates a positive influence of the treatment on the specific receptor- or immunoglobulin-dependent first step of phagocytosis as well as on the second step, the ingestion of the absorbed cells.

References

Bentley-Phillips CB, Cooper RC, Hallet AF (1982) Pharmacological modulation of neutrophil phagocytic function in a patient with recurrent sepsis, pyoderma gangrenosum and impaired phagocytosis. Br J Dermatology 106:687–695

Bergham L, Ahlgren T, Lahnborg G (1977) Heparin induced impairment of phagocytic and catabolic functions of the reticulo-endothelial system in rats. In: Wisse E, Knook DL (eds) Kupffer cells and other sinusoidal cells. Elsevier, North-Holland Biomedical Press, Amsterdam

Gerhardt P (1972) Über den Einfluß einer unspezifischen Reiztherapie mit Esberitox auf die Leukopoese bei der Anwendung ionisierender Strahlen. Strahlentherapie 143(5):549–558
Guillouzo A, Lement B, Bogue JM, Gugum-Guillouzo C (1983) Functional capacities of adult human and rat hepatocytes maintained in a co-culture system. In: van Bezooijen CFH (ed) Pharmacological, morphological and physiological aspects of liver aging. Eurage Rijswijk
Hager K (1983) Untersuchungen zur Phagozytoseaktivität isoliert perfundierter Rattenlebern. Biochemische und ultrastrukturelle Untersuchungen zur Frage der altersabhängigen Erythrozytenphagozytose. Dissertation, Erlangen
Hopf U, Ramadori G (1980) Physiologie und Pathophysiologie des reticuloendothelialen Systems der Leber. Leber, Magen, Darm 10/5:277–283
Horwitz MA (1982) Phagocytosis of microorganisms. Review of Infectious diseases 4/1:104–123
Hunt JS, Beck ML, Wood GW (1981) Monocyte-mediated erythrocyte destruction. A comparative study of current methods. Transfusion 21/6:735–738
Ito S, Karnovsky (1968) Formaldehyde-glutaraldehyde fixatives containing trinitro compounds. Journal of Cell Biology 39:168–169
Katz DH (1980) Cellular and genetic basis of immunologic responses. In: Kay MMB, Galpin J, Makinodan T (eds) Aging, immunity and arthritic diseases (Aging, vol 11). Raven Press, New York
Kay MMB (1980) Immunological aspects of aging. In: Kay MMB, Galpin J, Makinodan T (eds) Aging, immunity and arthritic disease (Aging, vol 11). Raven Press, New York
Lehninger AL (1972) Biochemistry. Worth Publishers, Inc New York, 6th ed.
Makinodan T, Good R, Kay MMB (1976) Cellular basis of immunosenescence. In: Makinodan T, Yunis E (eds) Immunology and aging. Plenum, New York London
Milatovic D (1983) Antibiotics and phagocytosis. Eur J Clin Microbiol 2/5:414–425
Miller SC, Meinykovych G (1982) Inhibition by glucocorticoids of endocytosis in a macrophage like cell line. Journal of Cellular Biochemistry 18:423–431. Cellular Recognition 703–711
Price GB, Makinodan T (1972) Immunologic deficiencies in senescence: I. Characterization of intrinsic deficiencies. J Immunol 108:403–412
Quadripur SA (1976) Medikamentöse Beeinflussung der Phagozytosefähigkeit der Granulozyten. Therapie der Gegenwart 6:115, 1072–1078
Sanui H, Yoshida SI, Nomoto K, Ohara R, Adachi Y (1982) Peritoneal macrophages which phagocytose autologous polymorphonuclear leucocytes in guinea-pigs I: Induction by irritants and microorganisms and inhibition by colchicine. Br J Exp Path 63:278
Schauer R, Franco M, Müller E (1982) Involvement of a macrophage lectin in the phagocytosis of sialidase-treated erythrocytes. Clin Chem Clin Biochem 20,3:130
Scholz R (1968) Untersuchungen zur Redoxkompartimentierung bei der hämoglobinfrei perfundierten Rattenleber. In: Staib W, Scholz R (eds) Stoffwechsel der isoliert perfundierten Leber. Springer, Heidelberg Berlin New York
Vömel Th (1984) The influence of piracetam on the age-dependent phagocytosis of the RHS in the isolated perfused rat liver. In: van Bezooijen CFA (ed) Pharmacological, morphological and physiological aspects on liver ageing. Eurage, Rijswijk
Vömel Th, Platt D (1982) Age-dependent red cell phagocytosis and activity of the rabbit reticulohistiocytic system. Gerontology 28:144–155
Vömel Th, Platt D (1983) Phagozytoseaktivität der Leber bei verschiedenen Perfusionstemperaturen. Aktuelle Gerontologie 13/3:122–124
Weisdorf DJ, Chaddock PR, Jacob HS (1982) Glycogenolysis versus glucose transport in human granulocytes: differential activation in phagocytosis and chemotaxis. Blood 60/4:888–893
Whitelaw DM, Batho HF (1975) Kinetics of monocytes. In: van Furth R (ed) Mononuclear phagocytes in immunity, infection and pathology. Blackwell Scientific Publications, Oxford

Age-Dependent Differences of the Therapeutic Effect on Experimental Liver Fibrosis and Cirrhosis (Morphology and Biochemistry)

J. LINDNER [1], R. EURICH [1], K. GRASEDYCK [2], P. SCHMIEGELOW [1], and A. NÜSSGEN [1]

Introduction

Little is known about the subject of this paper. This is why experimental investigations are so important, and means that in vitro and especially in vivo analysis has to be done. Therefore we have chosen the most appropriate model of chronic liver fibrosis and cirrhosis, thioacetamide intoxication, which is better than other experimental intoxication models for comparison with human disease. This is important because these investigations are of practical clinical significance for the therapy in all age groups, and in particular the elderly. Especially the age-dependent differences in therapeutic effects on the basic processes will be analyzed, e.g., the primary necrosis of hepatocytes,histologically quantified by estimating the necrosis index, their regeneration (= ^{3}H-thymidine indices), the remaining intact or destroyed basic structure, etc. In this context it is appropriate to point out the importance of endothelial cell damage, especially of centroacinar endothelia but also of sinus endothelia which can be regenerated from histiogenic and hematogenic origin. So, age-dependent drug effects on cell proliferation and production metabolism will be analyzed, especially drug influences on decreasing and increasing parameters of degradation, synthesis, turnover, and total content of mesenchymal structure macromolecules after injuries with development of liver fibrosis and cirrhosis. Nearly all cell populations of the liver are involved in these glycosaminoglycans and collagen processes, which are enhanced under pathological conditions: hepatocytes and connective tissue cells (sinus endothelia, Kupffer cells, Ito cells, and portal fibroblasts), and other epithelial cells like bile duct epithelia. The total content of connective tissue in liver is low, but its metabolism is high, even under physiological conditions. The increased metabolism under pathological conditions depends on the severity and duration of injury, resulting in reversible or irreversible hepatic fibrosis, in experimental animals as well as in humans. The investigations of age-dependent differences in therapeutic effects on experimental fibrosis and cirrhosis should augment our present knowledge with regard to the important problems of the reversibility and irreversibility of liver fibrosis, too. This is investigated and described morphologically and biochemically by way of examples, and shows that the research into age-dependent drug influences on the development and progression of liver fibrosis and cirrhosis is of theoretical and practical importance.

[1] Abteilung für Zellpathologie des Instituts für Pathologie und [2] Med. Klinik der Universität Hamburg, Martinistraße 52, D-2000 Hamburg 20/F.R.G.

Drugs and Aging
Ed. by D. Platt

Material and Methods

Wistar outbred rats, strain Chbb:THOM (SPF), and Sprague-Dawley albino rats, strain Sut:SDT (Chbb:SPF), were used. The rats were of both sexes, and their age ranged from mature to senile. Methods were as follows:
Acute, subacute, or chronic thioacetamide (TAA) intoxication, sometimes with discontinuation for investigation of reversibility and irreversibility, esp. of liver fibrosis and cirrhosis, with and without treatment (chronic TAA intoxication = 25 mg TAA/kg body weight, daily, 6 days a week, orally by a gastric tube; acute intoxication = 100 mg TAA/kg body weight i.p. injected over a period of 5 days) (Becker et al. 1964; Lindner and Grasedyck 1973; Grasedyck et al. 1974, 1980; Grasedyck 1976; Grasedyck and Lindner 1976; Bachmann et al. 1978; Friedrich et al. 1978; Farhat et al. 1979; Helle et al. 1979; Willemer et al. 1984)
Measurement of body weight and absolute and relative organ weights (Grasedyck 1976; Bachmann et al. 1978; Farhat et al. 1979; Helle et al. 1979)
Macro- and microscopic investigations:
Standardized stains for ground substance and fiber components; morphological staging (Lindner 1972; Lindner and Grasedyck 1973; Grasedyck and Lindner 1976; Bachmann et al. 1978; Helle et al. 1979)
Enzyme histochemical stains; lysosomal enzymes, especially β-glucuronidase for glycosaminoglycans (GAG) degradation, with biochemical quantitative analysis (Fishman 1974), and also β-*N*-acetyl-D-glucosaminidase and collagen peptidase (for collagen degradation) (Borooah et al. 1961; Woollen et al. 1961; Grasedyck et al. 1971; Lindner 1972; Lindner and Grasedyck 1973; Ernst 1983; Schönrock 1983)
^{3}H-thymidine, ^{3}H-proline-, and ^{35}S-sulfate autoradiography with assays of labeling, and also of silver grain indices (Lindner et al. 1968; Lindner 1972)
Radio- and biochemical investigations:
Analysis of ^{3}H-thymidine incorporation rates (Lindner 1972, 1981), of DNA content (Burton 1956), of specific DNA activity (Lindner 1972; Schütte et al. 1979/1980; Lindner 1981), and of nucleotides and lactate (Schmiegelow 1979)
Assays of hexosamines, uronic acids (Gatt and Berman 1966; Svejcar and van Robertson 1967; Blumenkrantz and Asboe-Hansen 1973), ^{35}S-sulfate incorporation rates, and the specific activities of sulfated GAG (Becker et al. 1964; Lindner 1972, 1975), in part after GAG fractionation (Willemer et al. 1984)
Analysis of labeled hydroxyproline (Juva and Prockop 1966) and of the specific activity of hydroxyproline (Grasedyck 1976; Grasedyck and Lindner 1976; Grasedyck et al. 1980), in part after fractionation in neutral soluble collagen, acid soluble collagen, insoluble collagen, or pepsin degraded material (Grasedyck 1976; Friedrich et al. 1978; Helle et al. 1979; Grasedyck et al. 1980)
Assays of nonlabeled hydroxyproline contents in tissues, serum, and urine (Stegemann and Stalder 1967; Langness 1970; Grasedyck 1976; Farhat et al. 1979), of collagen-like protein (CLP) in serum (Langness 1971; Grasedyck 1976; Farhat et al. 1979), of the protein content (Lowry et al. 1951), and of prolyl hydroxylase (PPH) activities (an indicator enzyme for collagen synthesis) in liver and serum (Hutton et al. 1966, 1967).

As a means of comparison, similar analyses were performed on some human liver biopsies.

Results and Discussion

First, age-dependent differences of therapeutic effects are demonstrated by means of examples of chronic TAA-liver intoxication, fibrosis, and cirrhosis, because this model is more suitable for these investigations than other experimental liver fibrosis and cirrhosis models (Becker et al. 1964; Langness et al. 1975; Grasedyck 1976, 1980; Grasedyck and Lindner 1976; Bachmann et al. 1978; Friedrich et al. 1978; Farhat et al. 1979; Helle et al. 1979).

Figures 1–5 show (as one example of our investigations) a comparison between 1.5- and 16-month-old rats at the start of the experiment. The therapeutic influence is demonstrated by the data collected following administration of penicillamine (PEN) and prednisolone (PRED) together with TAA or alone [25 mg TAA, 200 mg PEN, 2.5 mg PRED (per kg bw), orally with a stomach tube]. The physiological development of the body weight was inhibited by TAA intoxication with and without therapy for the first 3 months of the experiment in the young rats. Older rats showed a physiological decrease in body weight over the course of the experiment. The decrease was greater following PEN and PRED treatment (both with and without TAA intoxication) than in control animals or animals that had undergone TAA intoxication without any form of treatment (Fig. 1, right side).

The body weight of mice and rats differs between strains and according to sex. Sprague-Dawley rats [Sut:SDT (Chbb:SPF)] showed their highest values at the end of the 15th month of life in females, and at the end of the 20th month in males. The body weight dropped after this maximum point in both sexes (corresponding

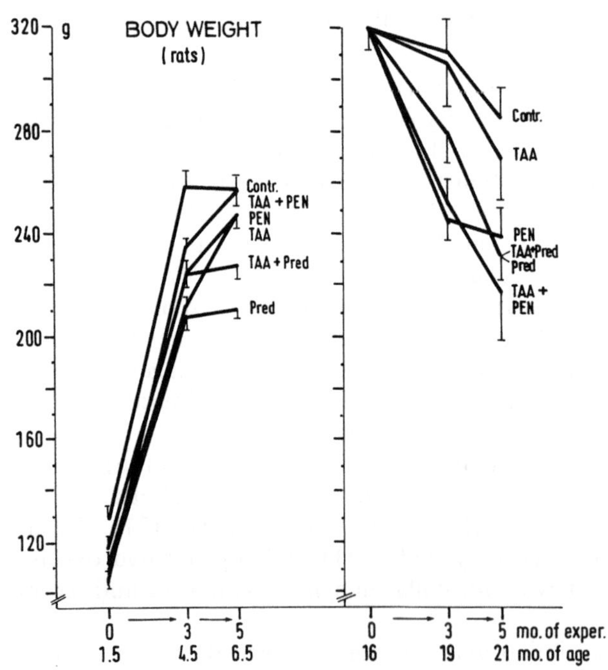

Fig. 1. Age-dependent changes of body weight of rats intoxicated by TAA and/or treated with PEN or PRED respectively (further details: see text)

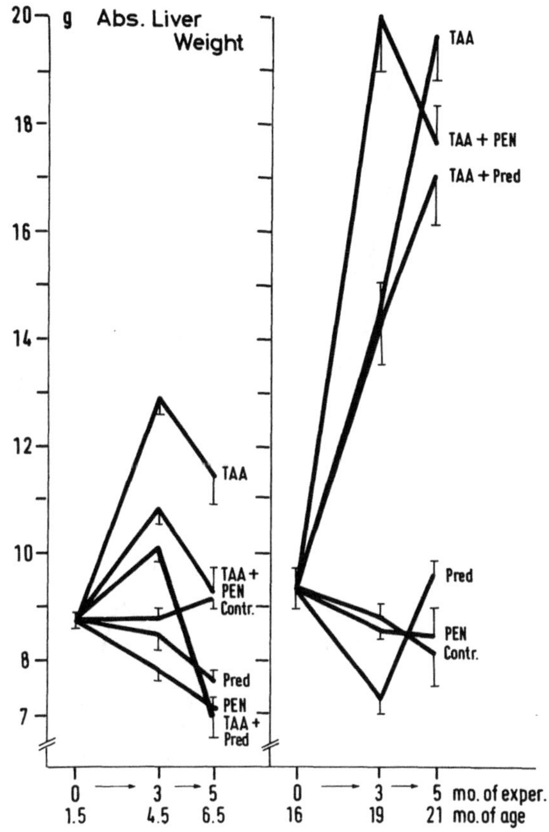

Fig. 2. Age-dependent changes of absolute liver weight of rats intoxicated by TAA and/or treated with PEN or PRED respectively (further details: see text)

to earlier findings: Lindner 1975, 1981; Kewitsch et al. 1978; Schütte et al. 1979/1980; Eurich and Lindner 1984). This is important for these and further investigations, and has a bearing on the absolute and especially relative liver weight.

In Fig. 2 the age-dependent differences in absolute liver weight by TAA injury and therapy with both drugs are demonstrated, but there were no age dependent differences in the drug effect without TAA injury in either age group considered. The absolute liver weight shows differences depending on the strain of rat, but also sex-dependent differences, like the body weight (Lindner 1975, 1981; Grasedyck 1976; Kewitsch et al. 1978; Farhat et al. 1979; Helle et al. 1979; Schütte et al. 1979/1980; Eurich and Lindner 1984). Similarities between the body and organ weights of humans and animals have been investigated (Rössle and Roulet 1932; Lindner 1975, 1981). These comparisons are essential for the analysis and the practical use of age-dependent differences in therapeutic effects, e.g. to fix more exact drug dosages in the elderly and children (= in relation to weight units). The age-dependent differences in the rat strain analyzed in Figs. 1–5, Sprague-Dawley strain Sut:SDT (Chbb:SPF), shows differences that can be compared with the findings in the Wistar outbred rat strain Chbb:THOM (SPF). Both strains have been well investigated by us (Lindner and Grasedyck 1973; Lindner 1975; Grasedyck 1976; Grasedyck and Lindner 1976; Bachmann et al. 1978;

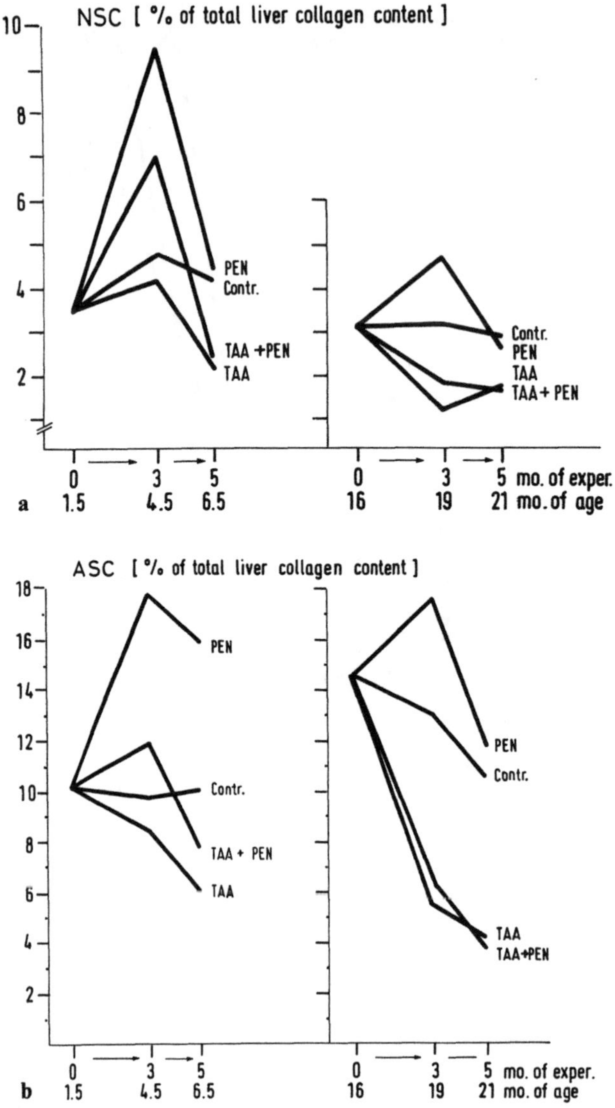

Fig. 3 a, b. Age-dependent changes of neutral soluble (**a**) and acetic acid soluble collagen (**b**) of rats intoxicated by TAA and/or treated with PEN (abbreviations and further details: see text)

Friedrich et al. 1978; Kewitsch et al. 1978; Farhat et al. 1979; Helle et al. 1979; Schütte et al. 1979/1980; Grasedyck et al. 1980; Lindner 1981; Ernst 1983; Schönrock 1983; Eurich and Lindner 1984; Willemer et al. 1984). The sex-dependent differences in body weight as well as in absolute liver weight are the reason why the relative liver weights (related to the body weight) are not quite suitable as an independent reference parameter for performances etc. The same is true for the relationship of the liver weight to the weight of the brain. This relationship is used for special reasons (Eurich and Lindner 1984) in some investigations of age-dependent differences in therapeutic effects in large series. The calculation of the relative liver weight (liver wet weight/body weight) still seems to be an easy

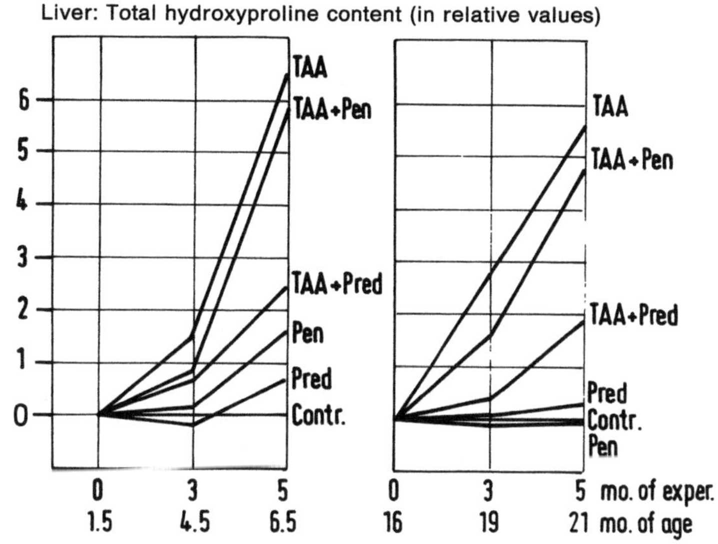

Fig. 4. Age-dependent changes of total hydroxyproline content (documented in relative values) of rats intoxicated by TAA and/or treated with PEN or PRED respectively (abbreviations and further details: see text)

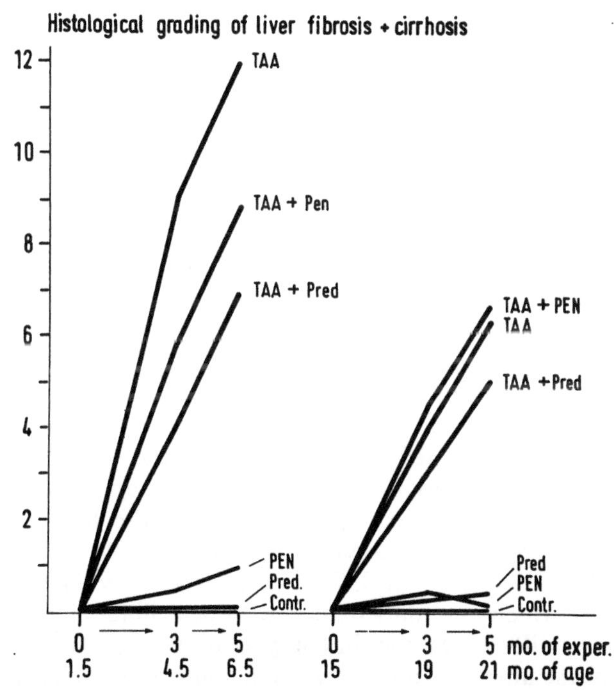

Fig. 5. Age-dependent changes of histological grading of liver fibrosis and cirrhosis (according to previous publications, further details: see text) of rats intoxicated by TAA and/or treated with PEN or PRED respectively

and reliable method for evaluating approximately the quantitative degree of age-dependent differences in therapeutic effects (especially the increase in liver collagen content), particularly for routine research in series (Bachmann et al. 1978). The age-dependent differences in relative liver weight by TAA injury and therapy are demonstrated, too, by our series: The values were higher in the older than in the younger animals, e.g., values of relative liver weight (in percent $\pm$ SD) for the untreated noninjured controls after 3 experimental months were 3.08 ± 0.17, for TAA 5.55 ± 1.36, and for TAA + prednisolone 5.21 ± 1.26. A further increase in the values was registered for the untreated TAA group at the 5th experimental month (7.55 ± 1.86) compared with the prednisolone-treated TAA group (3.92 ± 0.40), while the control group (without injury and treatment) showed the same relative liver weight as before.

Collagen fractionation was used in order to differentiate quantitatively neutral soluble collagen (NSC), acetic acid soluble collagen (ASC), and insoluble collagen (ISC) fractions (Grasedyck 1976; Friedrich et al. 1978; Helle et al. 1979; Grasedyck et al. 1980). In this way it is possible to identify drugs which hinder the maturation of collagen by inhibiting the transition of soluble to insoluble collagen. These substances are the subject of basic research into collagen biosynthesis and its disturbance (Becker et al. 1964; Hauss et al. 1968; Lindner 1972; Lindner and Grasedyck 1973; Chvapil 1975; Grasedyck 1976; Bachmann et al. 1978; Friedrich et al. 1978; Farhat et al. 1979; Helle et al. 1979; Ernst 1983).

Figure 3a demonstrates the clear age-dependent differences of therapy with penicillamine (PEN) alone or simultaneously with the TAA injury in the NSC fraction. The higher increase of NSC in percent of the total collagen in the younger age group in comparison to the older rat group is important, because NSC can be regarded as a parameter for the degree of synthesis, turnover, and metabolism of collagen, as shown by ^{3}H or ^{14}C labeling (Juva and Prockop 1966; Lindner 1972; Lindner and Grasedyck 1973; Chvapil 1975; Grasedyck 1976; Friedrich et al. 1978; Helle et al. 1979; Grasedyck et al. 1980).

Figure 3b demonstrates the percentual proportion of the ASC fraction. There are clear age-dependent differences in the single penicillamine effect compared with the control, and a stronger therapeutic penicillamine effect on TAA-induced liver fibrosis and cirrhosis in the younger than of the older age group In comparison with the TAA group, the rats which were intoxicated with TAA and additionally treated with penicillamine showed a significant difference in collagen maturation: The therapeutically desired decrease of collagen maturation was associated with an increase in the soluble collagen fractions (with easier and faster degradation), causing retardation or inhibition of the development of experimental fibrosis and cirrhosis of the liver (Lindner 1973; Lindner and Grasedyck 1973; Grasedyck et al. 1974, 1980; Grasedyck 1976; Bachmann et al. 1978; Friedrich et al. 1978; Farhat et al. 1979; Helle et al. 1979). Nonintoxicated rats, which were only treated with penicillamine or prednisolone, showed significant differences, too, in comparison with (a) livers predamaged with TAA and (b) the untreated and noninjured control rats. This again means a decrease in the synthesis, maturation, and deposition of collagen and thus in its total amount in the liver. These therapeutically positive effects of the two drugs are found only at the onset and during the early development of the disturbance of the normally high collagen metabolism of the liver. In progressive fibrosis and naturally in cirrhosis of the liver, these as well as other substances are not able to restore (or to normalize) the structural alterations, biochemically characterized by a high increase in the normally low total liver collagen content. Thus prompt treatment with these or other substances is desirable in human medicine. But the transfer of these or other results from animal experiments to human therapy is possible only with the usual restrictions (if it is at all possible) (Hauss et al. 1968; Lindner 1972; Grasedyck et al. 1974; Chvapil 1975; Langness et al. 1975; Bachmann et al. 1978; Friedrich et al. 1978; Farhat et al. 1979; Helle et al. 1979).

The ISC and the total collagen content of the liver are without essential age-dependent differences in the therapeutic effect of penicillamine. There was a positive quantitative correlation between the total collagen content and the morphological quantification of liver fibrosis and cirrhosis (see Fig. 5) in the younger rat group (Bachmann et al. 1978). Similar correlations were found by other groups, but without evaluation of age-dependent therapeutic influences (Kent et al. 1959).

The penicillamine and prednisolone effects are comparable with earlier findings by our and other groups, but in the past there has not been sufficient investigation of age-dependent differences in these and other therapeutic effects on the development of human and experimental liver fibrosis and cirrhosis (Becker et al. 1964; Koizumi et al. 1967; Hauss et al. 1968; Platt and Leinweber 1969; Takeuchi and Prockop 1969; Grasedyck et al. 1971; Lindner 1972; Galambos et al. 1973; McGee 1974; Chvapil 1975; Langness et al. 1975; Suzuki et al. 1975; Grasedyck and Lindner 1976; Risteli 1977; Bachmann et al. 1978; Friedrich et al. 1978; Farhat et al. 1979; Helle et al. 1979; Schmiegelow 1979; Stuhlsatz et al. 1980; Schönrock 1983; Willemer et al. 1984).

Figure 4 shows the percentual increase of the total collagen content compared with the controls (=0). This percentual increase is highest with TAA intoxication; no essential age-dependent differences are seen in the therapeutic effect of the drugs, given simultaneously or alone.

Age-dependent differences in the therapeutic effect of penicillamine and prednisolone on experimental TAA liver intoxication, fibrosis, and cirrhosis can be demonstrated by exact histological grading (Fig. 5). Histology can reveal fatty degeneration, further degenerative signs, and final necrosis of hepatocytes, which is quantified by the so-called necrosis-index of hepatocytes. The subsequent reactive infiltration and proliferation of hematogenic and histiogenic cells, with progression to "fat liver hepatitis," can be demonstrated and evaluated (the hematogenic and histiogenic origin of the cells is shown by special ^{3}H-thymidine-autoradiographic methods; for further details see Table 1). Semiquantitative evaluation of fatty degeneration, necrosis, and early fibrosis by TAA intoxication with and without prednisolone treatment – compared with untreated and prednisolone-treated control groups (without any intoxication) – shows that prednisolone can enhance the fatty degeneration of hepatocytes, besides some other injury effects on hepatocytes (Becker et al. 1964; Bachmann et al. 1978; Helle et al. 1979). The various signs of degradation of hepatocytes and the reactive processes around them (sinusoid cells and fibers), combined with mesenchymal cell proliferation and matrix deposits, can be demonstrated at higher magnification.

The role of degenerating and necrotizing hepatocytes as well as of proliferating epithelial cells of bile ductules in the disturbed collagen metabolism at the beginning of liver fibrosis is to be regarded as a process of induction and interaction between epithelial and mesenchymal cells of the liver. Furthermore, the epithelial cells of the liver have the capacity for collagen synthesis, which they do not use under essentially physiological conditions in adult life and aging. However, they can use this capacity under pathological conditions in vivo, besides other capacities of hepatocytes in culture (Ohuchi and Tsurufuji 1972; Sakakibara et al. 1977; Prinz et al. 1980). The epithelial cells of the liver, and especially the hepatocytes, are able to synthesize the various glycosaminoglycans (GAG) under normal and especially under pathological conditions in the organ in vivo. We differentiate between intraperi-, and intercellular GAG fractions of the several GAG types, in particular the GAG of intracellular organelles, including the nuclei, and the GAG secreted by cells in the peri- and intercellular space for further turnover and/or extracellular deposition.

The role of the GAG content in the nuclei of hepatocytes must be investigated under normal and pathological conditions (Furukapa and Terayama 1979; Willemer et al. 1984). Age-dependent drug effects on the different GAG localizations are now being analyzed. Such differentiation is necessary, because besides the epithelial cells, all mesenchymal cells of the liver are engaged with the GAG and the collagen metabolism: sinusoid cells, perisinusoid cells, Kupffer cells, endothelial cells, and Ito cells (for further details see Table 1). The localization and to some extent, the quantification of the disturbed and drug-influenced GAG and collagen metabolism in the liver cell populations is demonstrated by ^{35}S-sulfate and ^{3}H-proline autoradiographic results (Becker et al. 1964; Lindner et al. 1968; McGee and Patrick 1969, 1972; Lindner 1972; McGee et al. 1974). Radiobiochemical assays of the disturbed and drug-influenced GAG and collagen metabolism (using the suitable labeled precursors: ^{35}S-sulfate, ^{14}C-glucosamine, ^{3}H- or ^{14}C-proline, and others) carried out between experimental acute, subacute or chronic liver injury until the development of liver fibrosis ultimately show the same processes as in wound healing and other kinds of new formation of connective tissue in a granulation tissue: The GAG metabolism reacts before the collagen metabolism, both in degradation and in de novo synthesis (Becker et al. 1964; Hauss et al. 1968; Lindner 1972, 1975, 1981; Lindner and Grasedyck 1973; Chvapil 1975); this is also true in aging.

Synthesis, degradation, metabolism, and the total content of sulfated GAG are increased by acute, subacute, and chronic experimental and human liver injury and active fibrosis (Becker et al. 1964; Hutterer 1966; Koizumi et al. 1967; Hauss et al. 1968; McGee and Patrick 1969; Platt and Leinweber 1969; Takeuchi and Prockop 1969; Galambos and Shapira 1973; Lindner and Grasedyck 1973; McGee et al. 1974; Okazaki and Maruyama 1974; Suzuki et al. 1975; Pott et al. 1979; Edward et al. 1980; Gressner et al. 1980; Stuhlsatz et al. 1980; Willemer et al. 1984). In preliminary studies we have shown that the total ^{3}H-glucosamine incorporation in the quantitatively determined GAG fraction does not alter with age, but is significantly increased by acute TAA injury; this increase is much more evident in younger than in older rats, especially significantly for dermatan sulfate. In older rats the amount of incorporated radioactivity and especially hyaluronic acid increase after acute TAA intoxication. Thus the increased quantity and turnover of GAG following acute TAA intoxication run parallel, with differences for each specific GAG fraction. This is shown in more detail after different liver injuries, too (McGee and Patrick 1969; Suzuki et al. 1975; Edward et al. 1980; Gressner et al. 1980), and in human material (Koizumi et al. 1967; Galambos and Shapira 1973; McGee et al. 1974; Galambos et al. 1977; Stuhlsatz et al. 1980). Without TAA intoxication we found the well known age-dependent alterations in the GAG fractions in the liver: a relative increase in the percentage of dermatan and heparan sulfate (as in both human and experimentally induced liver fibrosis), partly decreasing during further development (Koizumi et al. 1967; Galambos and Shapira 1973; Suzuki et al. 1975; Gressner et al. 1980; Stuhlsatz et al. 1980). This is important with regard to age-specific therapeutic influences. The increase in the total GAG content in the liver with aging contrasts with its age-dependent decrease in other organs, whereas the age-dependent quantitative shifting of the GAG spectrum in the liver is very similar to that in other organs (Lindner 1975, 1981). Thus, the hepatic GAG metabolism in prenatal and postnatal maturation as well as in aging, with and without injuries (=disturbances of the physiological development and aging), needs to be analyzed in detail (see the following paper by Gressner). This is the prerequisite for investigations of age-dependent differences in therapeutic effects on the experimentally intoxicated liver with fibrosis and cirrhosis (Becker et al. 1964; Lindner 1972, 1975; Schmiegelow 1979; Schütte et al. 1979/1980; Lindner 1981; Ernst 1983; Schönrock 1983; Willemer et al. 1984). The uronic acid and hexosamine contents increase less than the hydroxyproline content in developing liver fibrosis and cirrhosis, with some age-dependent differences (in the proteoglycan, glycoprotein, and collagen contents). The DNA content increases faster in younger than in older rats during this process after acute and chronic injuries (independent on the aging polyploidization). Elevation of hydroxyproline/DNA ratio is demonstrated during the development of liver fibrosis and cirrhosis, with age-dependent therapeutic influences; this contrasts with our results to date in respect of the uronic acid/DNA and hexosamine/DNA ratios. Generally, there are stronger drug effects in younger than in older age groups (regarding these performance parameters). The data on the disturbed GAG metabolism in the development of liver fibrosis are still insufficient to explain the basic processes involved in reasonable and effective therapeutic influences, including age-dependent differences.

Besides GAG, all populations of liver cells, including hepatocytes, are able to synthesize collagen, with the capacity to produce collagen types I, III, and IV (Kent et al. 1976; Voss et al. 1980). But physiologically the capacity of collagen synthesis seems to be limited in fibroblasts and fibroblast-like cells in the liver. Under pathological conditions, hepatocytes can produce collagen. Hepatocytes in culture as well as hepatocytes isolated from injured liver contain large amounts of the indicator enzyme for collagen synthesis, i.e., prolyl hydroxylase (Ohuchi and Tsurufuji 1972). This enzyme activity is increased by injuries of the liver within 1–2 days, if fibroblasts are activated but not yet proliferating. Thus injury of the hepatocytes seems to be the primary reason for the immediate increase in prolyl hydroxylase activity following acute intoxication and injuries of the liver in humans and animals, as suggested by the results of our and other groups and by correlations of these enzyme findings with other indicators of the disturbed GAG and collagen metabolism (Hutterer 1966; Koizumi et al. 1967; Takeuchi and Prockop 1969; Langness 1970, 1971; Galambos and Shapira 1973; Grasedyck et al. 1974; Risteli and Kivirikko 1974; Langness et al. 1975; Grasedyck 1976; Grasedyck and Lindner 1976; Risteli 1977; Furukawa and Terayama 1979; Pott et al. 1979; Schmiegelow 1979; Edward et al. 1980; Gressner et al. 1980; Lindner 1981). Furthermore, activated macrophages stimulate perisinusoidal cells, which stimulate fibroblasts and fibroblast-like cells of the liver. The number of collagen-producing cells is further enhanced by the collagenase effects of Kupffer cells and other histiogenic and hematogenic macrophages (Lindner 1972; Lindner and Grasedyck 1973; Okazaki and Maruyama 1974; Lindner 1975; Knook et al. 1977; Wisse and Knook 1979). So, the primary increase in degradation (and degradation products) of collagen and GAG can stimulate the division and the production metabolism, esp. of mesenchymal cells in the liver after injuries, with age-dependent differences and with and without therapeutical influencibility (as in other organs displaying inflammation: review, Lindner 1972).

Besides autoradiographic localization and quantification, the increased GAG and collagen biosynthesis after injuries can be determined and quantified radiochemically, e.g., labeled soluble collagen increases to a value 8 times higher than that of control levels in early liver fibrosis (Grasedyck et al. 1974; Grasedyck 1976; Grasedyck and Lindner 1976). The same holds true for the labeled hydroxyproline in the insoluble collagen fraction. Thus the radioactivity of the collagen fractions is increased by TAA intoxication. Age-dependent therapeutic influences have been insufficiently investigated until now (Lindner and Grasedyck 1973; Grasedyck et al. 1974; Grasedyck 1976; Grasedyck and Lindner 1976; Helle et al. 1979; Grasedyck et al. 1980).

In early stages of fibrosis, the prolyl hydroxylase activity (according to Hutton et al. 1966, 1967) is increased, in part with a positive correlation of this indicator enzyme activity for the collagen synthesis from liver tissue to serum, and also with a correlation to the hydroxyproline content in the serum in comparison to the NSC content of the liver, which has previously been described as a special parameter for the collagen metabolism (Grasedyck et al. 1974; Langness et al. 1975; Grasedyck 1976; Grasedyck and Lindner 1976; Friedrich et al. 1978; Farhat et al. 1979; Helle et al. 1979; Grasedyck et al. 1980). Similar results have been reported by other authors (Takeuchi and Prockop 1969; Risteli and Kivirikko 1974; Risteli 1977). The prolyl hydroxylase activities in the liver decrease with aging, as in other organs, concomitant with the age-dependent decline in the connective tissue metabolism (Lindner 1975, 1981). The activity of this indicator enzyme for collagen synthesis is enhanced by TAA intoxication in the liver and in serum [e.g., it is three times elevated compared with control values during 3, 5, and 7 months of experimental TAA liver intoxication with fibrosis and cirrhosis: prolyl hydroxylase/liver (cpm/mg protein) in control vs. TAA intoxication = 3000 : 10950 at 3 months, 2200 : 9000 at 5 months, and 2000 : 7500 at 7 months]. Penicillamine and prednisolone treatment reduce the pathologically elevated prolyl hydroxylase activity (Langness et al. 1975; Grasedyck 1976). Age-dependent differences in these and other drug effects on prolyl hydroxylase are unclear at present; this is to be further investigated, because this enzyme activity is a very sensitive parameter that can be specifically used as an index of collagen synthesis. We demonstrated (like other groups) a correlation between this enzyme activity in the liver and the biochemically determined liver collagen content but not the prolyl hydroxylase activity in serum, and in part a correlation of this enzyme with other serum enzyme activities or parameters (Takeuchi and Prockop 1969; Ohuchi and Tsurufuji 1972; Grasedyck et al. 1974; McGee et al. 1974; Risteli and Kivirikko 1974; Langness et al. 1975; Grasedyck 1976; Farhat et al. 1979; Pott et al. 1979; Okazaki and Maruyama 1979; Grasedyck et al. 1980).

By biochemical determination, changes in the collagen content can be estimated earlier and more precisely than by routine histomorphology, where predominantly the insoluble collagen is stained and determined. The estimation of the specific activity of hydroxyproline is much more sensitive and determines the de novo synthesized part of collagen from the collagen pool (=ratio of labeled collagen to the total collagen content). By means of this ratio, the physiologically high collagen turnover (normally resulting in a relatively low total collagen content) as well as disturbances of liver collagen caused by injuries and therapeutical influences can be determined more exactly than by prolyl hydroxylase activity. All these measurements can also be made from small tissue particles like human biopsy material and are therefore very important for clinical questions (Takeuchi and Prockop 1969; McGee et al. 1974; Grasedyck 1976; Grasedyck et al. 1980).

The immediate increase in the anabolic mesenchymal processes following the increased catabolism of the liver normally having a high turnover of connective tissue can be determined by these methods (Hutterer 1966; Platt and Leinweber 1969; Lindner 1972; Lindner and Grasedyck 1973; Grasedyck et al. 1974; Langness et al. 1975; Lindner 1975; Grasedyck 1976; Grasedyck and Lindner 1976; Grasedyck et al. 1980; Lindner 1981). The activities of nonspecific protease and of lysosomal β-glucuronidase (Fishman 1971), an indicator enzyme for the final degradation of GAG, are to some extent enhanced in the liver by chronic TAA and/or penicillamine administration, without significant age-dependent differences (Lindner and Grasedyck 1975). The collagen peptidase activity (used in large routine series) shows a similar behavior and can be reduced by penicillamine in young and older chronically TAA-injured rats (Grasedyck and Lindner 1975, 1976). The serum values of this enzyme are nonspecific and without any age-related differences in animals and humans (Grasedyck et al. 1971, 1974; Grasedyck 1976; Grasedyck and Lindner 1976).

Another serum parameter of collagen metabolism is CLP (collagen-like protein). Figure 6 shows age-dependent differences: the control values are higher in older than in younger rats. The percentual increase by chronic TAA and/or penicillamine administration is higher in older than in younger rats, as are the absolute values. The total hydroxyproline content in serum is the sum of CLP, free hydroxyproline, and other hydroxyproline peptides, depending on collagen synthesis and degradation. The predictive value of this parameter for diagnosis, prognosis, and therapy of liver fibrosis and cirrhosis is low (Becker et al. 1964; Langness 1971; Chvapil 1975; Grasedyck 1976; Farhat et al. 1979; Grasedyck et al. 1980).

Penicillamine, glucocorticoids, and other drugs suppress (like lathyrogens) the proliferation of fibroblasts (see Table 1) and partly the degradation but especially

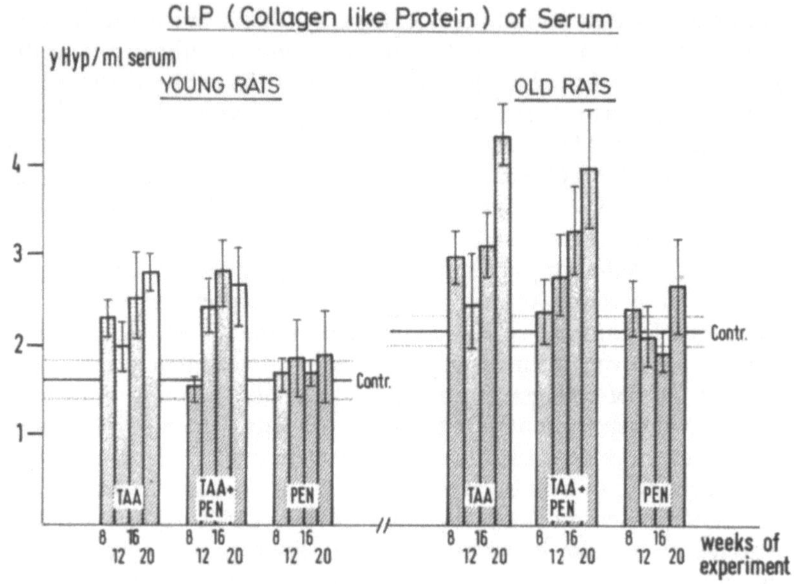

Fig. 6. Age-dependent changes of collagen like protein of serum of rats intoxicated by TAA and/or treated with PEN with regard to duration of the experiments

the synthesis of GAG and collagen. They inhibit ribosomal synthesis and the prolyl hydroxylase activity. Penicillamine inhibits aldehyde groups which are necessary for the cross-linking process of collagen and splits unstable cross-linked intermediates. In contrast to this effect of penicillamine, lathyrogens prevent the collagen cross-linking processes by inhibition of lysyl oxidase with depletion of aldehyde group formation. The results are ultimately the same in both cases: less insoluble collagen is formed, more of the enhanced soluble collagen fractions are degraded, and the development of fibrosis and cirrhosis can be depressed (Becker et al. 1964; Hauss et al. 1968; Lindner 1972; Lindner and Grasedyck 1973; Chvapil 1975; Grasedyck 1976; Bachmann et al. 1978; Friedrich et al. 1978; Farhat et al. 1979; Helle et al. 1979). We have shown that corticosteroids, estrogen, and progesterone can partially inhibit the collagen aggregation and thereby increase the amount of soluble collagen fractions, in particular of NSC (Bachmann et al. 1978; Friedrich et al. 1978; Helle et al. 1979). All these drugs show age-dependent differences in the inhibition of ^{35}S-sulfate, ^{3}H-proline incorporation rates, and GAG and collagen synthesis (Lindner 1972; Lindner and Grasedyck 1973; Grasedyck et al. 1974; Grasedyck 1976; Grasedyck and Lindner 1976; Bachmann et al. 1978; Friedrich et al. 1978; Farhat et al. 1979; Helle et al. 1979; Grasedyck et al. 1980). The significant increase in the NSC fraction due to TAA and penicillamine is more apparent in young animals (1.5 months old at the start of the experiment) than in the older rats (at least 16 months of age at the start of the experiment) (see Fig. 3 a). More than twice the total amount of collagen in the rat liver was produced by the younger group after extended TAA intoxication (which was tolerated much better by these animals than by older rats) but less by embryonic than by young adult rats. The same is true for the toleration of the drugs mentioned previously (Becker et al. 1964; Lindner 1972; Grasedyck 1976; Bachmann et al. 1978; Friedrich et al. 1978; Farhat et al. 1979; Helle et al. 1979; Grasedyck et al. 1980; Lindner 1981; Ernst 1983; Schönrock 1983).

Without going into detail, it may be concluded that after the embryonic development, growing, maturing, and adult rats have better regulating capacities for tolerating exogenous intoxication, injuries, disturbances, and drug treatments than rats at higher or senile age (Platt and Leinweber 1969; Platt and Katzenmeier 1970; Adelman 1972; Lindner 1972; Platt and Pauli 1972; Lindner and Grasedyck 1973; Chvapil 1975; Grasedyck 1976; Bachmann et al. 1978; Friedrich et al. 1978; Farhat et al. 1979; Helle et al. 1979). These age-dependent differences in therapeutic effects are demonstrated by the examples of penicillamine and prednisolone, but also by estrogen and progesterone therapy of TAA-induced liver injury, fibrosis, and cirrhosis. This is important for the age dependency of the reversibility and irreversibility of experimental and human liver fibrosis with and without treatment (Becker et al. 1964; Lindner 1972; Lindner and Grasedyck 1973; Grasedyck et al. 1974; Grasedyck 1976; Grasedyck and Lindner 1976; Bachmann et al. 1978; Friedrich et al. 1978; Farhat et al. 1979; Helle et al. 1979; Grasedyck et al. 1980; Willemer et al. 1984). Besides age, the drug effect depends on the dosis, duration of treatment, etc. (reviews: Hauss et al. 1968; Lindner 1972; Chvapil 1975). For further evaluation, the determination of age-dependent differences in therapy effects have to be investigated step by step, including the proof of inhibition of fibroblast proliferation and function in cell cultures of human fetal livers and of the inhibition of ^{3}H-thymidine labeling indices of these and other mesenchymal cells as well as of epithelial cells prenatally and postnatally, e.g., with and without the enhancing influence of kallikrein (Lindner 1972; McGee and Patrick 1972; Ohuchi and Tsurufuji 1972; Galambos and Shapira 1973; Risteli and Kivirikko 1974; Risteli 1977; Sakakibara et al. 1977). These and other groups have also investigated the age-dependent therapeutic effects on the various steps of GAG and collagen metabolism – that is, besides cell division, the performance steps of the cells, e.g., incorporation rates, transformation of proline to hydroxyproline, enzyme activities (prolyl hydroxylase, lysyl hydroxylase, galactosyl, and glycosyl transferase activities), and other steps of synthesis as well as of degradation of collagen and GAG (Becker et al. 1964; Takeuchi and Prockop 1969; Langness 1971; Lindner 1972; McGee and Patrick 1972; Lindner and Grasedyck 1973; Grasedyck et al. 1974; Risteli and Kivirikko 1974; Langness et al. 1975; Grasedyck 1976; Grasedyck and Lindner 1976; Risteli 1977; Sakakibara et al. 1977; Bachmann et al. 1978; Friedrich et al. 1978; Farhat et al. 1979; Helle et al. 1979; Grasedyck et al. 1980). Thus the further investigation of age-dependent differences in the therapeutic effects on experimental liver fibrosis and cirrhosis is the analysis just of the first steps by basic research.

For this purpose we investigated in particular acute TAA intoxication (100 mg/kg bw i.p. for 3 days) with resulting age-dependent differences in body weight as well as in absolute and relative liver weights: The physiological body weight increase was reduced by TAA application from +62.0% to +44.5% within 7 days in 1-month-old rats. 9.5-month-old rats showed a body weight decrease of 5.4% within 7 days after 4 days of TAA intoxication. Simultaneous prednisolone administration resulted in a greater weight depletion of 11.5% in 9.5-month-old rats and a greater inhibition of weight increase in 1-month-old rats (to only +36.0%). These are significant age-dependent differences.

TAA intoxication for 4 days resulted in an increase in relative liver weight (related to the body weight): In 1-month-old rats the increase from 5.5% to 6.8% was more significant than in 9.5-month-old rats, in which it was elevated from 3.7% to 4.0%. Simultaneous prednisolone administration caused a slightly greater increase in relative liver weight, to 6.9% in the younger and 4.5% in the older group. Four days after acute TAA intoxication, DNA was increased in 1-month-old as well as in 9.5-month-old Wistar rats (strain CHbb:THOM). Figure 7 shows that simultaneously administered prednisolone decreases DNA significantly more in 9.5-month-old rats compared with the younger age group. The older rats show parallel curves in ^{3}H-thymidine incorporation rate and in specific DNA activity, whereas in the younger ones this is not so. Summarizing, the older age group showed a more significant effect of TAA intoxication and corticoid administration, especially on the DNA content, with concomitant graphs of the specific activity than the younger animals.

A few samples are now given of the age-dependent differences in therapeutic effects on the basic processes:

Table 1 summarizes the results of quantitative autoradiography of ^{3}H-thymidine labeling indices. Remarkable is the decrease of these indices from the higher prenatal values during the postnatal maturation until its end – and until

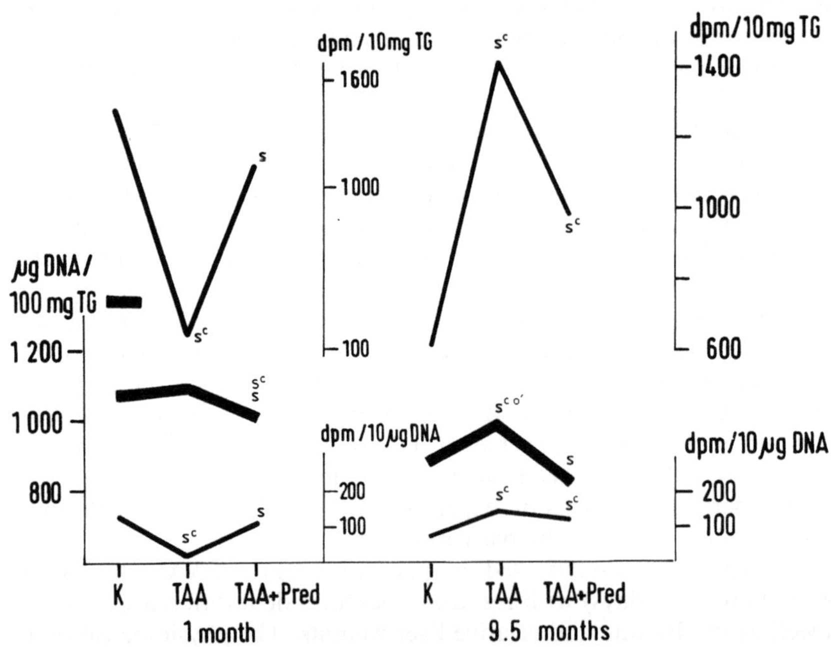

Fig. 7. Age-dependent changes of DNA, ^{3}H-thymidine incorporation rate, and specific DNA-activity of rat livers intoxicated by TAA or simultaneously treated with PRED (abbreviations and further details: see text)

Table 1. Age dependent differences of ^{3}H-thymidine-labeling indices (L. I. in %) of various cells of the liver without and after TAA injury (⬈, ↗). ▲ and ▼ = age dependent differences of further increase or decrease of L. I. by treatments (further details: see text)

	1 day prenatal	1.5 mo	5.5 mo	22 mo
Hepatocytes	4.05	0.5–0.84 ⬈ 5–10% ▲	0.2–0.34 ⬈ 4–8% ▲	0.05–0.1 ↗ 3–5% ▲
Sinus endothelial cells	1.0–1.1	1.8–2.2 ⬈ 3–6% ▲	1.5–1.75 ⬈ 3–5% ▲	0.05–0.1 ↗ 2–3% ▲
Periportal fibroblasts	1.0–1.5	2.0–2.5 ⬈ 15–30% ▼	1.5–2.0 ⬈ 10–15% ▼	0.05–0.1 ↗ 5–10% ▼
Portal bile-duct-epithelia	1.5–2.0	0.5–1.0 ⬈ 20–40% ▼	0.2–0.3 ⬈ 10–15% ▼	0.05–0.1 ↗ 5–8% ▼
Central venous endothelia	1.0–1.5	0.2–0.5 ⬈ 3–6%	0.1–0.3 ⬈ 2–4%	0.05–0.1 ↗ 2–3%

the comparatively low stable values, which we also see, for example, in 22-month-old rats (Table 1). The age-dependent increase in the ^{3}H-thymidine labeling indices caused by injuries, here by TAA, is very fast at younger ages (demonstrated by nearly vertical arrows). These findings are in contrast to the results at higher ages (more horizontal arrows; see right side of Table 1). This indicates that at higher ages the increase in the proliferation of the cell populations caused by injuries starts more slowly and later but is in part relatively higher than at younger ages. This is fundamental for the further investigation of age-dependent differences in therapeutic effects on the proliferation of these cell types (as well as their performance, discussed before). This is especially true for the promoting influence on the proliferation of hepatocytes and sinus endothelial cells as well as for the inhibition of proliferation (and performance) of fibroblasts and fibroblast-like cells in the liver, desirable because their proliferation (—increase of division and performance metabolism) is responsible for the progression of liver fibrosis and cirrhosis (Becker et al. 1964; McGee and Patrick 1969, 1972; McGee et al. 1974; Ohuchi and Tsurufuji 1972; Galambos et al. 1973, 1977; Kent et al. 1976; Knook et al. 1977; Sakakibara et al. 1977; Wisse and Knook 1979; Grasedyck et al. 1980; Prinz et al. 1980; Voss et al. 1980; Lindner 1981; Willemer et al. 1984).

In Table 1, our results and those of other groups are summarized for five liver cell populations (two epithelial, three mesenchymal cells). In microscopic ^{3}H-thymidine autoradiographs it is impossible to differentiate the several kinds of liver sinus endothelial cells, and in particular to separate the so-called Ito cells, the number of which varies, especially under pathological conditions. Several injuries and intoxications and administration of radioactive labeled vitamin A (orally or parenterally) rapidly increase the number of lipid-storing cells (the morphological descriptive name of the so-called Ito cells) according to the results of our and other groups about the structure, function, and variation in number of these cells, which show age-dependent differences under normal and pathological conditions, with and without treatment by drugs (Kent et al. 1976; Knook et al. 1977; Wisse and Knook 1979). Preliminary results show that the more the typical lipid storage of Ito cells increases, the less they are labeled by radioactive precursors for the localization and identification of GAG and collagen synthesis. Similar observations have been made by our and other groups regarding the same problem with smooth muscle cells: The more they become foam cells by lipid storing and/or lipid synthesis, the less they are able to synthesize the vascular GAG and collagen types (review: Lindner 1975, 1981). There are comparable findings on Kupffer cells, too: they can simultaneously express both processes, phagocytosis and collagen synthesis, like other mesenchymal cells of the liver and other organs, as demonstrated by simultaneous phagocytosis and autoradiographic localization of collagen as well as of GAG synthesis by suitable labeled precursors (see above). Like other liver mesenchymal cells which are responsible for the development of liver fibrosis, Kupffer cells proliferate especially after certain kinds of injury.

In particular, Kupffer cells activate collagenase. But all the mesenchymal cells of the liver (as well as of other organs) which are able to synthesize connective tissue structure macromolecules (proteoglycans, GAG, collagen, elastin) are also able to degrade these macromolecules. So each of the cells is responsible for degradation *and* synthesis under normal and much more intensively under pathological conditions (review: Lindner 1972, 1975, 1981).

The longer liver injuries last and the more serious they are, the more hematogenic cells participate in the mesenchymal cell pool (proliferation *and* production outside and inside the portal areas). As Table 1 shows, the sinusoid cells (Kupffer cells, endothelial cells, and Ito cells) can be injured and proliferate. The histiogenic and hematogenic origin of mesenchymal cells after acute and chronic injuries of the liver (for the function of macrophages and fibroblasts) depends finally on the kind, strength, and duration of intoxication and injury of the liver (Becker et al. 1964; Lindner et al. 1968; Lindner 1972; Lindner and Grasedyck 1973; Lindner 1975; Kent et al. 1976; Galambos et al. 1977; Knook et al. 1977; Bachmann et al. 1978; Wisse and Knook 1979; Schütte et al. 1979/1980; Lindner 1981).

Thus the discussion of the findings in Table 1 is more simple regarding the age-dependent differences in the ^{3}H-thymidine labeling indices of the various cell populations of the liver without and after TAA injury, as well as the age-dependent differences in a further decrease or increase of these ^{3}H-thymidine labeling indices following drug treatment. One of the first pathological collagen deposits takes place around the sinusoids by the cells named before. Hence the formation of basement membranes of sinusoids (with so-called capillarization) is one of the first responses to chronic liver injuries before and during the development of fibrosis (Kent et al. 1959; Becker et al. 1964; Cossel 1966; McGee and Patrick 1972; Lindner and Grasedyck 1973; Grasedyck et al. 1974; Chvapil 1975; Grasedyck 1976; Bachmann et al. 1978; Helle et al. 1979). Also one of the first features in this process is the increase of myofibroblasts in the perivenolar area, which are able to synthesize collagen types I, III, and IV and elastin as well as GAG types, especially after injuries of the centrolobular endothelial and mesenchymal cells.

This is demonstrated by immunofluorescence and by autoradiographic methods. The increase of GAG and collagen is preceded by the increase in cell proliferation (see Table 1). These findings are proven by experimental research and in part by human biopsy material (incubated and incorporated with the suitable radioactive labeled precursors in vitro). In human liver biopsies, the increased division and production metabolism in the development of liver fibrosis and cirrhosis is demonstrated by autoradiographic, biochemical, and radiochemical methods (Kent et al. 1959; Becker et al. 1964; Koizumi et al. 1967; Lindner et al. 1968; McGee and Patrick 1969; Lindner 1972; McGee and Patrick 1972; Galambos and Shapira 1973; Lindner and Grasedyck 1973; McGee et al. 1974; Risteli and Kivirikko 1974; Suzuki et al. 1975; Grasedyck 1976; Kent et al. 1976; Galambos et al. 1977; Knook et al. 1977; Bachmann et al. 1978; Pott et al. 1979; Wisse and Knook 1979; Edward et al. 1980; Gressner et al. 1980; Stuhlsatz et al. 1980; Voss et al. 1980; Lindner 1981; Willemer 1984). The increase in the division and production metabolism declines in late stages of cirrhosis and can increase again during repeated damage and recurrences (Becker et al. 1964; Lindner and Grasedyck 1973; Grasedyck et al. 1974; Grasedyck 1976; Grasedyck and Lindner 1976; Bachmann et al. 1978; Willemer et al. 1984).

Figure 8 a–c demonstrate final examples of the exact analysis of the influence of 6-methyl-prednisolone (6 mg/kg bw). The 10th day of life is compared with the

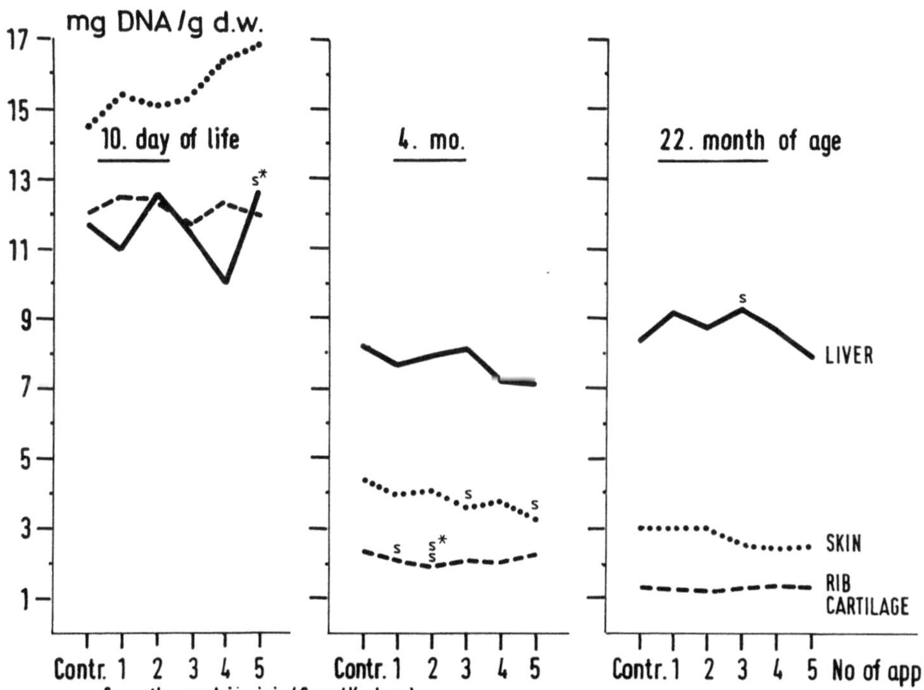

8a

Fig. 8 a–c. Age-dependent changes of DNA (**a**), β-glucuronidase (**b**) and β-N-acetyl-glucosaminidase (**c**) of rats treated with 1–5 applications of 6-methyl-prednisolone comparing rib cartilage, skin, and liver (further details: see text)

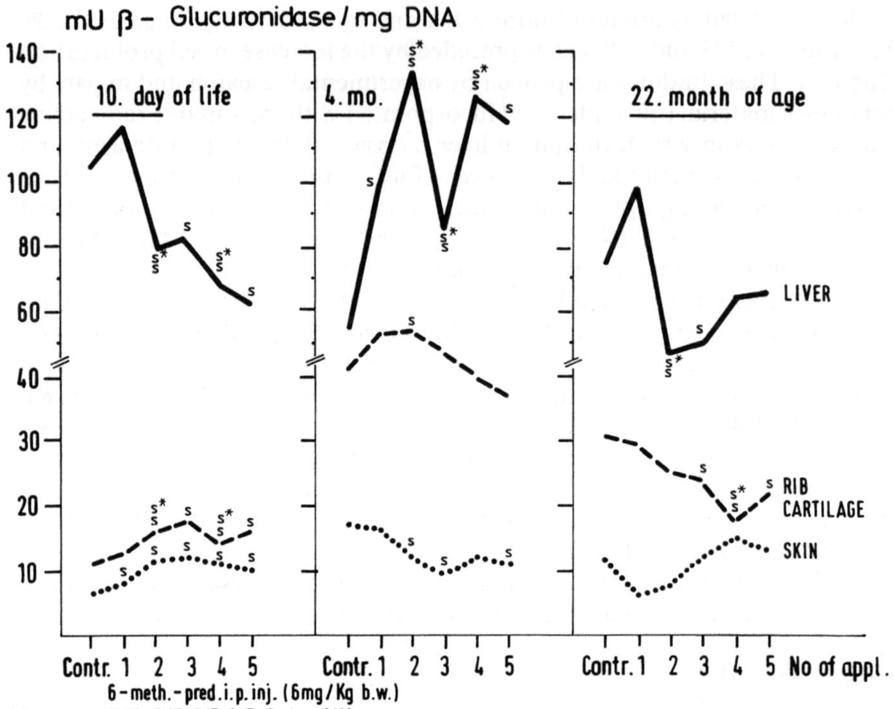
mU β - Glucuronidase / mg DNA
140
120
100
80
60
40
30
20
10
10. day of life
4. mo.
22. month of age
LIVER
RIB
CARTILAGE
SKIN
Contr. 1 2 3 4 5
Contr. 1 2 3 4 5
Contr. 1 2 3 4 5 No of appl.
6-meth.-pred. i. p. inj. (6mg / Kg b.w.)
5./5.-6./5.-7./5.-8./5.-9. day of life

8b

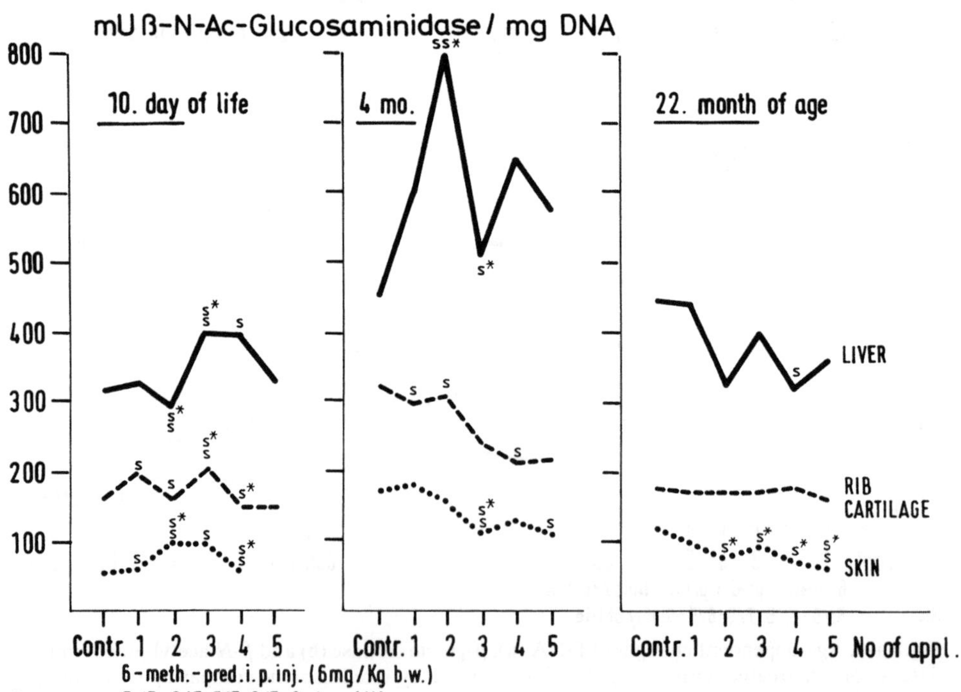
mU β-N-Ac-Glucosaminidase / mg DNA
800
700
600
500
400
300
200
100
10. day of life
4 mo.
22. month of age
LIVER
RIB
CARTILAGE
SKIN
Contr. 1 2 3 4 5
Contr. 1 2 3 4 5
Contr. 1 2 3 4 5 No of appl.
6-meth.-pred. i. p. inj. (6mg / Kg b.w.)
5./5.-6./5.-7./5.-8./5.-9. day of life

8c

4th and 22nd months of age (one to five administrations, in the youngest group starting at the 5th day of life), without significant alterations in the DNA content of the liver (Fig. 8 a) [Wistar outbred rats, strain Chbb:THOM (SPF)]. This is why the DNA content is used as a good reference for the indicator enzymes of GAG degradation: β-glucuronidase (Fig. 8 b) and β-*N*-acetyl-D-glucosaminidase (Fig. 8 c), with age dependent differences of this drug influence. Significant decreases of enzymes were evident at the early age of 10 days, compared with the group before (=s*) and with the control value (=s). 4-month-old rats showed a significant increase by 2 days of application, with a subsequent decrease and increase. 22-month-old rats showed similar results after only one application. The results concerning cartilage are particularly important because of its uniform cell population (Fig. 8 b). The age-dependent differences in the prednisolone influence on the GAG-degrading enzyme β-*N*-acetyl-D-glucosaminidase are similar to those in respect of β-glucuronidase (Fig. 8 c). So, the first two glucocorticoid dosages caused a significant increase in both enzyme activities per mg DNA and per g dry weight in the liver (as well as in the spleen, kidney, and other investigated organs) of 4-month-old rats. The results are to be discussed as an acceleration of maturation, enzyme induction, and age-dependent differences in adaptation, which is of theoretical and clinical importance (Platt and Katzenmeier 1970; Adelman 1972; Platt and Pauli 1972; Lindner 1981; Ernst 1983; Schönrock 1983). The enzyme activities were also calculated in relation to dry weight, absolute liver weight, and protein content, regarding questions of polyploidization in some organs, especially the liver, with aging (=increasing DNA content of the liver at higher age: Lindner 1975, 1981; Schütte et al. 1979/1980; Ernst 1983; Schönrock 1983). The age-dependent alterations of the activities of both enzymes were independent of age-polyploidization: significantly higher β-glucuronidase activity per mg DNA *and* per g dry weight in the livers of 22-month-old than of 4-month-old animals, but significantly lower activity in skin and rib cartilage (control values: Fig. 8 b). The β-*N*-acetyl-D-glucosaminidase activity per mg DNA *and* per g dry weight was significantly lower in the skin and cartilage of 22-month-old rats than in those 4 months old (Fig. 8 c).

So, the different influences of drugs on the lysosomal enzyme activities depend on the age of the animals, on the enzymes and organs tested, on the dosage, and on the time span between administration and enzyme analysis. The initial drug (glucocorticoid)-caused alteration in the enzyme activity can already be compensated when the estimation is done a few days later. Consideration must be given to the possibility of cell reactions such as rebound effects causing the approximation of the initially glucocorticoid-induced increase or decrease in enzyme activity to the level of the controls in spite of increasing glucocorticoid application or dosages.

These examples (Fig. 8) demonstrate the enzyme induction, maturity and age-dependencies: different periods between last corticoid application and time of killing or enzyme estimation, with compensating mechanisms, time of observation, circadian rhythms etc.

Adaptation capacities decrease with aging, especially regarding enzyme induction (Platt and Katzenmeier 1970; Adelmann 1972; Platt and Pauli 1972; Lindner 1981; Ernst 1983; Schönrock 1983).

Summary

Age-dependent differences in therapeutic effects on experimental liver fibrosis and cirrhosis are investigated. The morphological and autoradiographic but also the biochemical and radiochemical findings obtained with the most suitable experimental model show similarities to the basic processes of human liver fibrosis and cirrhosis. There are valid results concerning age-dependent differences in therapeutic effects on the experimental liver fibrosis, too. The enhanced GAG and collagen biosynthesis is variously influenced by drugs, according to the age of the animals. This is demonstrated by the most sensitive parameters, e.g., labeled soluble collagen (increasing to values 8 times the control levels in early fibrosis) and labeled hydroxyproline in the insoluble collagen fraction. The indicator enzyme for collagen synthesis, prolyl hydroxylase, can be influenced by drugs, depending on age, especially in the early stages of experimental and human liver fibrosis (partly with positive correlation of the results from liver tissue to serum). Before or simultaneous with the increased synthesis processes, the GAG and collagen degradation is enhanced, with age-dependent differences in mesenchymal-suppressing drug influences. Further parameters of the GAG metabolism are demonstrated, with regard being paid to age differences in therapeutic effects. Investigations based on experimental TAA liver intoxication and fibrosis model can explain and support findings in human liver fibrosis and cirrhosis.

Thus liver injuries are followed by an increase in hepatic mesenchymal metabolism. Depending on the severity and duration of the liver intoxication and injury, reversible and at last irreversible collagen depositions occur, with resulting liver fibrosis and cirrhosis, which are influenced by drugs with age-dependent differences. These findings are of theoretical and clinical interest, because they show the importance of experimental investigations for better understanding of the causal and formal pathogenesis of liver fibrosis, its treatment, and questions of reversibility.

Concomitant with polyploidization and simultaneously increased function of hepatocytes, there is less sensitivity to hepatotoxic agents, but at the same time drugs are less effective (TAA, prednisolone etc.). This seems to be the explanation for our results: *less* toxicity at higher than at younger ages and *more* reactive liver connective tissue proliferation, production, and deposition in younger than in older animals. Drugs are also *more* effective on the liver connective tissue processes in younger than in older animals, as analyzed by morphological and biochemical methods. The capacity of adaptation *decreases* with aging, also regarding the well-known biochemical model of enzyme induction (Platt and Katzenmeier 1970; Adelmann 1972; Platt and Pauli 1972; Lindner 1981; Ernst 1983; Schönrock 1983). Regarding acute, subacute, and chronic TAA intoxication, as well as drug influences, 1- and 1.5-month-old rat livers are more tolerant than the embryonic liver and also more so than 9½- and 12-month-old rat livers, which are, on the other hand, more tolerant than 16-, 17-, 18-, or 19-month-old rat livers (=age at the start of our experiments). This is demonstrated by the mortality rates of the rats, too.

These results concerning age-dependent therapeutic effects on experimental liver fibrosis and cirrhosis are due to the drug, the dosis, the duration of application, and the experimental material and methods. The examples given of necessary basic research into fundamental processes and of possibilities of influencing these processes demonstrates the theoretical and practical importance of our investigations for clinical hepatology.

References

Adelman RC (1972) Age dependent control of enzyme adaptation. In: Strehler BL (ed) Adv. in Gerontol. Res, vol 4. Academic Press, New York London, p 1–21

Bachmann E, Lindner J, Grasedyck K, Eurich R (1978) Rattenleberkollagen bei protrahierter Thioacetamid-Intoxikation. 1. Mitt.: Vergleichende quantifizierende biochemische und histologische Untersuchungen (mit und ohne medikamentöse Beeinflussung). Arzneim Forsch/Drug Res 28 (II):2260–2274

Becker K, Szarvas F, Lindner J (1964) Untersuchungen zum Sulfateinbau bei experimenteller Leberzirrhose. Med Welt 1:1622–1625

Blumenkrantz N, Asboe-Hansen G (1973) New method for quantitative determination of uronic acids. Ann Biochem 54:484–489

Borooah J, Leaback DH, Walker PG (1961) Studies on glucosaminidase. II. Substrates for β-*N*-acetyl-D-glucosaminidase. Biochem J 79:106–110

Burton K (1956) A study of the condition and mechanism of the diphenylamine reaction for the colorimetric estimation of desoxyribunucleic acid. Biochem J 62:315–322

Chvapil M (1975) Pharmacology of fibrosis: definitions, limits and perspectives. Life Science 16:1345–1362

Cossel L (1966) Über akutes Auftreten von Basalmembranen an den Lebersinusoiden. (Beitrag zur Kenntnis der kapillären Basalmembranen). Beitr Pathol Anat 134:103–122

Edward M, Long WF, Watson HHK, Williamson FB (1980) Sulphated glycosaminoglycans in regenerating rat liver. Biochem J 188:769–773

Ernst P (1983) Vergleichende Untersuchung zum Einfluß postnataler 6-Methylprednisolon-Applikation unterschiedlicher Dosierung auf die Aktivität der β-Glucuronidase, der β-*N*-Acetyl-D-Glucosaminidase sowie auf den DNA-Gehalt bindegewebiger und parenchymatöser Organe der neugeborenen Ratte (zur Frage der Reifungsabhängigkeit). Inaug Diss Univ Hamburg

Eurich RE, Lindner J (1984) Body weights, absolute and relative organ weights by maturation and ageing (with sexual differences), and their importance as measures of reference for metabolic investigations. Z Gerontol 17:60–68

Farhat K, Grasedyck K, Lindner J, Schütte B, Okpanyi SN, Eurich R (1979) Rattenleberkollagen bei protrahierter Thioacetamid-Intoxikation. 4. Mitt.: Zur Bestimmung des Collagen-like-protein (CLP) und des Hydroxyprolingehaltes im Serum als Parameter für Kollagenstoffwechselstörungen der Leber. Arzneim Forsch/Drug Res 29 (I):82–90

Fishman WH (1974) β-Glucuronidase. In: Bergmeyer HE (Hrsg) Methoden der enzymatischen Analyse, Bd. 2. Chemie, Weinheim, S 885–900

Friedrich O, Grasedyck K, Lindner J, Eurich R, Okpanyi SN (1978) Rattenleberkollagen bei protrahierter Thioacetamid-Intoxikation. 2. Mitt.: Untersuchungen zur Kollagenneubildung, seiner Löslichkeit und deren Beeinflussung durch Penicillamin. Arzneim Forsch/Drug Res 28 (II):2275–2281

Furukawa K, Terayama H (1979) Pattern of glycosaminoglycans and glycoproteins associated with nuclei of regenerating liver of rat. Biochim Biophys Acta 585:575–588

Galambos JT, Shapira R (1973) Natural history of alcoholic hepatitis. IV. Glycosaminoglycuronans and collagen in the hepatic connective tissue. J Clin Invest 52:2952–2962

Galambos JT, Hollingsworth MA Jr, Falek A, Warren WD, McCain JR (1977) The rate of synthesis of glycosaminoglycans and collagen by fibroblasts cultured from adult human liver biopsies. J Clin Invest 60:107–114

Gatt R, Berman ER (1966) A rapid procedure for the estimation of amino sugars on micro scale. Anal Biochem 15:873–876

Grasedyck K (1976) Untersuchungen der Leberfibrose und -zirrhose anhand des Kollagenstoffwechsels, speziell der Kollagensynthese. Habil Schrift Univ Hamburg

Grasedyck K, Lindner J (1976) Die chronische Thioacetamid-Intoxikation als Modell einer experimentellen Leberzirrhose. Verh Dtsch Ges Inn Med 82:374–376

Grasedyck K, Ropohl D, Szarvas F, Lindner J (1971) Kollagenpeptidaseaktivität menschlicher Seren bei Lebercirrhose. Klin Wochenschr 49:163–164

Grasedyck K, Helle M, Lindner J, Langness U (1974) Kriterien der Aktivität einer pathologischen Bindegewebsvermehrung bei chronischen Lebererkrankungen. Verh Dtsch Ges Inn Med 80:503–506

Grasedyck K, Friedrich O, Thäter G, Lindner J, Langness U (1980) The collagen metabolism during development of liver cirrhosis. In: Robert AM, Robert L (eds) Biochimie des tissues conjonctifs normaux et pathologiques. Centre Nat Recherche Scient, Paris, p 279–280

Gressner AM, Köster-Eiserfunke W, van der Leur E, Greiling H (1980) Metabolic and structural studies on serum and liver-glycosaminoglycans in normal and liver-injured rats. J Clin Chem Clin Biochem 18:279–285

Hauss WH, Junge-Hülsing G, Gerlach U (1968) Die unspezifische Mesenchymreaktion. Thieme, Stuttgart

Helle M, Grasedyck K, Lindner J, Okpanyi SN, Eurich R (1979) Rattenleberkollagen bei protrahierter Thioacetamid-Intoxikation. 3. Mitt.: Die Kollagenfraktionierung zur Untersuchung des pathologisch gestörten Kollagenstoffwechsels der Leber. Arzneim Forsch/Drug Res 29 (I):71–80

Hutterer F (1966) Degradation of mucopolysaccharides by hepatic lysosomes. Biochim Biophys Acta 115:312–317

Hutton JJ, Tappel AL, Udenfriend S (1966) A rapid assay for collagen proline hydroxylase. Anal Biochem 16:384–394

Hutton JJ, Tappel AL, Udenfriend S (1967) Cofactor and substrate requirements of collagen proline hydroxylase. Arch Biochem Biophys 118:231–240

Juva K, Prockop DJ (1966) Modified procedure for the assay of ^{3}H- or ^{14}C-labeled hydroxyproline. Anal Biochem 15:77–83

Kent G, Fels IG, Dubin A, Popper H (1959) Collagen content based on hydroxyproline determination in human and rat livers. Its relation to morphologically demonstrable reticulum and collagen fibers. Lab Invest 8:48–56

Kent G, Gay S, Inouye T, Bahu R, Minick OT, Popper H (1976) Vitamin A-containing lipocytes and formation of type III collagen in liver injury. Proc Natl Acad Sci (USA) 73:3719–3722

Kewitsch F, Schütte B, Eurich R, Lindner J (1978) Beitrag zur Frage des Wassergehaltes (mit Untersuchungen von Frisch- und Trockengewicht) mesenchymaler und parenchymatöser Organe von Mensch und Ratte im Lebensablauf. Akt Gerontol 8:303–316

Knook DL, Blansjaar N, Sleyster ECh (1977) Isolation and characterization of Kupffer and endothelial cells from the rat liver. Exp Cell Res 109:317–329

Koizumi T, Nakamura N, Abe H (1967) Changes in mucopolysaccharides in the liver in hepatic fibrosis. Biochim Biophys Acta 148:749–752

Langness U (1970) Hydroxyprolinausscheidung und Kollagenstoffwechsel. Dtsch Med Wochenschr 95:1530–1535

Langness U (1971) Collagen-like protein. Dtsch Med Wochenschr 96:475–477

Langness U, Grasedyck K, Borgmann J, Lindner J (1975) Collagen prolyl hydroxylase activity in experimental cirrhosis. In: Popper H, Becker K (eds) Collagen metabolism in the liver. Stratton, New York, p 73–77

Lindner J (1972) Die posttraumatische Entzündung und Wundheilung. In: Gohrband E, Gabka J, Berndorfer A (Hrsg) Handbuch der plastischen Chirurgie, vol I, Beitr. 6. W. de Gruyter, Berlin New York, S 1–153

Lindner J (1975) Zur Alterung der Organe. Verh Dtsch Ges Path 59:181–242

Lindner J (1981) Zur Entwicklung und Alterung von Binde- und Stützgeweben. Verh Anat Ges 75:61–98

Lindner J, Grasedyck K (1973) Experimental fibrosis in liver and other organs. In: Kulonen E, Pikkarainen J (eds) Biology of fibroblast. Academic Press, London New York, p 539–557

Lindner J, Grasedyck K, Johannes G (1968) Beitrag zu quantitativen Untersuchungen an Autoradiographien. Verh Dtsch Ges Path 52:533–541

Lowry OH, Rosenbrough NJ, Farr AL, Randall RJ (1951) Protein measurement with the folin phenol reagent. J Biol Chem 193:265–275

McGee JO'D, Patrick RS (1969) The synthesis of sulphated mucopolysaccharide in mouse liver following carbon tetrachloride injury. I. Autoradiographic studies. Br J Exp Path 50:521–526

McGee JO'D, Patrick RS (1972) The role of perisinusoidal cells in hepatic fibrogenesis. Lab Invest 26:429–440

McGee JO'D, Patrick RS, Rodger MC, Luty CM (1974) Collagen proline hydroxylase activity and S^{35} sulphate uptake in human liver biopsies. Gut 15:260–267

Ohuchi K, Tsurufuji S (1972) Protocollagen proline hydroxylase in isolated rat liver cells. Biochim Biophys Acta 258:731–740

Okazaki I, Maruyama K (1974) Collagenase activity in experimental hepatic fibrosis. Nature (London) 252:49–50

Platt D, Leinweber B (1969) Untersuchungen zum katabolen Mucopolysaccharidstoffwechsel bei Lebererkrankungen. (Catabolic mucopolysaccharide metabolism in liver diseases). Acta Hepatogastroenterol 16:324–330

Platt D, Katzenmeier U (1970) Untersuchungen zur Frage der Induzierbarkeit lysosomaler Enzyme der Rattenleber durch Phenobarbital. 1. Mitt.: β-glucuronidase, β-Acetylglucosaminidase und Kollagenase. Arzneim Forsch/Drug Res 20:258–261

Platt D, Pauli H (1972) Age dependent determination of lysosomal enzymes in the liver of spironolactone and aldosterone pretreated rats. Exp Geront 7:1–11

Pott G, Eberhardt G, Gerlach U (1979) Activity of procollagen-prolyl-hydroxylase and *N*-Acetyl-β-glucosaminidase in human fibrosis. Klin Wochenschr 57:587–588

Prinz R, Klein U, Sudhakaran PR, Sinn W, Ullrich K, v. Figura K (1980) Metabolism of sulfated glycosaminoglycans in rat hepatocytes. Biochim Biophys Acta 630:402–413

Risteli J (1977) Effect of prednisolone on the activities of the intracellular enzymes of collagen biosynthesis in rat liver and skin. Biochem Pharmacol 26:1295–1298

Risteli J, Kivirikko KI (1974) Activities of prolyl hydroxylase, lysyl hydroxylase, collagen galactosyltransferase and collagen glucosyltransferase in the liver of rats with hepatic injury. Biochem J 144:115–122

Rössle R, Roulet F (1932) Maß und Zahl in der Pathologie. Springer, Berlin

Sakakibara K, Umeda M, Saito S, Nagase S (1977) Production of collagen and acidic glycosaminoglycans by an epithelial liver cell clone in culture. Exp Cell Res 110:159–165

Schmiegelow P (1979) Nucleotidstoffwechsel (ATP, ADP, AMP), Brenztraubensäure- und Milchsäurestoffwechsel der gesunden und der zirrhotischen Leber unter Hypoxie. Inaug Diss Univ Hamburg

Schönrock P (1983) Untersuchung zum Einfluß unterschiedlich häufiger 6-Methylprednisolon-Applikationen auf die Aktivität der β-Glucuronidase und der β-*N*-Acetyl-D-Glucosaminidase sowie auf den DNA-Gehalt ausgewählter bindegewebiger und parenchymatöser Organe 4 und 22 Monate alter Ratten (Frage der Altersabhängigkeit). Inaug Diss Univ Hamburg

Schütte B, Ziebell K, Zerbst B, Bock PR, Bittmann S, Mangold I, Lindner J (1979 u. 1980) Untersuchungen von Gewichten und Wassergehalt sowie von DNA-Synthese und -Gehalt bindegewebiger und parenchymatöser Organe der Ratte prä- und postnatal. Akt Gerontol 9:527–531; 573–583; 10:37–43

Stegemann H, Stalder K (1967) Determination of hydroxyproline. Clin Chim Acta 18:267–273

Stuhlsatz HW, Vierhaus S, Greiling H (1980) Analyse der Glykosaminoglykantypen in der normalen und cirrhotischen Leber des Menschen. Fresenius Z Anal Chem 301:102–108

Suzuki Su, Suzuki Sa, Nakamura N, Koizumi T (1975) The heterogenity of dermatan sulfate and heparan sulfate in rat liver and shift in the glycosaminoglycan contents in carbon tetrachloride-damaged liver. Biochim Biophys Acta 402:167–181

Svejcar J, van Robertson WIB (1967) Micro separation and determination of mammalian acidic glycosaminoglycans (mucopolysaccharides). Anal Biochem 18:333–350

Takeuchi T, Prockop DJ (1969) Protocollagen proline hydroxylase in normal liver and in hepatic fibrosis. Gastroenterol 56:744–750

Voss B, Rauterberg J, Allam S, Pott G (1980) Distribution of collagen type I and type III and of two collagenous components of basement membranes in the human liver. Pathol Res Pract 170:50–60

Willemer S, Sames K, Lindner J, Schmiegelow P (1984) Die Altersabhängigkeit der frühen Reaktion im Glycosaminoglycan-Stoffwechsel der Rattenleber auf eine einzeitige Thioacetamidschädigung. Z Gerontol 17:150–156

Wisse E, Knook DL (1979) The investigation of sinusoidal cells: a new approach to the study of liver function. In: Popper H, Schaffner F (eds) Progress in liver disease, vol VI. Grune & Stratton, New York, p 153–171

Woollen JW, Heyworth R, Walker PG (1961) Studies on glucosaminidase. 3. Testicular *N*-acetyl-β-glucosaminidase and *N*-acetyl-β-galactosaminidase. Biochem J 78:111–116

Developmental and Age-Dependent Changes of Proteoglycan Metabolism in Normal and Experimentally Injured Liver and the Effects of Drugs

A. M. GRESSNER [1]

Both human and rat livers contain only small amounts of connective tissue (extracellular matrix) components; they are restricted to less than 1% of total liver weight and account for about 1% of liver volume. Besides collagens and structural glycoproteins (fibronectin, laminin), the main constituents of the extracellular matrix are proteoglycans, i.e., complex glycoprotein-like molecules consisting of unbranched polyanionic (i.e., sulfated) heteropolysaccharides covalently linked to the seryl-residues of a core protein moiety (with the exception of hyaluronate) (Gressner 1983). The predominant type is a proteoheparan sulfate (molecular mass 80000 daltons) consisting of a core protein moiety (20000 daltons) and four heteropolysaccharide chains [=glycosaminoglycans (GAG), 14000 daltons] (Oldberg et al. 1977). Under physiologic conditions the parenchyma–stroma (extracellular matrix) ratio remains constant, and only two pathologic conditions are associated with loss of this homeostatic mechanism:

1. Fibrosis of the liver, characterized by a strong increase in the total amount of GAG and elevation of chondroitin sulfate and dermatan sulfate, accompanied by a decrease in heparan sulfate (Stuhlsatz et al. 1982).
2. Liver cell carcinoma, characterized by an excessive increase in chondroitin sulfate and a decrease in heparan sulfate (Kojima et al. 1975).

In the following experiments developmental and age-related changes of hepatic proteoglycan metabolism were investigated to decide whether disease-related loss of proteoglycan–parenchyma homeostasis mimics developmental and age-related changes. The effects of a hepatotoxic compound, D-galactosamine (Decker and Keppler 1974), on hepatic proteoglycan metabolism in embryonic, adult, and senescent liver and of some hepatocytoprotective drugs were studied in detail.

As reported previously (Gressner et al. 1979), the synthesis rate of hepatic proteoglycans remains nearly constant during the life span of an adult rat (Table 1). There is also no change in the proportion of synthesized heparan sulfate and chondroitin sulfate between young and senescent rats (Table 2). D-Galactosamine, a hepatocytotoxic compound which acts by trapping UTP in the cell, decreases in a dose-dependent manner total GAG synthesis in young, adult, and senescent rats, showing no significant differences between the age groups (Fig. 1). In addition, the fraction of newly synthesized heparan sulfate is decreased by D-galactosamine independently of the age of the animal. This implies that D-galac-

[1] Department of Clinical Chemistry and Central laboratory, Philipps University Marburg, D-3550 Marburg/F.R.G.

Drugs and Aging
Ed. by D. Platt

Table 1. Synthesis of total glycosaminoglycans in liver slices from rats of various age groups[a]

Age (days)	Incorporation (dpm/mg protein)	
	[^{14}C]-glucosamine	**[^{35}S]-sulfate**
9 ± 0	3,460 ± 500 (n = 10)	–
140 ± 17	1,650 ± 350 (n = 12)	1,770 ± 290 (n = 4)
490 ± 60	1,470 ± 500 (n = 12)	1,300 ± 380 (n = 4)
940 ± 60	1,550 ± 400 (n = 12)	1,480 ± 360 (n = 4)

[a] The rate of synthesis was determined either by the incorporation of [^{14}C]-glucosamine or [^{35}S]-sulfate into cetylpyridinium chloride precipitable glycosaminoglycans. The values are the mean ± SD of n rats

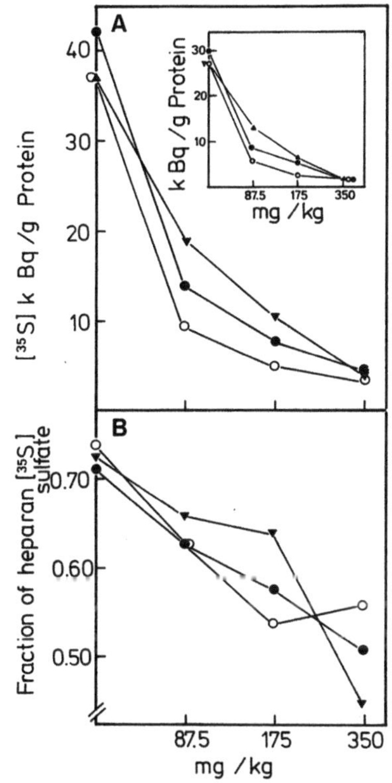

Fig. 1 A, B. Dose-dependent inhibition of the incorporation of [^{35}S]sulfate into total glycosaminoglycans (**A**) of young rats (aged 140 ± 17 days) (●), adult rats (aged 490 ± 60 days) (○), and senescent rats (aged 940 ± 60 days) (▼). In **B** the fractional synthesis of heparan sulfate of the various age groups under the influence of D-galactosamine is illustrated. The *inset* in **A** represents the synthesis of total protein under the influence of D-galactosamine in the liver of various age groups

tosamine reduces mainly the synthesis of heparan sulfate, and that of chondroitin sulfate and dermatan sulfate to a much lesser extent. Experiments with the artificial carbohydrate chain acceptor β-D-xyloside suggest that the mechanism of D-galactosamine-induced inhibition is an impairment of glycosaminoglycan chain initiation and/or elongation rather than an inhibition of core protein synthesis, because β-D-xylosides are unable to restore GAG synthesis inhibited by the

Table 2. The proportional rates of synthesis of specific types of hepatic GAG in aging rats as determined by the incorporation of [^{14}C]-glucosamine[a]

Age (days)	Percentage of total glycosaminoglycan synthesis			
	Heparan sulfate	Chondroitin sulfate	Hyaluronic acid	"Keratan sulfate"
9 ± 0 (n = 10)	79 ± 3.8	14.3 ± 2.1	9.1 ± 1.9	–
140 ± 17 (n = 12)	86 ± 3.1	8.1 ± 3.6	1.9 ± 1.8	1.1 ± 0.6
490 ± 60 (n = 12)	85 ± 4.6	8.8 ± 4.2	1.3 ± 1.3	2.5 ± 2.0
940 ± 60 (n = 12)	80 ± 9.8	7.9 ± 3.8	1.3 ± 1.1	1.2 ± 0.6

[a] The values are expressed as percentage of the incorporation into total glycosaminoglycans (including the keratan sulfate-like fraction). They are the mean ± SD of n separate experiments

Table 3. The effect of diethyldithiocarbamate and of (+)cianidanol-3 on the galactosamine-induced inhibition of glycosaminoglycan synthesis in liver[a]. (Gressner et al. 1982)

Source of liver		Total glycosaminoglycan synthesis (kBq/g protein)	Heparan sulfate (fraction of total glycosaminoglycans)
	Diethyldithiocarbamate		
Control rat		40.7 ± 0.9 (1.0)	0.75 ± 0.01
	+	24.8 ± 0.1 (0.61)	0.81 ± 0.03
Galactosamine rat		3.3 ± 0.4 (0.08)	0.52 ± 0.02
	+	15.4 ± 0.6 (0.38)	0.69 ± 0.003
	(+) Cianidanol-3		
Control rat		37.6 ± 7.4 (1.0)	0.80 ± 0.01
	+	35.8 ± 10.4 (0.95)	0.82 ± 0.05
Galactosamine rat		21.4 ± 8.2 (0.56)	0.73 ± 0.04
	+	28.8 ± 10.2 (0.77)	0.78 ± 0.06

[a] Rats were injected in vivo with 700 mg/kg body weight of D-galactosamine (diethyldithiocarbamate experiment) or 450 mg/kg body weight (cianidanol experiment), or a similar volume of saline instead of galactosamine (control rats). Diethyldithiocarbamate (300 mg/kg body weight) was administered 45 min before the application of galactosamine. 2 h after injection of galactosamine the rats were sacrificed. (+) Cianidanol-3 (a suspension of 250 mg/kg body weight in saline) was applied intraperitoneally 48 h, 24 h, and 3 h before injection of D-galactosamine into the rats. 3 h after administration of galactosamine the animals were decapitated. The liver slices were prepared and incubated with [^{35}S] sulfate as described. The values are the mean ± SD of 3 experiments. The relative changes of total glycosaminoglycan synthesis are listed in parentheses

amino sugar (Gressner et al. 1982). As demonstrated in Table 3, treatment of rats with some hepatocytoprotective compounds, i.e., diethyldithiocarbamate (Homann et al. 1977) and the natural flavonoid (+)cianidanol-3, prior to the application of D-galactosamine partially restores total GAG synthesis and the fraction of proteoheparan sulfate diminished by D-galactosamine. The dose-dependent response of young and senescent rats to the protective drugs was similar (not shown). It would be important to decide whether the partial restoration of hepatic GAG synthesis by the protective drugs is a consequence of less severe hepatic damage by D-galactosamine or vice versa.

As shown in Tables 1 and 2, neonatal rat liver exhibits a strong increase in the synthesis of total GAG and chondroitin sulfate. This is confirmed in a more detailed study in Fig. 2. The production of heparan sulfate and dermatan sulfate remains constant in embryonic and early postnatal liver (Fig. 2). This implies dramatic changes in the proportions of synthesized chondroitin sulfate and heparan sulfate (Fig. 3). The former decreases from about 50%–60% in the embryonic liver tissue to 2%–3% at the 7th day of postnatal life, whereas the proportion of heparan sulfate increases from about 40% in embryonic tissue to more than 80% in postnatal liver. Altogether, chondroitin sulfate synthesis in embryonic liver slices is about 30 times higher than in adult liver explants.

Previous reports have suggested a positive relation of chondroitin sulfate content and an inverse relation of heparan sulfate content in a tissue to the proliferation tendency of the cells (Kojima et al. 1975). In fact, we found a rather strong positive correlation ($r=0.95$) between the incorporation of [^{3}H]thymidine into DNA and (a) the synthesis rates of chondroitin sulfate and (b) the chondroitin sulfate/heparan sulfate ratio (Fig. 4).

In order to define the cell types responsible for the developmental changes of proteoglycan synthesis in neonatal liver, hepatocytes were separated from nonparenchymal cells, mainly erythroblasts. The latter cells accumulating in embryonic liver tissue synthesize nearly exclusively chondroitin sulfate (constituting about 92% of their total GAG synthesis), but their total GAG synthesis rate represents only about 13% of that of whole embryonic liver slices. Thus, erythro-

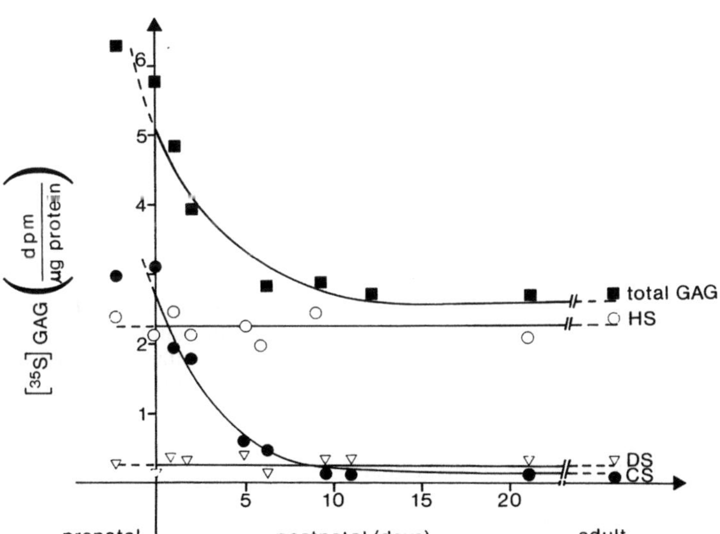

Fig. 2. Incorporation of [^{35}S]sulfate into total and specific types of glycosaminoglycans in rat liver slices at different developmental stages. *GAG*, glycosaminoglycans; *HS*, heparan sulfate; *DS*, dermatan sulfate; *CS*, chondroitin sulfate

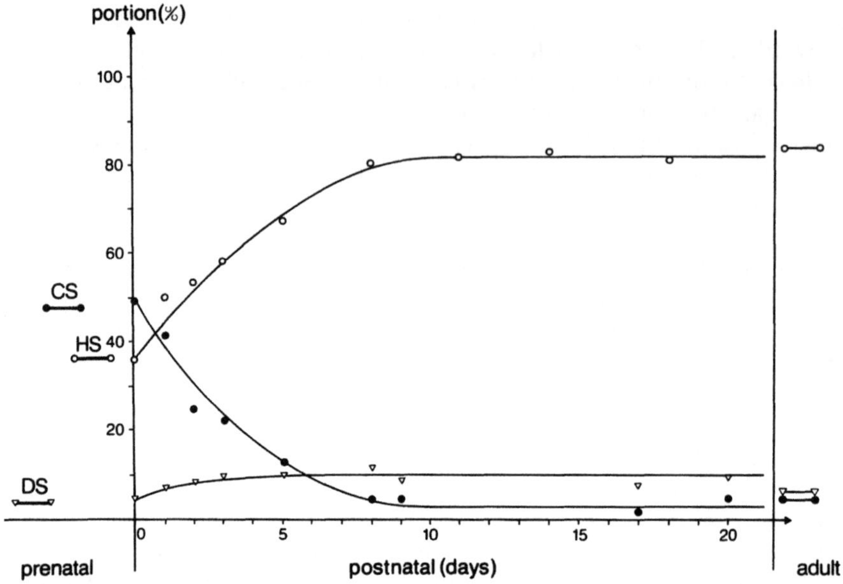

Fig. 3. Time curve of the relative incorporation of [^{35}S]sulfate into specific types of glycosaminoglycan in embryonic and early postnatal liver slices. *CS*, chondroitin sulfate; *HS*, heparan sulfate; *DS*, dermatan sulfate

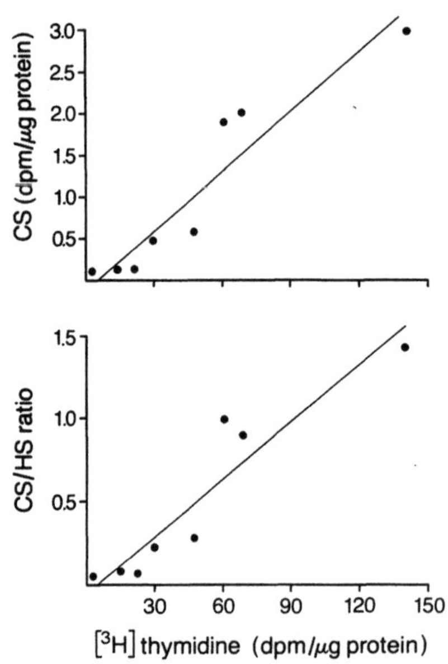

Fig. 4. Correlation between the synthesis of chondroitin sulfate and the chondroitin sulfate/heparan sulfate ratio with the synthesis of DNA (incorporation of [^{3}H]thymidine) in perinatal liver

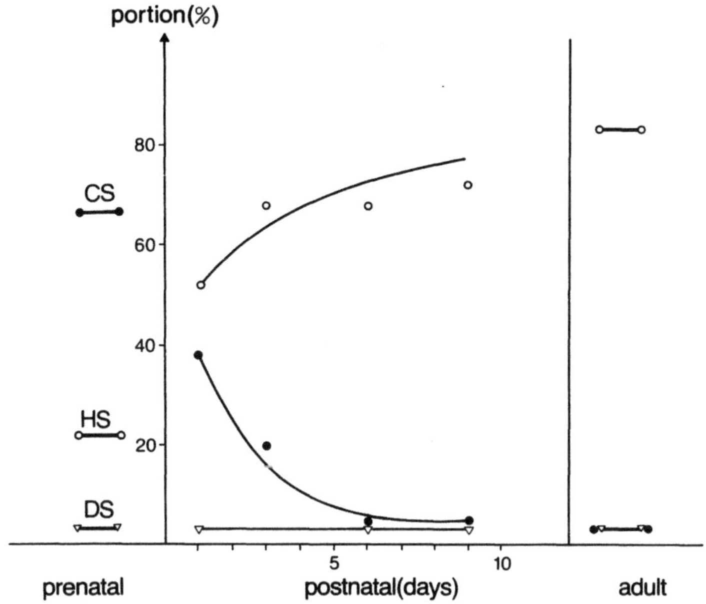

Fig. 5. Incorporation of [^{35}S]sulfate into heparan sulfate *HS*, chondroitin sulfate *CS*, and dermatan sulfate *DS* of late embryonic, early postnatal, and adult hepatocytes. The relative proportion in the synthesis of the various glycosaminoglycans is illustrated

blasts do not contribute significantly to the changes in proteoglycan metabolism described above for liver tissue. This is confirmed in Fig. 5, where similar changes in the proportion of heparan sulfate and chondroitin sulfate in isolated perinatal hepatocytes as in liver slices are illustrated.

Proteoglycan synthesis in both adult and embryonic liver is dependent on protein synthesis. Puromycin inhibits strongly total GAG synthesis without changing the proportion of chondroitin sulfate and heparan sulfate (Table 4). Glycosaminoglycans incorporate both [^{3}H]serine and [1^{4}C]glucosamine, which indicates their synthesis as a proteoglycan both in adult and embryonic liver tissue. D-Galactosamine (0.5 mmol/liter) inhibits in adult and embryonic liver slices the incorporation of both [^{3}H]serine and [^{14}C]glucosamine into peptido-glycosaminoglycans, but the degree of inhibition is less in embryonic liver slices (about 60%) than in adult liver tissue (about 85%) (Table 5). This points to a reduced sensitivity of the embryonic tissue against D-galactosamine. As already mentioned, the inhibition of peptido-glycosaminoglycan synthesis by D-galactosamine is independent of general protein synthesis, which was not affected by the amino sugar (Table 5).

It was described above how chondroitin sulfate synthesis in adult liver is (nearly) refractory to D-galactosamine. The same is true in embryonic rat liver slices, in which the synthesis of heparan sulfate but not that of chondroitin sulfate was strongly diminished by D-galactosamine (Table 6). Thus, the portion of chondroitin sulfate, labeled either with [^{35}S]sulfate or [^{14}C]glucosamine, is enhanced in D-galactosamine exposed embryonic liver tissue (Table 6). Furthermore, the

Table 4. Inhibition by puromycin of the incorporation of [^{35}S]sulfate (25 μCi) into total and specific glycosaminoglycans of adult and embryonic rat liver slices. The slices were incubated for 3 h in presence of 0.39 mmol/liter puromycin

Rat liver	Puromycin	Total glycos-aminoglycans (dpm/mg protein)	Heparan sulfate	Chondroitin sulfate
			(%)	
Adult	−	380	81	8.7
	+	39	83	5.7
Embryonic	−	1,190	30	64
	+	150	29	67

Table 5. Incorporation of [^{3}H]serine and [^{14}C]glucosamine into peptidoglycosaminoglycans of adult and embryonic rat liver slices in the absence and presence of D-galactosamine (0.5 mmol/liter). In parallel incubations the incorporation of [^{14}C] valine into protein was determined. 5 μCi of each isotopic precursor was used; the time of incubation was 3 h; mean values ± SD of 3 experiments

Rat liver	D-Galactos-amine	Peptido-glycosaminoglycans		[^{14}]-Glucosamine	Total protein synthesis (dpm/mg protein)
		[^{3}H]-Serine (dpm/mg protein)	[^{14}C]-Glucosamine (dpm/mg protein)	[^{3}H]-Serine	
Adult	−	342∓19	867∓ 34	2.56	28,620∓2,430
	+	55∓ 8	131∓ 11	2.38	29,890∓2,150
Embryonic	−	545∓31	1,180∓108	2.16	36,430∓3,800
	+	256∓18	427∓ 34	1.66	38,860∓4,900

Table 6. Effect of D-Galactosamine (0.5 mmol/liter) on the incorporation of [^{35}S] sulfate (25 μCi) and [^{14}C] glucosamine (2.5 μCi) into total and specific glycosaminoglycans (GAG) of embryonic rat liver slices. Mean values ± SD of 3 experiments are given

Radio-active precursor	D-Galactos-amine	Total glycos-aminoglycans (dpm/mg protein)	Heparan sulfate	Chondroitin sulfate	Heparan sulfate	Chondroitin sulfate
			(dpm/mg protein)		(% of total GAG)	
[^{35}S]-Sulfate	−	2,000±160	802	1,022	40±3	51±6
	+	1,520±140	260	1,120	17±4	74±4
[^{14}C]-Glucos-amine	−	320± 35	200	75	64±2	24±1
	+	120± 10	65	55	46±4	44±3

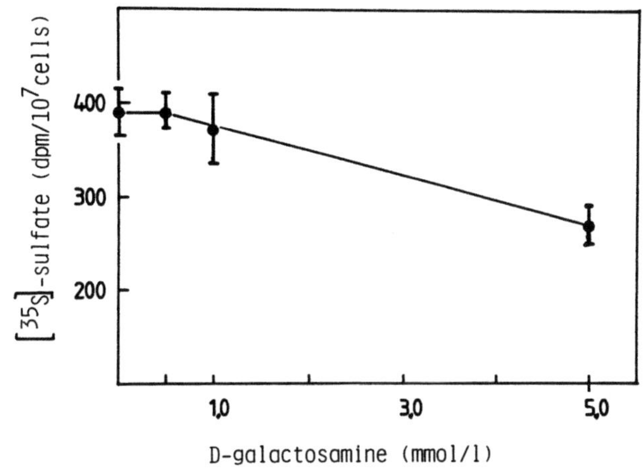

Fig. 6. Dose-dependent effects of D-galactosamine on the synthesis of chondroitin sulfate in erythroblasts from late embryonic rat liver. [^{35}S]sulfate was used as the radioisotopic precursor

synthesis of chondroitin sulfate in erythroblasts is reduced only slightly by high concentrations of D-galactosamine (Fig. 6).

Proteoglycans are distributed in three main compartments (intra-, peri-, and extracellularly). We studied their distribution on the plasma membranes of liver cells in adult and embryonic liver and the effect of D-galactosamine. In adult liver the amino sugar induces a time-dependent decrease in total GAG synthesis and in the glycosaminoglycans, nearly exclusively heparan sulfate, associated with the plasma membranes (Fig. 7). There are two fractions of membrane-associated proteoheparan sulfate; one is displaced by heparin, while the other can be liberated from the membranes only by treatment with detergents (triton X-100) (Fig. 8) (Kjellen et al. 1981). We found that the portion of plasma membrane heparan sulfate liberated by heparin and triton X-100, respectively, was unaffected by D-galactosamine (Fig. 7). Early postnatal liver cell plasma membranes contain a significant portion of [^{33}S]labeled chondroitin sulfate which decreases during the first 10 days of postnatal life (Table 7). Thus, chondroitin sulfate is expressed on the cell membrane of embryonic but not of adult liver. The portion of cell membrane-associated chondroitin sulfate proved to be insensitive to the action of D-galactosamine.

The results of this study allow us to conclude that:

- Chondroitin sulfate is the main proteoglycan synthesized in embryonic and early postnatal liver tissue. It decreases rapidly during the first 6 days of postnatal life and reaches adult levels at about the 10th day of life.
- The synthesis rate of chondroitin sulfate has a positive statistical correlation with the synthesis of DNA (or [^{3}H]thymidine incorporation).
- Proteochondroitin sulfate is expressed on the plasma membranes of embryonic liver cells but not on those of adult hepatocytes.
- The pattern of glycosaminoglycans, i.e., decrease of heparan sulfate and increase of chondroitin sulfate, in embryonic liver tissue ressembles that in malignant and fibrotic liver.
- D-Galactosamine, a hepatotoxic compound with a well defined mechanism of action, inhibits similarly in adult, postnatal, and embryonic liver the synthesis

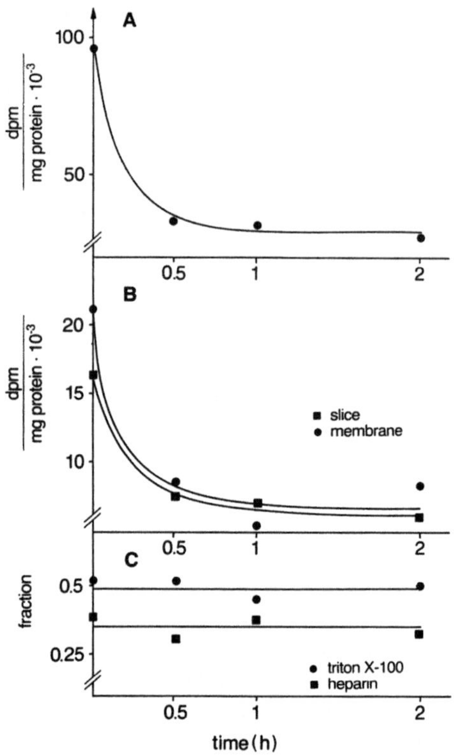

Fig. 7 A–C. General protein synthesis **A**, incorporation of [^{35}S]sulfate into total glycosaminoglycans and liver cell membrane-associated heparan sulfate **B**, and the proportion of heparin-sensitive and triton X-100-sensitive fractions of membrane-associated heparan sulfate **C** in slices from livers injured in vivo for various times with 700 mg D-galactosamine/kg body weight

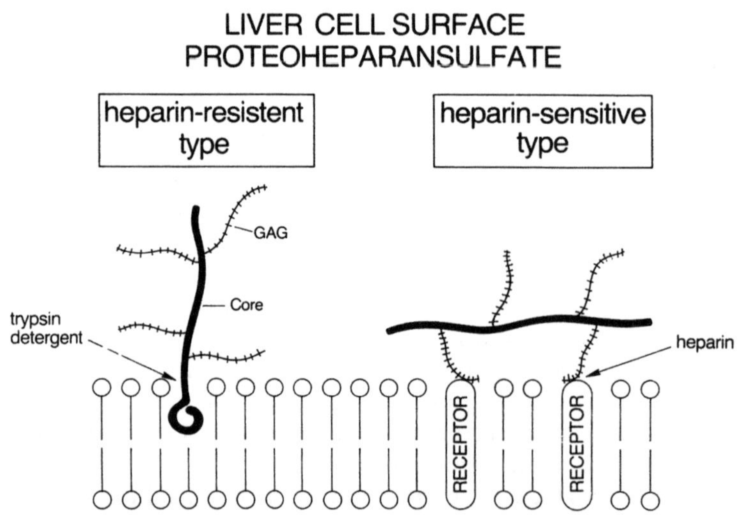

Fig. 8. Schematic representation of the two types of liver cell surface proteoheparan sulfate (Kjellen et al. 1981). The heparin-sensitive fraction (about 30%) can be displaced from the "receptors" by treatment with heparin; the heparin-resistant fraction (about 65%) is liberated by detergent or proteolytic treatment. In liver cell injury there is a concomitant decrease of both subfractions

Table 7. Incorporation in vivo of [^{35}S] sulfate into specific types of glycosaminoglycans associated with plasma membranes from adult and postnatal rat livers. Adult rats received i. p. 300 μCi, neonatal rats 25 μCi [^{35}S] sulfate 1 h before exitus. Plasma membranes were isolated by centrifugation in a discontinuous sucrose gradient. The data represent mean values ± SD of 3 experiments

Source of plasma membranes	Relative distribution of glycosaminoglycans (%)		
	Heparan sulfate	Chondroitin sulfate	Dermatan sulfate
Adult liver	72±1.6		2.7±1.1
Postnatal liver			
1 day	60±2.0	23.0±4.6	4.0±1.4
2 days	66±3.4	15.5±3.3	–
10 days	64±2.8	5.8±4.2	–

of heparan sulfate, but (nearly) not that of chondroitin sulfate. The mechanism of inhibition is independent of its effect on general protein synthesis.
- The sensitivity of GAG synthesis in young, adult, and senescent liver to D-galactosamine is similar, but embryonic and early postnatal liver seems to be less sensitive than adult liver tissue.

References

Decker K, Keppler D (1974) Galactosamine hepatitis: key role of the nucleotide deficiency period in the pathogenesis of cell injury and cell death. Rev Physiol Biochem Pharmacol 71:78–106

Gressner AM (1983) Hepatic proteoglycans – a brief survey of their pathobiochemical implications. Hepatogastroenterology 30:225–229

Gressner AM, Schulz W, Greiling H (1979) The synthesis of glycosaminoglycans in ageing rat liver. Med Ageing Develop 10:445–450

Gressner AM, Heinrig S, Grouls P (1982) The sequence of changes in the biosynthesis of sulfated glycosaminoglycans in acute, experimental liver disease. J Clin Chem Clin Biochem 20:15–24

Homann J, Gerhardt H, Hopf F (1980) Protektiver und kurativer Effekt von Diethyldithiocarbamat auf die Galaktosamin-Hepatitis der Ratte. Arzneim Forsch/Drug Res 30:645–647

Kjellen L, Oldberg A, Höök M (1981) Cell surface heparan sulfate: an intercalated membrane proteoglycan. Proc Natl Acad Sci USA 78:5371–5375

Kojima J, Nakamura N, Kanatani M, Ohmori K (1975) The glycosaminoglycans in human hepatic cancer. Cancer Res 35:542–547

Oldberg A, Höök M, Öbrink B, Pertoft H, Rubin K (1977) Structure and metabolism of rat liver heparan sulfate. Biochem J 164:75–81

Perrissoud D, Weibel I (1980) Protective effect of (+)cyanidanol-3 in acute liver injury induced by galactosamine or carbon tetrachloride in the rat. Naunyn-Schmiedeberg's Arch Pharmacol 312:285–291

Stuhlsatz HW, Vierhaus S, Gressner AM, Greiling H (1982) The distribution pattern and structural differences of the glycosaminoglycans in normal and cirrhotic human liver. In: Popper H, Reutter W, Gudat F, Köttgen E (eds) Structural carbohydrates in the liver. MTP Press, Lancaster, p 542–547

Age Dependence of the Structure and Metabolism of Joint Cartilage and the Influence of Drugs

H. GREILING [1]

The connective tissue is a target organ in the body, in which the age-dependent changes can be seen with our eyes. The wrinkling of skin is one piece of evidence of the physiological aging process, especially of connective tissue. The turgor and the skin elasticity are correlated with the chronological age and alterations in them are caused by definite biochemical and morphological changes in the connective tissue. The father of gerontology, the Swiss Verzar, first observed the age dependence of heat-induced shrinkage in rat tail tendons. On the basis of these observations, the cross-linkage theory was postulated, i.e., that aging is caused by increased cross-linking of proteins, especially collagens. But until now there has been no experimental evidence to support this theory, especially with the new knowledge about collagen types I–X.

Besides the various collagens and the elastins, the so-called ground substance (composed of GAGs and proteoglycans) is produced by specific cells in connective tissue. They are developed from a primitive mesenchymal cell. Specific cells, fibroblasts, chondrocytes etc., produce specific tissue types which have a characteristic composition of macromolecules and also GAGs and proteoglycans, which determine the biomechanical properties of the tissues.

Figure 1 shows the structure of the proteoglycans in cartilage. A proteoglycan subunit consists of CS and KS chains connected to a protein core. Numerous proteoglycan subunits are aggregated by means of a hyaluronate chain. Since the early report of Kaplan and Meyer, which described for the first time age-dependent changes in the composition of the glycosaminoglycans in human costal cartilage, further studies have confirmed both in animal and human cartilage an age-dependent decrease of total chondroitin sulfate (Fig. 2), combined with an increase in the proportion of chondroitin 6-sulfate to chondroitin 4-sulfate. In addition to the decrease in the total glycosaminoglycan concentration with age, the number of unsulfated disaccharide units present in chondroitin sulfate is reduced. Mathews and Glagov found in human costal cartilage a relative increase in keratan sulfate with age.

Roughley and White found that the proteoglycan content of human articular cartilage decreases with age; the same is true for the size of the proteoglycan subunit (Fig. 1). These authors confirmed our findings in human knee joint cartilage concerning the proportion of the chondroitin sulfate to keratan sulfate: an increase in keratan sulfate relative to chondroitin sulfate, and an increase in chon-

[1] Department of Clinical Chemistry and Pathobiochemistry, Technical University, D-5100 Aachen/F.R.G.

Drugs and Aging
Ed. by D. Platt

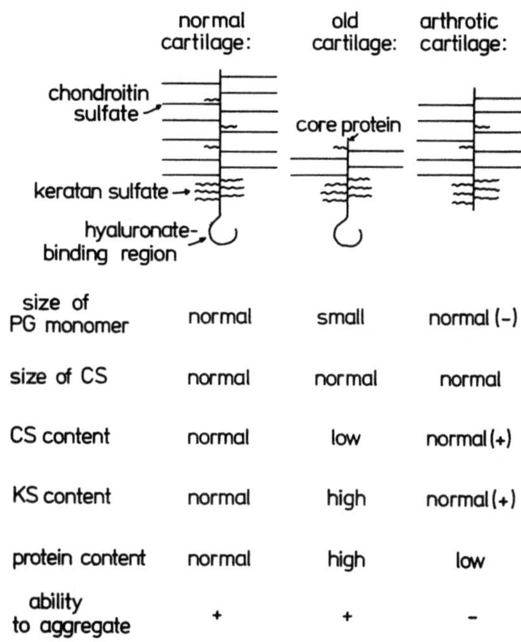

Fig. 1. Changes in the structure of the proteoglycan subunit in normal, old, and arthrotic cartilage. *PG*, proteoglycan; *CS*, chondroitin sulfate; *KS*, keratan sulfate. [Modified from Inerot S, Heinegard D, Andell L, Olsson SE (1978) Articular cartilage proteoglycans in aging and osteoarthritis. Biochem J 169:143–156]

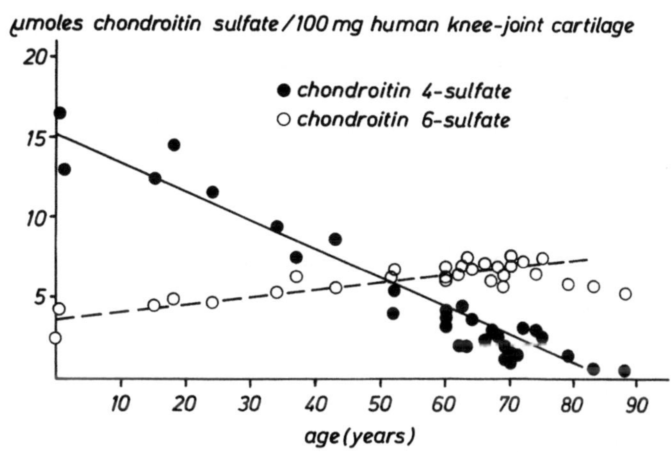

Fig. 2. Age-dependent chondroitin 4-sulfate and chondroitin 6-sulfate composition of human knee joint cartilage

droitin 6-sulfate relative to chondroitin 4-sulfate. In addition, Roughley and White observed an increase in protein relative to glycosaminoglycans, and a decrease in serine and glycine in relation to an increase in arginine of the core protein with age. Similar results had also been obtained previously by Inerot, Heinegard, Audell, and Olsson in canine hip articular cartilage. They found that the extracted proteoglycans were smaller in the older proteoglycan monomers. The hyaluronate binding region and the region rich in keratan sulfate were increased, and the molar concentration of proteoglycan probably increased with age. One also sees that the old cartilage has a structural tendency to turnover to osteoarthrosis in which the binding region is lost (Fig. 1).

How can we explain the age-dependent changes of decreased chondroitin sulfate and increased keratan sulfate on a molecular level? Whereas experimental evidence is lacking for a possible increase in the catabolic rate, some studies indicate an age-associated depression in the biosynthesis of proteochondroitin sulfate in both animal and human cartilage. The enzyme activity, catalyzing the covalent attachment of xylose to the seryl residues of the core protein, has been suggested to be rate limiting in the biosynthesis of the glycosaminoglycan chain of proteochondroitin sulfate. Therefore we studied the activity of UDP-xylose:core protein xylosyltransferase in the costal cartilage of young and senescent rats.

The activity of xylosyltransferase, measured in samples of old and young costal cartilage, is summarized in Fig. 3. Related to cartilage wet weight and protein, enzyme activity is decreased about 70% in the tissue of old rats.

In old cartilage, there was a reduction in cell number, as checked by the decline of extractable DNA to about 30%. However, the decrease in the activity of xylosyltransferase in relation to the concentration of DNA in old cartilage was similar to that reported above (about 70%). Thus, loss of xylosyltransferase activity in old tissue is not due to a higher reduction in the number of chondrocytes in the cartilage of old rats.

The results suggest that the reduced xylosyltransferase activity might lead to a diminished concentration of proteochondroitin sulfate in the cartilage of old animals. Therefore, the proteoglycans were isolated from the tissues and analyzed for their composition. In fact, the content of chondroitin sulfate, extractable with guanidinium chloride and represented by the amounts of uronic acid and (to exclude hyaluronic acid as a source of uronic acid) galactosamine, decreases from young to old animals by about 80%.

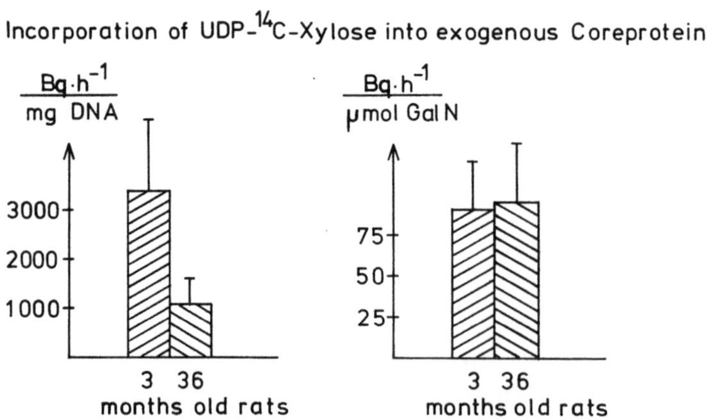

Fig. 3. Activity of UDP-xylose:core protein xylosyltransferase in costal cartilage of 3-month-old ($n = 16$) and 36-month-old ($n = 15$) rats. The activity ($Bq \cdot h^{-1}$) is related to either the concentration of DNA in tissue or to the amount of galactosamine-containing, guanidinium chloride-extracted proteoglycans in cartilage. The values represent the mean $\pm$SD of independent experiments in each age group

When the activity of xylosyltransferase is related to galactosamine as a measure of the concentration of chondroitin sulfate, no significant differences between young and old rats are detectable. Thus, there is a coordinate decrease in both xylosyltransferase activity and chondroitin sulfate content in the cartilage of old rats in comparison to that of young animals.

Our findings point to xylosyltransferase as a possible regulator of proteochondroitin sulfate synthesis at the posttranslational level. This is in agreement with the findings of Schwartz, which show the independence of proteochondroitin sulfate synthesis from the biosynthetic rate of the respective core protein. The rather short half-life of xylosyltransferase as compared with other enzymes involved in the glycosaminoglycan chain synthesis indicates the possible regulatory role of this enzyme in chondroitin sulfate proteoglycan production.

Since our experiments also showed a reduction in xylosyltransferase activity, if related to the concentration of DNA, a loss of chondrocytes as a cause of this change is excluded. The activity of another cytosolic enzyme, LDH, was found to be nearly unaffected by the age of the animals, if related to DNA. Therefore it is conceivable that, due to the strong reduction of xylosyltransferase activity in old cartilage, the enzymatic attachment of xylose to the seryl residues of core protein becomes rate limiting under such conditions. In accordance with this assumption, Inerot has shown similar chain lengths (molecular weights) of chondroitin sulfate in old and young cartilage, and Honda has presented evidence that the glycosaminoglycan chain elongation reaction is not impaired in the cartilage of senescent rats. Thus, the age-dependent diminution of total chondroitin sulfate is due to a reduced number of initiated carbohydrate side chains along the core protein, which is likely to be caused by the lower amounts of xylosyltransferase in old tissue.

Our results do not answer the question of whether there is a decrease in the specific activity of this enzyme or a diminution of enzyme protein. The nature of the primary event that causes diminished xylosyltransferase activity is not yet known and needs further investigation. Of particular importance might be the changing composition of hormones with age, since Schiller has shown that in diabetic thyroidectomized and hypophysectomized rats, the reduced synthesis of proteoglycans is due to decreased xylosyltransferase activity. She observed that in hormone-deficient animals, the enzymatic attachment of xylose to seryl residues of the core protein becomes the rate-limiting step in the synthesis of proteochondroitin sulfate. Other authors have shown that hormones involved in the sulfation of proteoglycans, e.g., somatomedin and thyroxine, specifically affect the activity of xylosyltransferase.

In Fig. 4 we propose a model for the mechanism of the age-related decrease of proteochondroitin sulfate content in cartilage. Accordingly, the activity of UDP-xylose:core protein xylosyltransferase controls the number of initiated chondroitin sulfate side chains. This explains the constant ratio between enzyme activity and proteochondroitin sulfate content in young and old cartilage.

I have shown that with increasing age, thyroxine and triiodothyronine concentrations in blood serum decrease. Table 1 shows the stimulation of chondroitin sulfate synthesis by triiodothyronine in chondrocyte cultures. In the presence of rT_3, the antagonist of T_3, the galactosamine/glucosamine ratio diminishes,

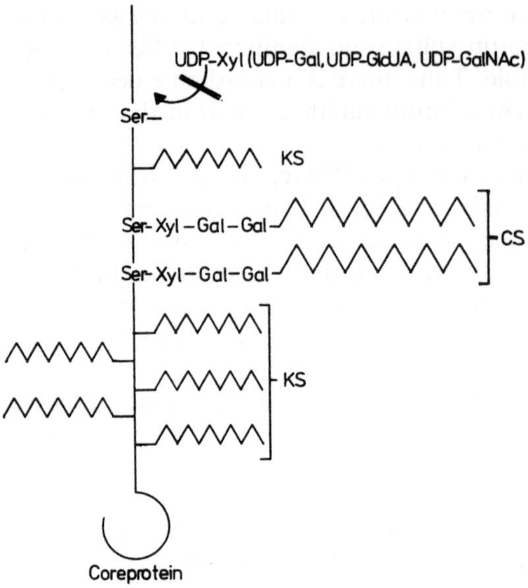

Fig. 4. Reduced chondroitin sulfate synthesis in old cartilage as the result of decreased activity of UDP-xylose: core protein xylosyltransferase

Table 1. Effect of L-3,5,3′-triiodthyronine (T_3) and L-3,3′5′-triiodthyronine (r.T_3) on the synthesis of proteoglycans in bovine chondrocytes

T_3	rT_3	Specific activity [Bq/nmol]		$\frac{GalN}{GlcN}$
(nmol/liter)		HexN	Ser	
–	–	29.6	7.9	0.51
–	–	29.9	8.7	0.47
0.05	–	28.6	7.2	0.98
0.1	–	38.2	12.2	1.92
0.2	–	60.2	20.8	2.15
0.4	–	46.0	11.9	1.23
0.8	–	32.9	8.3	0.72
0.4	0.2	34.9	10.9	1.02
0.4	0.4	32.4	8.7	0.74
0.4	0.8	26.8	7.1	0.89
0.4	1.6	27.3	7.2	0.84

which means an increase in keratan sulfate synthesis. Also, the incorporation of ^{14}C-serine into the core protein increases with T_3.

The same also occurs with thyroxine (T_4) and 3′,5′-diiodothyronine, which means an activation of chondroitin sulfate synthesis with T_4 and an inhibition with 3′,5′-diiodothyronine. In addition, in human blood serum there is an increase in the rT_3/T_3-ratio after 60 years (Table 2).

We postulate the following regulatory mechanism (Fig. 5): T_4 and T_3 stimulate the number of serine acceptors for xylose and therefore the xylosyltransferase

Table 2. Effect of thyroxine and L-3′,5′-diiodthyronine on the biosynthesis of proteoglycans in bovine chondrocytes

T_4	3′,5′-T_2	Specific activity [Bq/nmol]		GalN/GlcN
(nmol/liter)		HexN	Ser	
–	–	8.2	0.58	0.27
–	–	11.8	0.81	0.59
26	–	12.8	1.04	1.70
64	–	16.4	1.48	2.36
–	–	13.2	1.19	2.04
193	–	11.1	1.01	1.40
–	–	10.4	0.90	1.42
64	0.096	9.7	0.96	0.51
–	–	11.7	1.03	0.79
64	0.287	7.6	0.64	0.33
–	–	8.3	0.64	0.55
64	2.87	7.6	0.52	0.28
–	–	8.8	0.67	0.32

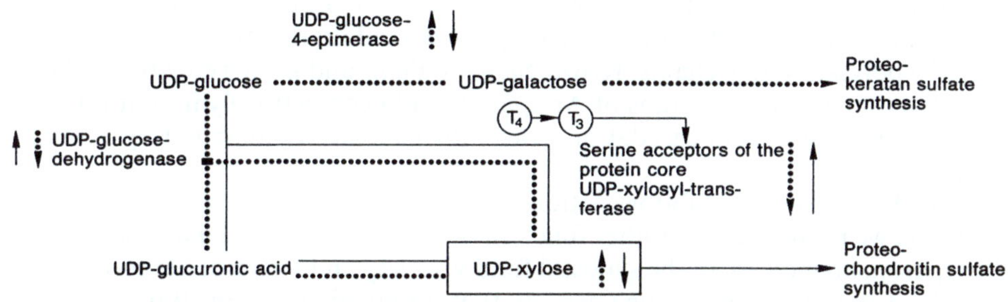

Fig. 5. Postulated action of thyroid hormones and their analogues on the distribution and biosynthesis of chondroitin sulfates and keratan sulfates in joint cartilage

activity. This results in a diminished UDP-xylose pool. UDP-xylose is a feedback inhibitor of UDP-glucose dehydrogenase. A decreased UDP-xylose concentration stimulates the UDP-glucose dehydrogenase and, therefore, the proteochondroitin sulfate synthesis. Decreased concentrations of T_4 and T_3 in blood serum found in older animals or an increase in 3′,5′-diiodothyronine or rT_3 have the inverse effect and stimulate the proteokeratan sulfate synthesis, as seen in the elderly. Thus we can explain from the regulatory enzyme level the characteristic changes in connective tissue with increasing age.

Influence of the So-called Chondroprotective Drugs on Cartilage Metabolism

In summary, with increasing age the glycosaminoglycan content of cartilage is decreased and the proteoglycan molecules are changed. Are there therapeutic possibilities to counteract this change and the degradation of proteoglycans?

In recent years there has been much discussion about the so-called chondroprotective drugs which are in therapeutic use for the treatment of osteoarthrosis.

Which qualities do we now expect in an antidegenerative, antiarthrotic chondroprotective drug?

1. It must normalize and stabilize the structure and the metabolism of proteolycans and collagens.
2. It should be capable of inhibiting the proteoglycan and collagen degradation in the cartilage.
3. It must also inhibit the inflammatory reactions which are present during the activated phase of arthrosis.

One of the so-called chondroprotective drugs is the glycosaminoglycan polysulfate Arteparon. Arteparon inhibits the degradation of the polysaccharide chains competitively, as we have shown for *β-N*-acetylglucosaminidase and *β*-glucuronidase. This competitive inhibition by Arteparon will be better understood when one examines its molecular structure, which contains the same constituents as the polysaccharide chains of cartilaginous proteoglycans, which in turn contain chondroitin sulfate and keratan sulfate, though both are oversulfated.

Arteparon is also an inhibitor of elastase. First the protein core of the proteoglycan molecules is degraded, followed by the degradation of the binding regions and the polysaccharide chains. Kruze, Salgam, Fehr, and Böni were able to show that even small concentrations of Arteparon could competitively inhibit this destructive process. This degradation is also physiologically inhibited by α_1-antitrypsin.

In addition to the inhibitory action of Arteparon on glycosaminoglycan degradation we must discuss another function. Following intra-articular injection of Arteparon, an increase in the synovial fluid viscosity and hyaluronate concentration is observed. Generally one can say that a reduction in joint fluid viscosity goes hand in hand with inflammatory processes and an increased lysosomal enzyme activity. We have shown a steady elevation of hyaluronate concentration in the joint fluid after an intra-articular injection of Arteparon while its total quantity decreases.

The lower polymerization degree of hyaluronate caused by an increase in the concentration of the hyaluronate-degrading lysosomal enzymes is one of the factors causing diminished synovial fluid viscosity in active arthrosis.

Another depolymerization factor is the superoxide radical. The hyaluronate-degrading enzymes are hyaluronate glycanohydrolase, *β*-glucuronidase, and *β-N*-acetylglucosaminidase. We assume that the Arteparon mechanism results in a competitive inhibition of the enzymes *β-N*-acetylglucosaminidase, *β*-glucuronidase, and hyaluronate glycanohydrolase, blocking the catabolic pathway of hyaluronate degradation. In compensation, synovial cells synthesize highly polymerized hyaluronic acid from UDP-*N*-acetylglucosamine and UDP-glucuronic acid. The normalization of the hyaluronate degradation is possibly followed by the normalization of its biosynthesis (Fig. 6).

We are also able to show the Arteparon is a very potent inhibitor of DNA-polymerase, RNA-polymerase, and "reverse transcriptase." It is, therefore, quite conceivable that a normalization of the biosynthetic processes takes place follow-

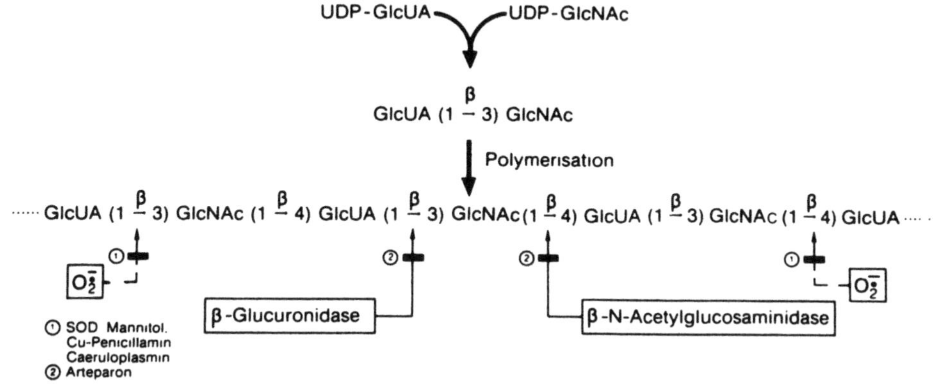

Fig. 6. Action of various drugs on the biosynthesis and degradation of hyaluronate

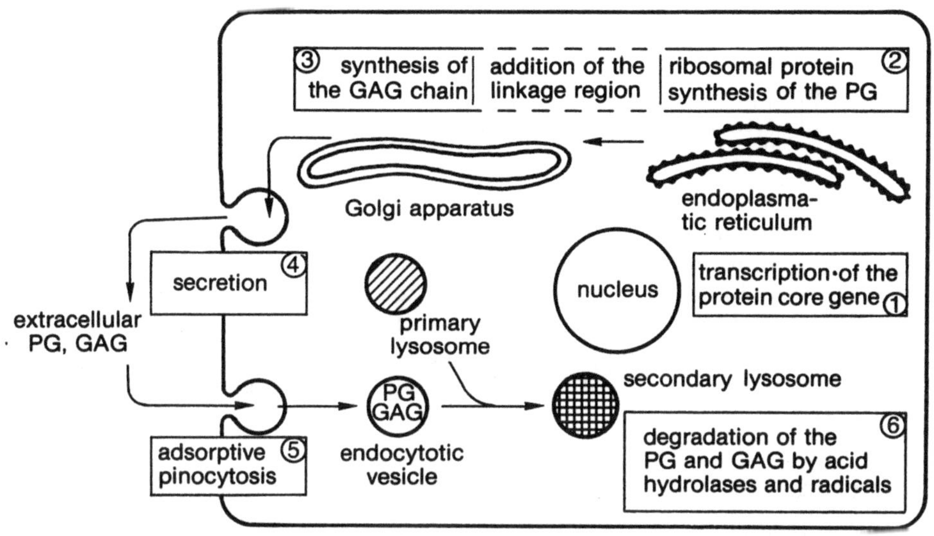

Fig. 7. Intracellular compartments and biosynthesis of proteoglycans. Possible actions of drugs. Benzarone, flufenamic acid, proquazone, glycosaminoglycan polysulfate (high concentrations); colchicine; glycosaminoglycan polysulfate

ing the interference of Arteparon with the information network between the nucleus, the endoplasmic reticulum, and the Golgi apparatus. These procedures, however, depend on the intracellular concentration of Arteparon (Fig. 7).

In synovia fibroblasts at concentrations between 10^{-7} and 10^{-5} mol/liter an increase in ^{14}C-GlcN incorporation in the total GAGs of the extracellular medium can be ascertained, with the maximum at low concentrations. We find an inhibition of the incorporation at concentration of 10^{-4} mol/liter. The ^{14}C-GlcN incorporation into the GAGs of the cell is increased with increased Arteparon concentration (Fig. 8).

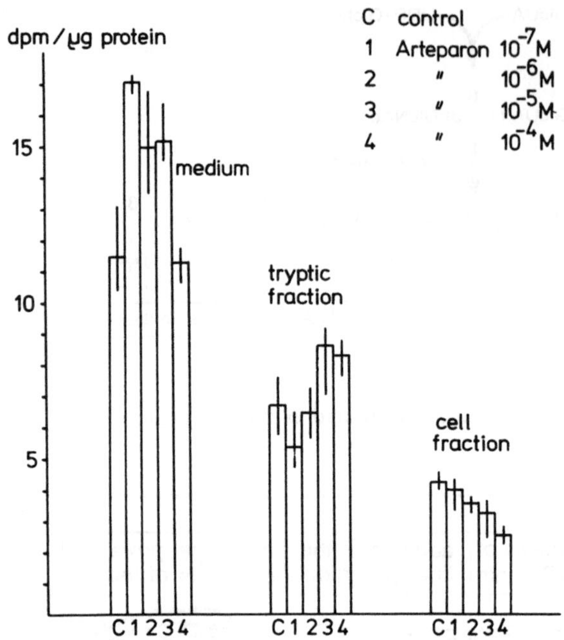

Fig. 8. Influence of Arteparon on the ^{14}C-glucosamine incorporation into glycosaminoglycans by synovial fibroblasts

A disadvantage of Arteparon, especially after intramuscular injection, is its low concentration in the synovial system and the "heparinoid" effect on blood coagulation, and in a few cases a shock reaction.

At the moment we have no chondroprotective drugs which fulfill the requirements mentioned above. In future we will have to search for such chondroprotective substances, which will stabilize the cartilage system in aged patients.

References

Greiling H (1982) Biochemical investigations of the mode of action of Arteparon. In: Dettmer N, Greiling H (eds) International drug symposium. Basle, Eular Publishers, p 11–18

Greiling H (1983) Biochemische Untersuchungen über mögliche antiarthrotisch-wirksame Medikamente. Z Rheumatologie 42:153–158

Greiling H, Gressner A, Kleesiek K (1983) Pathobiochemie und Pathophysiologie des Bindegewebes. In: Handbuch der Inneren Medizin, Bd VI/2A, Rheumatologie A. Springer, Berlin Heidelberg New York Tokyo, S 29–171

Kleesiek K, Brackertz D, Greiling H (1984) Pathobiochemische Mechanismen bei chronisch-entzündlichen Gelenkerkrankungen. In: Lang H, Greiling H (Hrsg) Pathobiochemie der Entzündung. Springer, Berlin Heidelberg New York Tokyo, S 203–225

Hypoxia and Ischemia of the Aged Brain: Pharmacotherapeutic Implications

S. HOYER [1]

The prevalence of most cerebral disorders in middle and old age is now known. Illnesses such as brain infarction, Parkinson's disease and the dementias, to mention the most important ones, are found to be most frequent in late life. They are often caused by hypoxic/ischemic events producing abnormalities in brain oxidative and energy metabolism. Therefore, with respect to the disorders mentioned, it would seem necessary to evaluate the effects of three factors on brain metabolism:

1. Age
2. Hypoxia
3. Ischemia

There has been prolonged discussion on the question of whether aging per se inevitably induces brain disorders such as those mentioned, particularly the dementias. The view has now been reached that normal cerebral aging is different from brain disorders in late life, particularly from dementia (for review, see Hoyer 1982b). For the normal brain, however, certain differences have been demonstrated between adulthood and senescence, e.g., mental capacities such as intelligence (Baltes and Schaie 1976; Baltes and Willis 1982; Horn and Cattell 1976; Horn and Donaldson 1976) and biological processes such as morphological and biochemical events (for review, see Hoyer 1982a).

Normal Cerebral Aging

Our studies demonstrated a general, more or less severe age-related reduction in the brain cortical concentrations of glucose, glucose-6-phosphate, fructose-1,6-phosphate, pyruvate, lactate, malate, creatine phosphate, and ATP, whereas an increase was found in ADP. This pattern was demonstrated as exponential fit curves (Fig. 1) (Hoyer 1983). However, the changes varied remarkably among different ages. Glucose, fructose-1,6-phosphate, and ATP dropped from 6 to 12 months of age, whereas the concentrations of pyruvate, malate, and creatine phosphate diminished between 12 and 24 months of age (Ulfert et al. 1982).

It has been well documented that rats may be designated as aged when their strain has a 50% survival rate and when their survival curve is more or less rectangular. In male Wistar rats this deflection point was found to be at the age of

[1] Institute of Pathochemistry and General Neurochemistry University of Heidelberg, Im Neuenheimer Feld 220, D-6900 Heidelberg/F.R.G.

Drugs and Aging
Ed. by D. Platt

Abbreviations Used in the Figures

Glu, Gl:	glucose	Succ:	succinate
G-6-P:	glucose-6-phosphate	Fum:	fumarate
F-6-P:	fructose-6-phosphate	Mal:	malate
F-1,6-P, FDP:	fructose-1,6-phosphate	OAA:	oxaloacetate
DHAP:	dihydroxyacetone phosphate	ATP:	adenosine triphosphate
Pyr:	pyruvate	ADP:	adenosine diphosphate
Lact:	lactate	AMP:	adenosine monophosphate
Citr:	citrate	CrP:	creatine phosphate
α-Keto:	α-ketoglutarate		

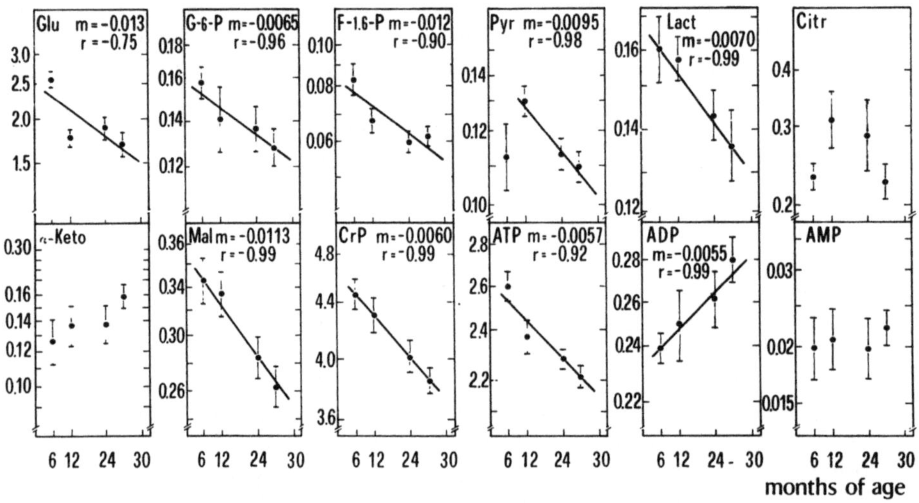

Fig. 1. Semilogarithmical graph of glucose and energy metabolite concentrations (in mol/g) in brain cortex of rats with increasing age

24 months (Hollander et al. 1983). Thus, adulthood is present at the age of 12 months and senescence at 24 months of age. In the following, these two ages are compared under normal and well-defined emergency conditions such as cerebral hypoxia and complete cerebral ischemia.

The results mentioned are in good agreement with the findings of other investigators, who showed a gradual decrease in oxidative processes in the brain cortex of rats from the age of 12 to 18 months and from 27 months onward (Peng et al. 1977), and a reduction of glucose oxidation in 2-year-old rats (Patel 1977). These findings are also consistent with the observation that the activities of hexokinase and phosphofructokinase are not reduced in rat brain cortex between 12 and 24 months of age (Iwangoff et al. 1980), that no differences exist in the enzyme activities of pyruvate carboxylase, citrate synthase, and NAD-isocitrate dehydrogenase during the same life span (Patel 1977), and that the enzyme activities of lactate dehydrogenase, pyruvate dehydrogenase, and NAD^+-malate dehydrogenase do not change in the brain cortex of rats between the ages of 3 months and 2 years, whereas fumarase significantly decreases during this time (Leong et al. 1981). These findings may suggest an only slightly reduced glucose and energy metabolism in rat brain cortex during aging from 12 to 24 months.

Cerebral Hypoxia

In cerebral hypoxia produced by severe arterial hypoxemia with a mean arterial pO_2 of 21 mmHg, significant increases in brain cortical concentrations of glucose, glucose-6-phosphate, fructose-1,6-phosphate, dihydroxyacetone phosphate, pyruvate, lactate, malate, ADP, and AMP and significant reductions in creatine phosphate and ATP could be observed in both age groups as compared with the respective controls. The metabolic pattern is characterized by an activation of glycolysis by means of the flux-controlling enzymes hexokinase, phosphofructokinase, and pyruvate kinase. Whereas the variations in glycolysis leading to massive lactate production were found to be major, only minor changes were observed in the tricarboxylic acid cycle (Fig. 2). This emergency condition may be counteracted by an increase in cerebral blood flow (Hamer et al. 1978).

However, it also becomes evident that the metabolic adaptation to the hypoxemic emergency conditions tends to become somewhat slower with aging. It may thus be assumed that the metabolic capacity to meet severe hypoxemic stress may be reduced with aging (Fig. 3). This also holds true for hypoxic ischemia, in which the increase in cerebral blood flow has been found to be less marked in aged than in young animals (Hoffman et al. 1984).

Hypoxia induced by cyanide in sublethal dosage caused metabolic variations in glycolysis which resembled those after severe arterial hypoxemia. The concentrations of glucose, fructose-1,6-phosphate, dihydroxyacetone phosphate, pyruvate, and lactate significantly increased. These variations point to an activation of glycolytic flux by means of increased phosphofructokinase activity. The changes in the tricarboxylic acid cycle were found to be most marked in a decrease in citrate and increase in succinate, fumarate, and malate, indicating the distur-

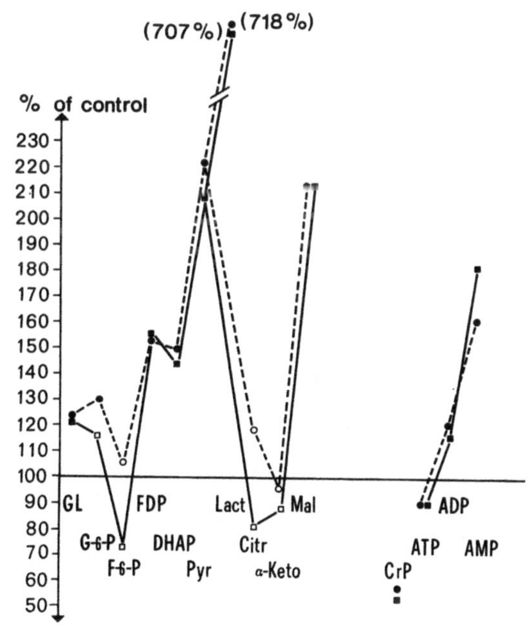

Fig. 2. Metabolites of glycolysis, tricarboxylic acid cycle, and energy rich compounds in brain cortex of 1- and 2-year-old rats after 15-min profound arterial hypoxemia (paO_2 20–25 mm Hg). The 100% level corresponds to the respective control group. *Filled symbols* represent statistically significant variations ($P \leqq 0.05$) o- - -o: hypoxemia in 1-year-old animals; □—□: hypoxemia in 2-year-old animals

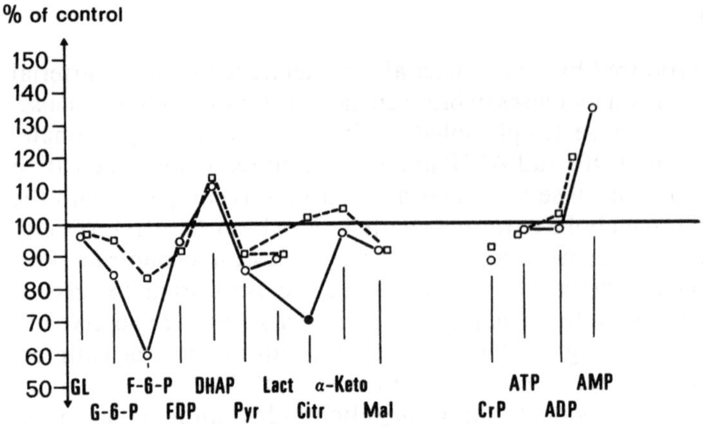

Fig. 3. Metabolites of glycolysis, tricarboxylic acid cycle, and energy rich compounds in brain cortex of 1- and 2-year-old rats. □---□: art. normotension, normocapnia, and normoxemia; 100% level corresponds to the 1-year-old group; ○—○: art. normotension, normocapnia, severe art. hypoxemia (paO_2 20–25 mm Hg); 100% level corresponds to the 1-year-old hypoxemia group. *Filled symbols* represents statistically significant difference ($P \leqq 0.05$)

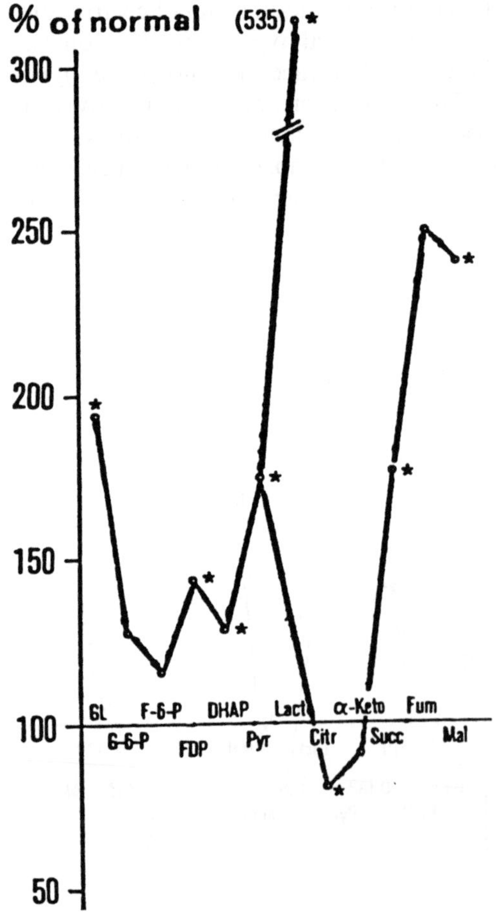

Fig. 4. Concentrations of glycolytic and tricarboxylic acid cycle intermediates in brain cortex of 2-year-old rats after infusion of 4 mg/kg b.w. cyanide. The 100% level corresponds to the control group. *, statistically significant difference from control

bance of NAD^+- and FAD^+-dependent redox reactions which also include the oxidation of pyruvate, thus increasing lactate formation (Fig. 4). Intoxication and damage to the respiratory chain by means of a sublethal dosage with cyanide did not result in variations of the tissue concentration of high-energy phosphates. Cyanide-induced hypoxia is also accompanied by an increase in cerebral blood flow, so that the emergency condition can be counteracted to some extent (Hoyer, unpublished data).

Hypoxic lesions of the brain induced by pure arterial hypoxemia may also produce changes in calcium and free fatty acid metabolism. However, brain damage by means of pure arterial hypoxemia is rather rare, and therefore the changes in calcium and free fatty acid metabolism will be discussed below in more detail. The cyanide model stands for a lesion not produced by a reduced substrate supply but induced by damage to a biological system, the respiratory chain, and normal oxygen availability. To some extent, it may resemble primary cell hypoxidosis (Strughold 1944).

Cerebral Ischemia

Complete cerebral ischemia produced almost complete depletion in the substrate concentration of glucose, oxaloacetate, ATP, and creatine phosphate, and a severe reduction in pyruvate, citrate, α-ketoglutarate, and malate, whereas fructose-1,6-phosphate, lactate, succinate, and AMP rose in both age groups studied. There were, however, some significant differences between the age groups concerning the substrates glucose, fructose-1,6-phosphate, lactate, succinate, malate, ADP, and AMP, suggesting that the biological plasticity of the glycolytic chain in the aging brain may be reduced to meet emergency conditions (Fig. 5). Anyway, ischemia induced a facilitation of the phosphofructokinase step and thus glycolysis in both age groups, resulting in a greatly elevated production of lactate and thus severe acidification of the brain (Ljunggreen et al. 1974).

Depletion of its physiological fuel glucose, depletion of the energy-rich compounds ATP and CrP, arrest of oxidative processes, and acidification of the tissue represent the pattern of oxidative brain metabolism in ischemia.

Beside the severe abnormalities found in glucose and energy metabolism, major disruptions of ion homeostasis occur. Potassium accumulates in the brain extracellular fluid, and extracellular sodium and calcium flood the cell interior, whereby calcium is also released from mitochondria and endoplasmic reticulum. The extremely elevated concentration of free calcium in the cytosol induce reactions which seem to damage the cell further. In peripheral nerves, neurofilaments and neurotubules are changed by proteases activated by an increased Ca^{2+} concentration (Schlaepfer 1971).

Furthermore, the rise in intracellular free calcium concentration causes the activation of membrane phospholipidase A and C, which degrade membrane phospholipids. Under physiological conditions, membrane phospholipids are recycled by some energy-dependent reactions. In ischemia, however, the brain is depleted of energy (see above), and phospholipids are broken down to free fatty acids, e.g., arachidonic acid. This free fatty acid accumulates in brain tissue in the absence

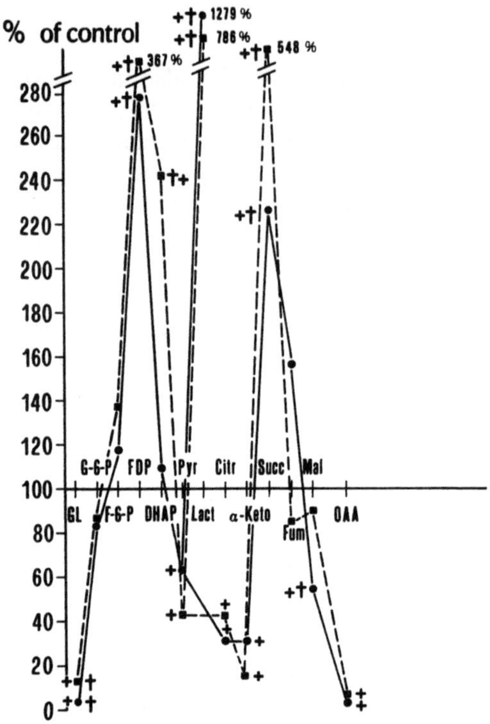

Fig. 5. Cerebral gray matter concentrations of glycolytic and tricarboxylic acid cycle intermediates after 15-min complete cerebral ischemia in 1-year-old (●) and 2-year-old (■) rats. The 100% level corresponds to the respective control groups. † = statistically significantly difference between the age groups; + = statistically significant difference from respective controls ($2P \leqq 0.05$)

of oxygen, i.e., in complete cerebral ischemia. In incomplete cerebral ischemia and in the recovery period of ischemia, however, arachidonic acid initiates a cascade of biochemical events leading to the formation of prostaglandins and thromboxanes. Associated with the formation of these compounds is the generation of active oxygen radicals. Thus, based on present knowledge, cerebral ischemia is not only associated with lacking or critically low tissue perfusion but also with detrimental changes in tissue metabolism. Since the latter may obviously outlast the period of complete or incomplete ischemia, it may also be assumed that ischemic tissue damage may be mainly characterized by the metabolic abnormalities in cellular and subcellular compartments.

Therapeutic Indications

What general consequences for the therapy of cerebral ischemic events can be inferred from these findings?

Zero or critically low cerebral blood flow may represent the first step in a sequence of events which may cause brain infarction. Therefore, improvement of the disturbed cerebral circulation should be started immediately to prevent further deterioration. In a second step, therapeutic efforts should be directed toward the different metabolic abnormalities: restitution of the oxidative pathway of glucose metabolism, restitution of ion homeostasis, particularly that of calcium, normalization of fatty acid metabolism, and reduction of the formation of active oxygen radicals.

What consequences can be inferred for the therapy of a brain-infarcted patient on the basis of therapeutic strategies so well documented that they can be applied in a patient with a certain chance of success?

In our studies in experimental rats, it could be shown that the metabolic changes induced by a sublethal dose of cyanide could be counteracted by naphtidrofuryl (Hoyer 1984). Findings from other investigations have demonstrated that this drug may also be able to reduce increased blood viscosity and thus improve the rheologic properties of the blood. This was also found to be true of drugs such as pentoxifyllin, piracetam, and Gingko biloba. The latter is presumed to scavenge active oxygen radicals (LePoncin-Lafitte et al. 1980, 1982; Herskovits et al. 1981; Etienne et al. 1984). It has become obvious that increased blood viscosity can also be counteracted by hemodilution (Gottstein 1984).

The information on drugs which may have effects on hypoxia/ischemia-induced metabolic abnormalities is very poor at present. Heiss et al. (1983) reported on an elevation of reduced glucose metabolism in brain infarction when piracetam was applied.

The administration of barbiturates to protect the brain from hypoxic/ischemic damage was recommended some years ago. However, more systematic studies in experimental and clinical fields unequivocally demonstrated that barbiturates did not improve the metabolic derangements in brain tissue and did not significantly improve the outcome of severe brain damage (Wiedemann and Hoyer 1983). The sole indication established for the administration of barbiturates was that they were found to decrease an increased intracranial pressure. The use of calcium antagonists might be helpful in reestablishing ion homeostasis in the brain cells damaged by hypoxia/ischemia. Whereas the effect of these drugs on calcium channels is well understood, there is little information on whether calcium antagonists also reduce the increased cytosolic Ca^{2+} concentration after hypoxia/Ischemia (van Reempts et al. 1984).

In general, many further efforts are required in both basic and clinical research to obtain more hard data that can serve as a rational basis for therapy of hypoxic/ischemic brain damage.

References

Baltes PB, Schaie KW (1976) On the plasticity of intelligence in adulthood and old age: Where Horn and Donaldson fail. Amer Psychologist 31:720–725

Baltes PB, Willis SL (1982) Plasticity and enhancement of intellectual functioning in old age. In: Craik FIM, Trehub EE (eds) Aging and cognitive processes. Plenum Press, New York, p 353–389

Etienne A, Chapelat MY, Braquet M, Clostre F, Drieu K, DeFeudis FV, Braquet P (1984) In vivo studies of free radical scavenging activity; relation to cerebral ischemia. In: Bes A, Braquet P, Paoletti R, Siesjö BK (eds) Cerebral ischemia. Excerpta Medica, Amsterdam, p 379–384

Gottstein U (1984) Hemodilution: Therapy in acute ischemic stroke. In: Bes A, Braquet P, Paoletti R, Siesjö BK (eds) Cerebral ischemia. Excerpta Medica, Amsterdam, p 311–324

Hamer J, Wiedemann K, Berlet H, Weinhardt F, Hoyer S (1978) Cerebral glucose and energy metabolism, cerebral oxygen consumption and blood flow in arterial hypoxemia. Acta Neurochir 44:151–160

Heiss WD, Ilsen HW, Wagner R, Pawlik G, Wienhard K (1983) Remote functional depression of glucose metabolism in stroke and its alteration by activating drugs. In: Heiss WD, Phelps ME (eds) Positron emission tomography of the brain. Springer, Berlin, p 162–168

Herskovits E, Famulari A, Tamaroff L, Gonzalez AM, Vazquez A, Smud R, Fraiman H, Vila J, Matera V (1981) Randomised trial of pentoxifylline versus acetylsalicylic acid plus dipyridamole in preventing transient ischaemic attacks. Lancet I:966–968

Hoffman WE, Pelligrino D, Miletich DJ, Albrecht RF (1984) Cerebrovascular and metabolic response of the aged rat to hypoxia. In: Fieschi C, Lenzi GL, Loeb CW (eds) Effects of aging on regulation of cerebral blood flow and metabolism. Karger, Basel, p 8–16

Hollander CF, van Zwieten MJ, Zurcher C (1983) The aged animal. In: Gispen WH, Traber J (eds) Aging of the brain. Elsevier, Amsterdam, p 187–196

Horn JL, Cattell RB (1976) Age differences in fluid and crystallized intelligence. Acta Psycholog 26:107–129

Horn JL, Donaldson G (1976) On the myth of intellectual decline in adulthood. Amer Psychologist 31:710–719

Hoyer S (1982a) The young-adult and normally aged brain. Its blood flow and oxidative metabolism. A review – part I. Arch Gerontol Geriatr 1:101–116

Hoyer S (1982b) The abnormally aged brain. Its blood flow and oxidative metabolism. A review – part II. Arch Gerontol Geriatr 1:195–207

Hoyer S (1983) Circulation and oxidative metabolism in the normally and abnormally aging brain. In: Gispen WH, Traber J (eds) Aging of the brain. Elsevier, Amsterdam, p 151–165

Hoyer S (1984) The effect of naftidrofuryl on cyanide-induced hypoxic damage to glucose and energy metabolism in brain cortex of rats. Arzneim Forsch/Drug Res 34:412–416

Iwangoff P, Enz A, Armbruster R, Emmenegger H, Pataki A, Sandoz P (1980) Der Einfluß von Alter. Zeitspanne bis zur postmortalen Isolierung des Gewebes sowie der Agonie auf einige glykolytische Enzyme in autoptischen Gehirnproben des Menschen. Akt Gerontol 10:203–212

Leong SF, Lai JCK, Lim L, Clark JB (1981) Energy-metabolizing enzymes in brain regions of adult and aging rats. J Neurochem 37:1548–1556

LePoncin-Lafitte M, Rapin J, Rapin JR (1980) Effect of Gingko biloba on changes induced by quantitative cerebral microembolization in rats. Arch Int Pharmacodyn 243:236–244

LePoncin-Lafitte M, Grosdemouge C, Roy-Billon C, Duterte D, Rapin JR (1982) Effects of naftidrofuryl on cerebral hemodynamic, metabolism and function after a retracted ischaemia. Arch Int Pharmacodyn 260:218–229

Ljunggren B, Norberg K, Siesjö BK (1974) Influence of tissue acidosis upon restitution of brain energy metabolism following total ischemia. Brain Res 77:173–186

Patel MS (1977) Age-dependent changes in the oxidative metabolism in rat brain. J Gerontol 32:643–646

Peng MT, Peng YI, Chen FN (1977) Age-dependent changes in the oxygen consumption of the cerebral cortex, hypothalamus, hippocampus, and amygdaloid in rats. J Gerontol 32:517–522

Schlaepfer WW (1971) Experimental alterations of neurofilaments and neurotubules by calcium and other ions. Exp Cell Res 67:73–80

Strughold H (1944) Hypoxydose. Klin Wochenschr 23:221–222

Ulfert G, Schmidt U, Hoyer S (1982) Glucose and energy metabolism of rat cerebral cortex during aging. In: Hoyer S (ed) The aging brain. Physiological and pathophysiological aspects. Exp Brain Res Suppl 5. Springer, Berlin, p 102–111

van Reempts J, Haseldonckx M, van de Ven M, Borgers M (1984) Morphology and ultrastructural calcium distribution in the rat hippocampus after severe transient ischemia. In: Bes A, Braquet P, Paoletti R, Siesjö BK (eds) Cherebral ischemia. Excerpta Medica, Amsterdam, p 113–118

Wiedemann K, Hoyer S (1983) Brain protection. Morphological, pathophysiological and clinical aspects. Springer, Berlin

Age-Dependent Actions of Benzodiazepines

U. Klotz [1]

Introduction

The elderly constitute approximately 20% of our population, and 50% or more of total drug consumption is by the elderly (WHO 1981). In view of the increased incidence of chronic illness and disability, these patients consume more than a proportionate share of drugs. In addition to the increased exposure to benzodiazepines, the elderly undergo a number of physiological changes that are likely to alter the response to benzodiazepines. As people grow older there is a wasting of muscle tissue, accumulation of fat, and a decrease in body water, liver mass, and brain weight. Progressive decreases with age are found for cardiac output (hepatic perfusion) and lung and kidney function. While there are many ways in which older patients respond differently from younger people, in many instances it is difficult to separate the overlapping effects of "normal" aging from the effects of degenerative diseases.

In geriatric clinical pharmacology age-related changes in drug disposition (absorption, distribution, elimination) and/or pharmacodynamics are considered as causative factors for an altered response to benzodiazepines. Thus, the purpose of this paper is to review the reasons for this phenomenon. First, some examples of the increased side-effect rate will be given which indicate the increased risks of toxicity in the elderly, followed by a section on age-related changes in pharmacodynamics. The second major part will deal with pharmacokinetic studies, with special emphasis on hepatic elimination and benzodiazepines. Finally, some experimental data will be discussed which might suggest age-induced alterations at receptor sites.

Increased Adverse Reaction Rate

Reports from the Boston Collaborative Drug Surveillance Program (see Table 1) have shown that older patients demonstrated an approximately two- to threefold higher incidence of side-effects with nitrazepam (Greenblatt and Allen 1978), flurazepam (Greenblatt et al. 1977), diazepam, and chlordiazepoxide. These data are derived from monitoring drug effects in actual clinical situations. Thus, the observed higher risks of toxicity cannot be solely attributed to aging per se; rather

[1] Dr. Margarete-Fischer-Bosch-Institut für Klinische Pharmakologie, Auerbachstr. 112, D-7000 Stuttgart 50/F.R.G.

Drugs and Aging
Ed. by D. Platt

Table 1. Increased toxicity of benzodiazepines in the elderly (data from the Boston Collaborative Drug Surveillance Program)

Drug	Patients studied	Adverse reactions	
		Normal patients	Elderly
Flurazepam	2,542	1.3% (<15 mg/day) 12.3% (>30 mg/day)	Drowsiness 2% 39%
Nitrazepam	2,111	3%	Drowsiness 11% CNS stimulation
Diazepam, chlordiazepoxide	270/186	5.6%	Drowsiness 12.9%

they must also be attributed to the severity and duration of concomitant disease(s) and comedications. However, it emphasizes the need for increased caution and careful monitoring of drug effects when treating the elderly.

The apparent increased frequency of adverse reactions to certain benzodiazepines in the elderly has stimulated research in investigating the mechanism(s) of altered drug response in old age. Several pharmacokinetic and/or pharmacodynamic studies have approached this clinically relevant problem.

Age-Related Changes in Pharmacodynamics

Pharmacodynamic causes would be responsible for an altered drug response if a given drug concentration yields a greater effect in an elderly person than in a young subject. Since in man drug levels at receptor sites cannot be measured, plasma concentrations have to be used as a substitute. Such a phenomenon could be observed with a single 10-mg oral dose of nitrazepam. Despite similar plasma concentrations of nitrazepam and elimination half-lives ($t_{1/2}$) in two groups of healthy young (mean age 25 years) and old people (mean age 75 years), the elderly made significantly more mistakes in a psychomotor test than did the young (Castleden et al. 1977). It could be concluded that the aging brain is more sensitive to nitrazepam.

Two different studies with diazepam indicate that the elderly are also more sensitive to the depressant effect of this benzodiazepine than the young. In patients undergoing elective cardioversion for treatment of arrhythmias, the response to painful and vocal stimulation was taken as a pharmacodynamic measurement. Elderly patients required lower doses and lower plasma levels of diazepam than younger patients to achieve the same degree of CNS depression (Reidenberg et al. 1978).

In patients aged 17–85 years intravenous diazepam was given for sedation prior to dental and endoscopic procedures. Plasma concentrations required for sedation fell two- to threefold between the ages of 20 and 80 years (Cook et al. 1984).

Body sway, choice reaction time, and critical flicker fusion threshold were used by Stevenson et al. (1982) as indices of the effect of a single oral dose of

20 mg temazepam. In the absence of appreciable differences in the plasma levels the immediate pharmacodynamic response (first 6 h postdosing) was more accentuated in the older (age range 68–75 years) than in the younger (age range 20–27) group.

Age-Related Changes in Pharmacokinetics

Several studies have focused on pharmacokinetic changes in the elderly. Since the benzodiazepines are mostly administered orally, strongly bound to plasma proteins, widely distributed within the body, and eliminated by hepatic metabolism, changes in the processes of drug absorption, distribution, and elimination have to be considered.

So far there is no evidence that absorption of benzodiazepines is impaired in old age. Theoretically, midazolam, a new hypnotic benzodiazepine with a relatively high, partly perfusion-dependent clearance and a considerable hepatic first pass effect (Allonen et al. 1981), might exhibit a higher oral bioavailability in the elderly, since cardiac output and consequently hepatic perfusion decline with age.

Age-related changes in body composition and the extent of plasma protein binding can influence the distribution of the benzodiazepines. This can indirectly be verified from the apparent volume of distribution (V) and the free fraction (fu) of the drug. Highly lipid-soluble benzodiazepines, such as chlordiazepoxide, clobazam, desmethyldiazepam, diazepam, midazolam, and nitrazepam, become more extensively distributed (increase in V) with age (see Table 2). Thereby differences in body composition between men and women also have to be taken into consideration.

The slight decrease in serum albumin, which might be larger in poorly nourished, ill, or severely debilitated elderly, can cause a minor increase in fu which could actually be observed only with very few benzodiazepines (see Table 3). Consequently, such compounds will be subject to more intensive distribution. However, it should be emphasized that the free steady state concentration remains the same, as does, therefore, the intensity of the clinical effect.

Benzodiazepines are exclusively metabolized in the liver, and total plasma/blood clearance (CL) is a model independent pharmacokinetic parameter best characterizing this elimination process. For a few oxidized/dealkylated benzodiazepines (phase I biotransformation steps) CL might be reduced in the elderly, suggesting some age dependency in drug metabolism. However, glucuronidated derivatives (phase II reaction) exhibit no age differences in their CL, indicating that such benzodiazepines are unaffected in their metabolism/hepatic elimination (see Table 4).

Often, especially in older studies, elimination half-life ($t_{1/2}$) has been considered an important pharmacokinetic variable. However, since according to the equation $t_{1/2} = 0.693 \times V/CL$ this constant depends on both the CL and V, it does not accurately describe drug elimination. Consequently, since V of many benzodiazepines increases with age (see Table 2), $t_{1/2}$ is prolonged in the elderly (Table 5). Again, benzodiazepines eliminated by glucuronidation exhibit no sig-

Table 2. Age and the apparent volume of distribution (V) of benzodiazepines

Benzodiazepine	V (liters/kg)[a]		References
	Young subjects	Elderly	
Alprazolam	1.02 (1.22)	0.89 (0.91)	Moschitto et al. (1981)
Bromazepam	0.7	1.1	Klotz and Brückel (1982)
Brotizolam	No significant differences		Jochemsen et al. (1983 a)
Chlordiazepoxide	0.42	0.52	Shader et al. (1977)
	0.26	0.38	Roberts et al. (1978)
Clobazam	0.87 (1.37)	1.40 (1.83)	Greenblatt et al. (1981)
Clotiazepam	Increase in elderly women		Ochs et al. (1984)
Desmethyldiazepam	0.64	0.85	Klotz and Müller-Seydlitz (1979)
	1.60 (2.11)	2.56 (3.01)	Allen et al. (1980)
	1.05 (1.28)	1.24 (1.54)	Shader et al. (1981)
Diazepam	0.6–1.0	1.5–2.0	Klotz et al. (1975)
	1.2 (1.4)	1.7 (2.5)	Divoll et al. (1983)
Flunitrazepam	No significant differences		Kanto et al. (1981)
Lorazepam	No significant differences		Kraus et al. (1978) and Greenblatt et al. (1979)
Lormetazepam	No significant differences		Hümpel et al. (1980)
Midazolam	1.7	2.5	Collier et al. (1982)
	(1.1)	(1.4)	Avram et al. (1983)
	1.34 (2.0)	1.64 (2.11)	Greenblatt et al. (1984)
Nitrazepam	2.7	2.9	Castleden et al. (1977)
	2.4	4.8	Kangas et al. (1979)
	1.9	2.9	Jochemsen et al. (1983)
Oxazepam	No significant differences		Shull et al. (1976) Greenblatt et al. (1980), and Klotz and Brückel (1982)
Temazepam	No significant differences		Divoll et al. (1981) and Smith et al. (1983)
Triazolam	No significant differences		Smith et al. (1983)

[a] Values in parentheses refer to women

Table 3. Age and plasma protein binding of benzodiazepines

Benzodiazepine	Free fraction (%)[a]		References
	Young subjects	Elderly	
Brotizolam	No significant differences		Jochemsen et al. (1983a)
Clobazam	11.2 (10.9)	11.9 (12.3)	Greenblatt et al. (1981a)
Desmethyldiazepam	3.0 (2.7)	2.9 (3.1)	Allen et al. (1980)
	2.6 (3.4)	3.2 (3.1)	Shader et al. (1981)
Diazepam	No significant differences		Klotz et al. (1975) and Ochs et al. (1981)
Lorazepam	10.5 (10.9)	11.6 (11.3)	Divoll and Greenblatt (1982)
Midazolam	No significant differences		Greenblatt et al. (1984)
Nitrazepam	No significant differences		Jochemsen et al. (1983b)
Oxazepam	No significant differences		Shull et al. (1976) and Greenblatt et al. (1980)
Temazepam	No significant differences		Divoll et al. (1981)
Triazolam	21.3	24.7	Greenblatt et al. (1983)

[a] Values in parentheses refer to women

Table 4. Age and clearance (CL) of benzodiazepines

Benzodiazepine	CL (ml/min)[a]		References
	Young subjects	Elderly	
Alprazolam	1.03 (0.85)[b]	0.64[b]	Moschitto et al. (1981)
Bromazepam	30.0	27.1	Klotz and Brückel (1982)
Brotizolam	109	40	Jochemsen et al. (1983)
Chlordiazepoxide	46.3	26.6	Shader et al. (1977)
	30	8	Roberts et al. (1978)
Clobazam	0.63 (0.56)[b]	0.36 (0.48)[b]	Greenblatt et al. (1981a)
Clotiazepam	No significant differences		Ochs et al. (1984)
Desmethyldiazepam	11.3	4.3	Klotz and Müller-Seydlitz (1979)
	0.35 (0.39)[b]	0.27 (0.46)[b]	Allen et al. (1980)
	0.22 (0.21)[b]	0.15 (0.27)[b]	Shader et al. (1981)
Diazepam	No significant differences		Klotz et al. (1975), Ochs et al. (1981), and MacLeod et al. (1979)
	0.46 (0.35)[b]	0.24 (0.29)[b]	Divoll et al. (1983)
Flunitrazepam	No significant differences		Kanto et al. (1981)
Lorazepam	No significant differences		Kraus et al. (1978) and Greenblatt et al. (1979)
	1.0 (0.98)[b]	0.8 (0.72)	Divoll and Greenblatt (1982)
Lormetazepam	No significant differences		Hümpel et al. (1980)
Midazolam	No significant differences		Collier et al. (1982), Avram et al. (1983), and Smith et al. (1984)
	534 (551)	339 (432)	Greenblatt et al. (1984)
Nitrazepam	No significant differences		Kangas et al. (1979) and Jochemsen et al. (1983b)
Oxazepam	No significant differences		Shull et al. (1976), Greenblatt et al. (1980), and Klotz and Brückel (1982)
Temazepam	No significant differences		Divoll et al. (1981) and Smith et al. (1983)
Triazolam	No significant differences		Smith et al. (1983)
	6.2 (8.8)[b]	3.2 (4.1)[b]	Greenblatt et al. (1983)

[a] Values in parentheses refer to women
[b] ml/min/kg

nificant changes in their $t_{1/2}$ with age. Thus, the "stable" pharmacokinetics of such derivatives might favor their use in the elderly.

If one tries to draw any conclusions from the numerous pharmacokinetic studies, it becomes obvious that the inconsistent age-induced changes in the distribution and/or elimination of the benzodiazepines can contribute only slightly to a better understanding of the higher sensitivity to these drugs in the elderly. A decreased CL will lead to a more intensive accumulation of the active compounds in the body, and a larger V indicates a higher drug uptake in certain tissue, including the brain. In addition to some peripheral binding changes, penetration

Table 5. Age and elimination half-life ($t_{1/2}$) of benzodiazepines

Benzodiazepine	$t_{1/2}$(h)[a]		References
	Young subjects	Elderly	
Alprazolam	13.6	19	Moschitto et al. (1981)
Bromazepam	19.8	35.1	Klotz and Brückel (1982)
Brotizolam	4.8	9.3	Jochemsen et al. (1983)
Chlordiazepoxide	10.1	18.2	Shader et al. (1977)
	7	40	Roberts et al. (1978)
Clobazam	17 (31)	48 (49)	Greenblatt et al. (1981a)
Clotiazepam	Increase in elderly women		Ochs et al. (1984)
Desalkylflurazepam	74 (90)	160 (120)	Greenblatt et al. (1981b)
Desmethyldiazepam	51	151	Klotz and Müller-Seydlitz (1979)
	62 (84)	128 (75)	Allen et al. (1980)
	64 (83)	120 (72)	Shader et al. (1981)
Diazepam	20–40	80–100	Klotz et al. (1975)
	32 (44)	101 (99)	Divoll et al. (1983
Flunitrazepam	No significant differences		Kanto et al. (1981)
Lorazepam	No significant differences		Kraus et al. (1978) and Greenblatt et al. (1979)
Lormetazepam	No significant differences		Hümpel et al. (1980)
Midazolam	2.8	4.3	Collier et al. (1982)
	2.7	3.2	Avram et al. (1983)
	2.1 (2.6)	5.6 (4.0)	Greenblatt et al. (1984)
Nitrazepam	No significant differences		Castleden et al. (1977)
	29	40	Kangas et al. (1979)
	26	38	Jochemsen et al. (1983)
Oxazepam	No significant differences		Shull et al. (1976), Greenblatt et al. (1980), and Klotz and Brückel (1982)
Temazepam	No significant differences		Divoll et al. (1981)
	(11.5)	(18.4)	Smith et al. (1983)
Triazolam	No significant differences		Smith et al. (1983), Dehlin et al. (1983), and Greenblatt et al. (1983)
Quazepam	25–41	53	Hilbert et al. (1984)
(*N*-desalkyl-2-oxoquazepam)	75–80	190	

[a] Values in parentheses refer to women

through the blood–brain barrier might be facilitated in the elderly. Consequently, all these phenomena would result in higher brain levels.

However, this is not directly measurable in man. Therefore some experimental data will be included to make possible a better discussion of the underlying mechanism(s) of the "age-sensitized" brain.

Experimental Age Studies

Pharmacokinetic studies with diazepam in rats demonstrated, in agreement with findings in man, an increased V and a prolonged $t_{1/2}$ in 18-month-old male Wistar rats compared with 6-month-old animals (Klotz 1979). A similar trend was observed when comparing 6- and 30-month-old Fisher-344 rats (Tsang and Wilkinson 1982).

In vitro binding experiments with ^{3}H-flunitrazepam in frontal cortex and cerebellum from young, mature, and senescent male Fisher-344 rats demonstrated no age-related changes in receptor density and affinity (Pedigo et al. 1981). Similarly, using washed membranes of female Fisher-344 rats' cerebral cortex, no age-related differences in the association, equilibrium, or dissociation binding characteristics of ^{3}H-diazepam were observed (Tsang et al. 1981). However, in the hippocampus of aged (26–28 months) Sprague-Dawley rats, receptor density (B_{max}), as measured from the ^{3}H-diazepam specific binding, was elevated if compared with that in mature animals (3–4 months). The affinity of binding (K_D) was not affected (Memo et al. 1981). Whether in other species or brain regions neurochemical and neurotransmitter receptor changes occur in the aged CNS remains to be elucidated. Since the benzodiazepine (BZD) binding sites are only one part of the GABA–benzodiazepine–ionophore receptor complex, it might be possible that in vivo age-related changes in the brain levels of GABA, chloride, or endogenous inhibitors/ligands (?) have also to be considered. In addition, the in vivo occupancy of the benzodiazepine recognition sites might be age dependent. It may well be that subpopulations of receptors exist which are regulated differently. Recently it was found that chronic and particularly acute exposure to diazepam elicits different responses in total receptor number and distribution of BZD_1 and BZD_2 subtypes between cortical membranes of 10- and 27-month-old male Fisher-344 rats (Reeves and Schweizer 1983).

In conclusion, the aging process is associated with complex pharmacokinetic and pharmacodynamic alterations resulting in a more pronounced CNS-depressant effect of the benzodiazepines. The different factors and the exact mechanism(s) of this phenomenon are still poorly understood.

Summary

Increased adverse reaction rates have been observed in the elderly with nitrazepam, flurazepam, chlordiazepoxide, and diazepam, and this increasing population seems to be more sensitive to the central nervous depressant effects of the benzodiazepines. Age-related pharmacokinetic changes have been demonstrated with numerous derivatives. The apparent volume of distribution of the lipophilic benzodiazepines increases with age, which causes prolongation of the elimination half-life. In addition, hydroxylation and dealkylation of some drugs (e.g., chlordiazepoxide, desmethyldiazepam) appear to be impaired. In contrast, the disposition of glucuronidated benzodiazepines (e.g., oxazepam, lorazepam, temazepam) is unaffected by age. In addition to pharmacokinetic changes, age-induced alterations at the receptor site have to be assumed, since lower plasma levels of the benzodiazepines are effective in the elderly.

Acknowledgments. The secretarial help of Mrs. I. Koch is gratefully acknowledged. The work was supported by the Robert Bosch Foundation Stuttgart, FRG.

References

Allen MD, Greenblatt DJ, Harmatz JS, Shader RI (1980) Desmethyldiazepam kinetics in the elderly after oral prazepam. Clin Pharmacol Ther 28:196–202

Allonen H, Ziegler G, Klotz U (1981) Midazolam kinetics. Clin Pharmacol Ther 30:653–661

Avram MJ, Fragen RJ, Caldwell NJ (1983) Midazolam kinetics in women of two age groups. Clin Pharmacol Ther 34:505–508

Clinical depression of the central nervous system due to diazepam and chlordiazepoxide in relation to cigarette smoking and age: a report from the Boston Collaborative Drug Surveillance Program (1973). N Engl J Med 288:277–280

Castleden CM, George CF, Marcer D, Hallett C (1977) Increased sensitivity to nitrazepam in old age. Brit Med J 1:10–12

Collier PS, Kawar P, Gamble JAS, Dundee JW (1982) Influence of age on pharmacokinetics of midazolam. Brit J Clin Pharmacol 13:602P–603P

Cook PJ, Flanagan R, James IM (1984) Diazepam tolerance: effect of age, regular sedation, and alcohol. Brit Med J 289:351–353

Dehlin O, Björnson G, Börjesson L, Abrahamsson L, Smith RB (1983) Pharmacokinetics of triazolam in geriatric patients. Eur J Clin Pharmacol 25:91–94

Divoll M, Greenblatt DJ (1982) Effect of age and sex on lorazepam protein binding. J Pharm Pharmacol 34:122–123

Divoll M, Greenblatt DJ, Harmatz JS, Shader RI (1981) Effect of age and gender on disposition of temazepam. J Pharm Sci 70:1104–1107

Divoll M, Greenblatt DJ, Ochs HR, Shader RI (1983) Absolute bioavailability of oral and intramuscular diazepam: effects of age and sex. Anesth Analg 62:1–8

Greenblatt DJ, Allen MD (1978) Toxicity of nitrazepam in the elderly: a report from the Boston Collaborative Drug Surveillance program. Brit J Clin Pharmacol 5:407–413

Greenblatt DJ, Allen MD, Shader RI (1977) Toxicity of high-dose flurazepam in the elderly. Clin Pharmacol Ther 21:355–361

Greenblatt DJ, Allen MD, Locniskar A, Harmatz JS, Shader RI (1979) Lorazepam kinetics in the elderly. Clin Pharmacol Ther 26:103–113

Greenblatt DJ, Divoll M, Harmatz JS, Shader RI (1980) Oxazepam kinetics: effects of age and sex. J Pharmacol Exp Ther 215:86–91

Greenblatt DJ, Divoll M, Puri SK, Ho I, Zinny MA, Shader RI (1981 a) Clobazam kinetics in the elderly. Brit J Clin Pharmacol 12:631–636

Greenblatt DJ, Divoll M, Harmatz JS, MacLaughlin DS, Shader RI (1981 b) Kinetics and clinical effects of flurazepam in young and elderly noninsomniacs. Clin Pharmacol Ther 30:475–486

Greenblatt DJ, Abernethy DR, Locniskar A, Harmatz JS, Limjuco RA, Shader RI (1984) Effect of age, gender and obesity on midazolam kinetics. Anesthesiol 61:27–35

Hilbert JM, Chung M, Radwanski E, Gural R, Symchowicz S, Zampaglione N (1984) Quazepam kinetics in the elderly. Clin Pharmacol Ther 36:566–569

Hümpel M, Nieuwebver B, Milius W, Hanke H, Wendt H (1980) Kinetics and biotransformation of lormetazepam. Clin Pharmacol Ther 28:673–679

Jochemsen R, Nandi KL, Corless D, Wesselman JGJ, Breimer DD (1983 a) Pharmacokinetics of brotizolam in the elderly. Brit J Clin Pharmacol 16:299S–307S

Jochemsen R, van Beusokom BR, Spoelstra P, Janssens AR, Breimer DD (1983 b) Effect of age and liver cirrhosis on the pharmacokinetics of nitrazepam. Brit J Clin Pharmacol 15:295–302

Kangas L, Iisalo E, Kanto J, Lehtinen V, Pynnönen S, Ruikka I, Salminen J, Sillanpää M, Syvälahti E (1979) Human pharmacokinetics of nitrazepam: effect of age and diseases. Eur J Clin Pharmacol 15:163–170

Kanto J, Kangas L, Aaltonen L, Hilke H (1981) Effect of age on the pharmacokinetics and sedative effect of flunitrazepam. Internat J Clin Pharmacol Ther Toxicol 19:400–404

Klotz U (1979) Effect of age on levels of diazepam in plasma and brain of rats. Naunyn-Schmiedeberg's Arch Pharmacol 307:167–169

Klotz U, Brückel KW (1982) Pharmacokinetics and pharmacodynamics in the elderly. In: Kitani K (ed) Liver and aging – liver and drugs. Elsevier Biomedical Press, Amsterdam, p 287–299

Klotz U, Müller-Seydlitz P (1979) Altered eliminiation of desmethyldiazepam in the elderly. Brit J Clin Pharmacol 7:119–120

Klotz U, Avant GR, Hoyumpa A, Schenker S, Wilkinson GR (1975) The effects of age and liver disease on the disposition and elimination of diazepam in adult man. J Clin Invest 55:347–359

Kraus JW, Desmond PV, Marshall JP, Johnson RF, Schenker S, Wilkinson GR (1978) Effects of aging and liver disease on disposition of lorazepam. Clin Pharmacol Ther 24:411–419

MacLeod SM, Giles HG, Bengert B, Liu FF, Sellers EM (1979) Age- and gender-related differences in diazepam pharmacokinetics. J Clin Pharmacol 19:15–19

Memo M, Spano F, Trabucchi M (1981) Brain benzodiazepine receptor changes during ageing. J Pharm Pharmacol 33:64

Moschitto LJ, Greenblatt DJ, Divoll M, Abernethy DR, Smith RB, Shader RI (1981) Alprazolam kinetics in the elderly: relation to antipyrine disposition. Clin Pharmacol Ther 29:267 (abstract)

Ochs HR, Greenblatt DJ, Divoll M, Abernethy DR, Feyerabend H, Dengler HJ (1981) Diazepam kinetics in relation to age and sex. Pharmacol 23:24–30

Ochs HR, Greenblatt DJ, Verburg-Ochs B, Harmatz JS, Grehl H (1984) Disposition of clotiazepam: influence of age, sex, oral contraceptives, cimetidine, isoniazid and ethanol. Eur J Clin Pharmacol 26:55–59

Pedigo NW, Schoemaker H, Morelli M, McDougal JN, Malick JB, Burks TF, Yamamura HI (1981) Benzodiazepine receptor binding in young, mature and senescent rat brain and kidney. Neurobiol Aging 2:83–88

Reeves PM, Schweizer P (1983) Aging, diazepam exposure and benzodiazepine receptors in rat cortex. Brain Res 270:376–379

Reidenberg MM, Levy M, Warner H, Coutinho CB, Schwartz MA, Yu G, Cheripko J (1978) Relationship between diazepam dose, plasma level, age and central nervous system depression. Clin Pharmacol Ther 23:371–374

Roberts RK, Wilkinson GR, Branch RA, Schenker S (1978) Effect of age and cirrhosis on the disposition and elimination of chlordiazepoxide. Gastroenterol 75:479–485

Shader RI, Greenblatt DJ, Harmatz JS, Franke K, Koch-Weser J (1977) Absorption and disposition of chlordiazepoxide in young and elderly male volunteers. J Clin Pharmacol 17:709–718

Shader RI, Greenblatt DJ, Ciraulo DA, Divoll M, Harmatz JS, Georgotas A (1981) Effect of age and sex on disposition of desmethyldiazepam formed from its precursor clorazepate. Psychopharmacol 75:193–197

Shull HJ, Wilkinson GR, Johnson R, Schenker S (1976) Normal disposition of oxazepam in acute viral hepatitis and cirrhosis. Annals Int Med 84:420–425

Smith MT, Heazlewood V, Eadie MJ, Brophy TO'R, Tyrer JH (1984) Pharmacokinetics of midazolam in the aged. Eur J Clin Pharmacol 26:381–388

Smith RB, Divoll M, Gillespie WR, Greenblatt DJ (1983) Effect of subject age and gender on the pharmacokinetics of oral triazolam and temazepam. J Clin Psychopharmacol 3:172–176

Stevenson IH, Hockings NF, Swift CG (1982) Pharmacokinetics and pharmacodynamics of single doses of hypnotic drugs in healthy elderly subjects. In: Kitani K (ed) Liver and aging – liver and drugs. Elsevier Biomedical Press, Amsterdam, p 317–328

Tsang C-F C, Wilkinson GR (1982) Diazepam disposition in mature and aged rabbits and rats. Drug Metab Disposition 10:413–416

Tsang CC, Speeg KV Jr, Wilkinson GR (1982) Aging and benzodiazepine binding in the rat cerebral cortex. Life Sci 30:343–346

World Health Organisation (1981) Health care in the elderly: Report of the technical group on use of medicaments by the elderly. Drugs 22:279–294

Influence of Age and Weight on Glycoside Therapy

A. Ruiz-Torres and R. Velasco [1]

It is known that old patients may develop digitalis toxicity when given amounts that are well tolerated by younger individuals. The reason for this can be increased sensitivity of the aged myocardium to a normal concentration, transformation of glycosides kinetics with aging that results in a higher myocardial concentration of digitalis, or a false estimation of dosages deduced from different body mass.

Aging and Digitalis Sensitivity

The aging process in humans reduces thyroid function, renal excretion, metabolic rate (i.e., drug elimination) and also body weight. All the mentioned pathogenic factors are present in the elderly patient and therefore they lead to the clinical impression that digitalis intoxication is more likely to occur in aged organisms. Gordon et al. (1969) have shown with tritiated digoxin given intravenously that the same dose leads to a higher blood concentration in old persons. Their results are due to the smaller body size and diminished urinary excretion. Some factors which may contribute to the true myocardial sensitivity have been determined in a range of digoxin serum levels less than 2 ng/ml; they are, besides electrolyte abnormalities, myocardial ischemia (Butler and Lindenbaum 1975) and hypothyroidism (Ruiz-Torres 1977).

Despite the relatively good explanation of why there is a tendency for elderly patients to require smaller doses to achieve adequate digitalization, the therapeutic problem remains, particularly in general practice. It is necessary to state the general criteria for the right individual dosage. Moreover, on the one hand the measurement of renal function cannot be recommended as a routing geriatric method, and on the other it has been found in elderly ambulant patients that the plasma digoxin levels are not correlated with blood urea concentrations or creatinine clearance (Baylis et al. 1972).

[1] Instituto Universitario de Investigación Gerontológica y Metabólica (Universidad Autónoma), in the Hospital de la Princesa, Madrid, Spain

Drugs and Aging
Ed. by D. Platt

Blood Levels and the Therapeutic Range

Studies by our group in Berlin – particularly by Schneider in 1977 – have found that digoxin levels clearly depend on body weight. In addition, we determined that the intoxication limit is above 2.0 ng/ml but the curve of blood levels does not correspond to a Gaussian distribution. Considering 93% of a total population of 317 patients with 1109 determinations, the therapeutic range varied between 1.2 and 1.7 ng/ml (Schneider and Ruiz-Torres 1977). The importance of the body weight as a parameter for dosages of digoxin was more evident in cases of underfeeding than in obesity. Consequently, we studied the intolerance rate of digitalis treatment in old patients in relation to their body weight and found that the tendency for intoxication to occur is strongly related to low body weight (Schneider and Ruiz-Torres 1978).

Blood Levels in Elderly Patients

Following a maintenance dose of 0.4 mg β-acetyldigoxin, concentrations of digoxin in blood were found to be higher in the elderly than in younger patients (Fig. 1, left). When digoxinemia was related to body weight by calculating the digoxin concentration per 70 kg body weight, the correlation with age was not significant (Fig. 1, right).

It is logical and predictable that higher blood concentrations of digoxin in old people may result in higher myocardial tissue concentrations. The results of Fig. 2 are in accordance with this. Patients with digitalis side-effects show a high blood concentration, but they are exceptions. The findings are probably related to the span of time between the beginning of intoxication and blood level determination. It is known that in intoxicated patients, digoxinemia decreases to normal range before adverse reactions have disappeared. In people more than 70 years old a big group of intoxicated patients can be noted, and yet greater digoxinemia that in younger ones.

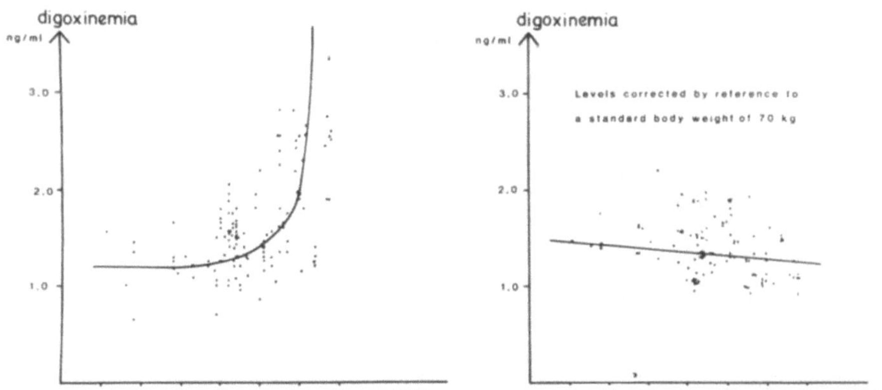

Fig. 1. Digoxin blood concentration depending on age 24 h after last maintenance dose of 0.4 mg β-acetyldigoxin (according to Schneider a. Ruiz-Torres (1977)).

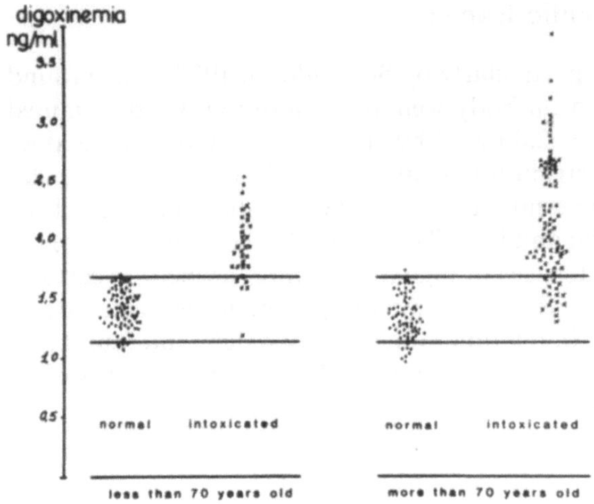

Fig. 2. Digoxin blood concentration, digitalis side-effects and their incidence in an elderly population

Practical Conclusions

Using these results in general practice, we have calculated a dose related to the body weight as an ideal dosage for maintenance therapy for heart failure in elderly patients without renal diseases. Our calculations (Table 1) have given a dosage for digoxin more or less corresponding to that recommended by Jelliffe and Brooker (1974) in their nomogram for patients with normal creatinin clearance. During the last 7 years we have applied this method in the treatment of our patients, and intoxications have rarely been observed. Moreover, the digoxinemia 24 h after oral administration has been determined weekly and also it showed the results that are expected. As counterproof we have readapted the digitalization

Table 1. Doses recommended for old patients[a]

Digoxin	~8 µg/kg b.w.
β-Acetyldigoxin	~5 µg/kg b.w.
β-Methyldigoxin	~4 µg/kg b.w.
Digitoxin	~1.5 µg/kg b.w.

[a] Note: Dose adaptation to pharmaceutical preparations in decreasing mode; PE in case of 60 kg = 480 µg, but only 375 (= 1 + $^1/_2$ tabl.) digoxin

Table 2. Selected examples of intoxication with digitalis

Case	Age	Recent dose	Body weight	Right dose
H.L.♀	68 yr	0.5 mg digoxin	42.2 kg	0.3 mg (≙1 tabl.)
M.G.♀	66 yr	0.2 mg digitoxin	51.7 kg	0.07 mg (≙$^1/_2$ tabl.)
E.F.♀	80 yr	0.5 mg digoxin	53.8 kg	0.4 mg (≙1 + $^1/_2$ tabl.)

of normal renal patients presenting with side-effects using the body weight as the only criterion. The digitalis therapy could be continued in every one without adverse reactions. Some examples are demonstrated in Table 2.

Summary

Adverse reactions to digitalis depend essentially on blood levels above the therapeutic range (up to 2 ng/ml). In the elderly patient several factors lead to a high blood concentration of glycosides when they are given in amounts that are well tolerated by younger persons. The factor of most importance is the lower body weight in old patients. Relating the dosage of digitalis to the body weight is a good method of counteracting the tendency of elderly patients to develop toxicity.

References

Baylis EM, Hall MS, Lewis G, Marks V (1972) Effects of renal function on plasma digoxin levels in elderly ambulant patients in domiciliary practice. Brit Med J 1:338–341

Butler VP, Lindenbaum J (1975) Serum digitalis measurements in the assessment of digitalis resistance and sensitivity. Am J Med 58:460–469

Gordon AE, Kapadia GG, Yao L, Lullin M, Marcus FI (1969) Digoxin metabolism in the elderly. Circulation 39:449–453

Jelliffe RW, Brooker G (1974) A nomogram for digoxin therapy. Am J Med 57:63–68

Ruiz-Torres A (1977) Änderung der Glykosidtoleranz durch hormonelle Faktoren. Verh Dtsch Ges Inn Med 83:91–99

Schneider J, Ruiz-Torres A (1976) Bedeutung des Körpergewichts bei der Digitalisierung des Herzkranken. Verh Dtsch Ges Inn Med 82:1709–1712

Schneider J, Ruiz-Torres A (1977) Digitalis effect and blood concentration. Int J Clin Pharmacol 15:424–427

Schneider J, Ruiz-Torres (1977) Bedeutung des Körpergewichts für die Therapie mit Digoxin und Digoxinderivaten. Dtsch Med Wochenschr 102:116–118

Schneider J, Ruiz-Torres A (1978) Zur Frage der vieldiskutierten Digitalisempfindlichkeit des alten Menschen: Die Digoxinserumkonzentration bei alten Menschen. Akt Geront 8:158–165

Pharmacokinetics of Acebutolol in the Elderly

W. MÖHRKE [1], E. MUTSCHLER [2], W. MÜHLBERG [4], and D. PLATT [3,4]

Introduction

β-Blockers are used as first-line drugs in the treatment of hypertension. Acebutolol has also been shown to be effective and safe in an elderly population (Guerin et al. 1981). After absorption acebutolol is metabolized by hydrolysis of the amide group to the amine (metabolite I) and conjugated to diacetolol (metabolite II). A second minor metabolic pathway involves the reduction of the acetyl moiety (metabolite III) (Fig. 1). It has been demonstrated that diacetolol is pharmacologi-

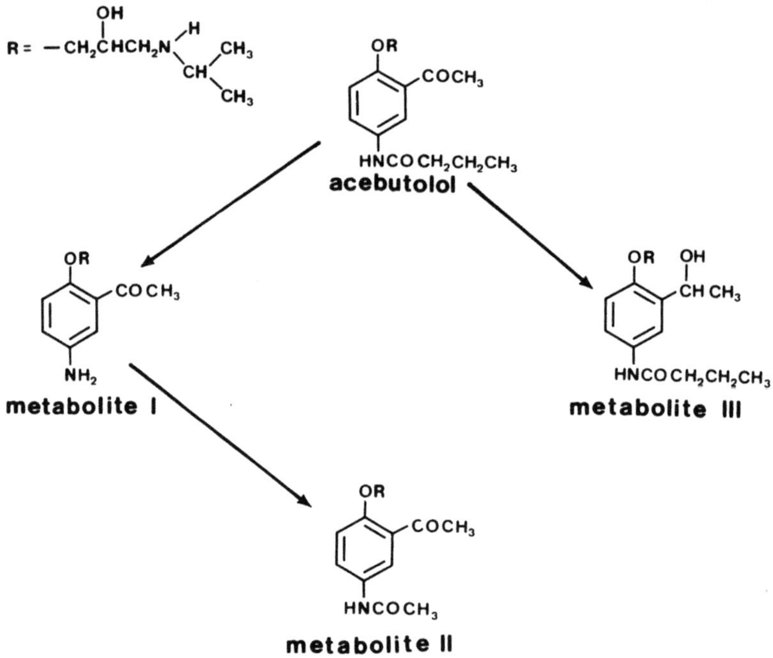

Fig. 1. Metabolic scheme of acebutolol

[1] Röhm Pharma, D-6108 Weiterstadt/F.R.G.
[2] Pharmakologisches Institut für Naturwissenschaftler der J.W. Goethe-Universität, D-6000 Frankfurt/Main/F.R.G.
[3] Institut für Gerontologie der Universität Erlangen-Nürnberg und
[4] 2. Medizinische Klinik, Klinikum Nürnberg, D-8500 Nürnberg/F.R.G.

Drugs and Aging
Ed. by D. Platt

cally as active as acebutolol. The elimination of acebutolol is independent of renal function, whereas the elimination of diacetolol is closely related to endogenous creatinine clearance. The terminal half-life of acebutolol is in the range of 7–12 h, while diacetolol possesses a $t_{1/2}$ of 11–13 h after oral administration (Gulaid et al. 1981; Kirch et al. 1982). The volume of distribution and total plasma clearance of acebutolol and diacetolol were reduced and the terminal half-lives prolonged in elderly female patients in comparison to healthy young male volunteers (Roux et al. 1983). No other age-dependent pharmacokinetic investigations have been published. We therefore considered it necessary to perform a pharmacokinetic study in male and female elderly multimorbid patients to extend our knowledge of the pharmacokinetics of acebutolol in this patient group.

Patients and Methods

Ten male patients aged 76.6±6.6 (mean ±SD) years (range 66–90 years) with a body weight of 67.6±8.9 kg (range 52–82 kg) and ten female patients aged 74.9±5.8 years (range 67±86 years) with a body weight of 59.0±8.5 kg (range 46–74 kg) were included in the study. All patients gave their informed consent.

They received a single dose of 400 mg acebutolol (Neptal 400) and 100 ml water in the morning after a standard breakfast. Blood samples were drawn just before and 0.5, 1, 2, 3, 4, 6, 8, 12, 24, 36, and 48 h after drug administration. Serum was separated by centrifugation and frozen until analysis. Urine was voided before drug administration and then collected in intervals from 0–2, 2–4, 4–6, 6–8, 8–12, 12–24, and 24–48 h; the volumes were measured and an aliquot frozen until analysis.

Serum was analyzed by a thin-layer chromatographic method. To 1 ml serum 0.2 ml 2 N NaOH was added and extracted with 2 ml ethylacetate. After centrifugation 1 ml of the supernatant was evaporated to dryness at 60 °C under nitrogen. The residue was dissolved in 0.05 ml ethylacetate and 0.04 ml was spotted on a thin-layer plate coated with silica gel. The TLC plate was developed with chloroform–methanol (85:10, v/v) in ammonia atmosphere. After air-drying for 15 min the plate was dipped in paraffin–cyclohexan (4:96, v/v) and the fluorescence measured at an excitation wavelength of 265 nm and an emission wavelength of 436 nm using a chromatògram spectrophotometer KM 3 (Zeiss, Oberkochen, West Germany).

Acebutolol and diacetolol were determined in urine (1 ml) by extraction with 0.5 ml ethylacetate after addition of 0.2 ml 2 N NaOH. 0.02 ml of the supernatant was applied on a TLC plate. Development and measurement followed the determination in serum. Pharmacokinetic parameters were estimated by standard methods (Wagner 1975).

The pharmacokinetic differences between young healthy volunteers and elderly patients were assessed by means of Wilcoxon's rank-sum test.

Results

The determination method outlined above was suitable for estimating the concentrations of acebutolol and diacetolol in the serum and urine of geriatric patients over a period of 48 h after a single oral dose of 400 mg acebutolol. In Fig. 2 the densitometer scans after extraction of blank serum, blank serum to which 500 ng/ml acebutolol and 500 ng/ml diacetolol were added, and a patient serum 3 h after the application of 400 mg acebutolol are shown.

The limit of determination was 10 ng/ml in serum for both acebutolol and diacetolol. In serum the coefficient of variation was 2.5% at 2000 ng/ml, 3.2% at 200 ng/ml, and 6.6% at 20 ng/ml. The calibration curve was linear up to 10 µg/ml with a correlation coefficient of $r = 0.998$.

In urine the limit of determination was 200 ng/ml and the relative coefficient of variation was 2.5% at 20 µg/ml and 7% at 400 ng/ml. No deviation of linearity of the calibration curve was observed up to 100 µg/ml.

Other drugs given concomitantly did not interfere with the determination of acebutolol or diacetolol, either in serum or in urine.

Serum concentrations of acebutolol and diacetolol in elderly patients and young volunteers after a single dose of 400 mg acebutolol are shown in Figs. 3 and 4. Relevant pharmacokinetic parameters are compiled in Table 1.

The rate of absorption of acebutolol is not influenced by age as the t_{max} values are not age dependent. C_{max} values of acebutolol but not diacetolol were significantly increased in some elderly patients compared to young volunteers (Fig. 4). Correspondingly, the AUCs of acebutolol were significantly increased in the elderly patients, whereas the AUCs of diacetolol were not altered in the aged group (Fig. 5). The terminal half-lives of acebutolol were not related to age (Fig. 6). The elimination of the main metabolite of acebutolol, diacetolol, was delayed in elderly patients, as indicated by the increased terminal half-lives.

The amount of acebutolol excreted renally was significantly decreased in elderly patients (Fig. 7). The difference in the elimination of diacetolol did not reach

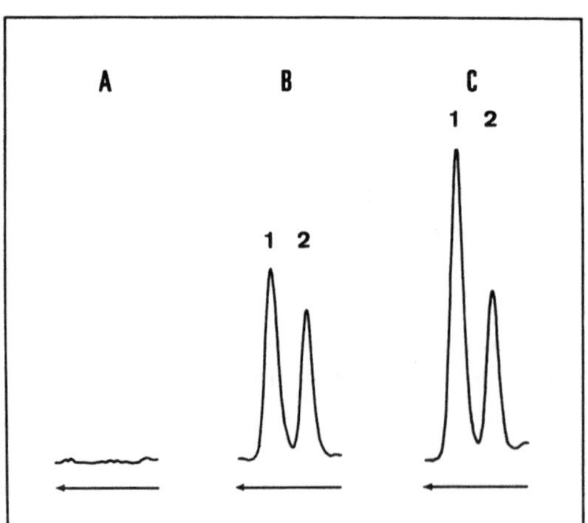

Fig. 2. Densitometer scans of blank serum (*A*), blank serum to which 500 ng/ml acebutolol (1) and diacetolol (*2*) were added (*B*), and a patient serum 3 h after receiving a single oral dose of 400 mg acebutolol (*C*)

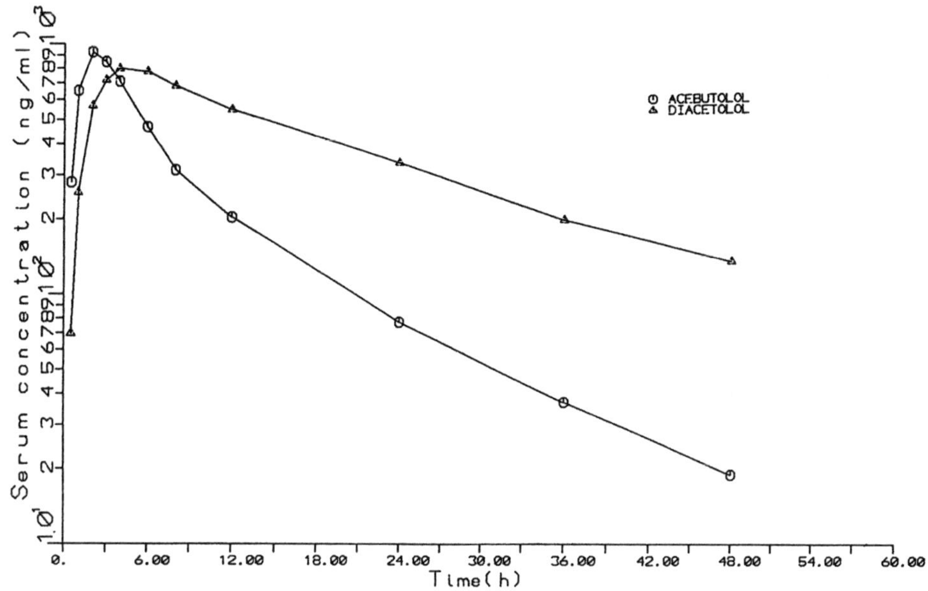

Fig. 3. Mean serum levels of acebutolol and diacetolol in 20 elderly patients after a single oral dose of 400 mg acebutolol

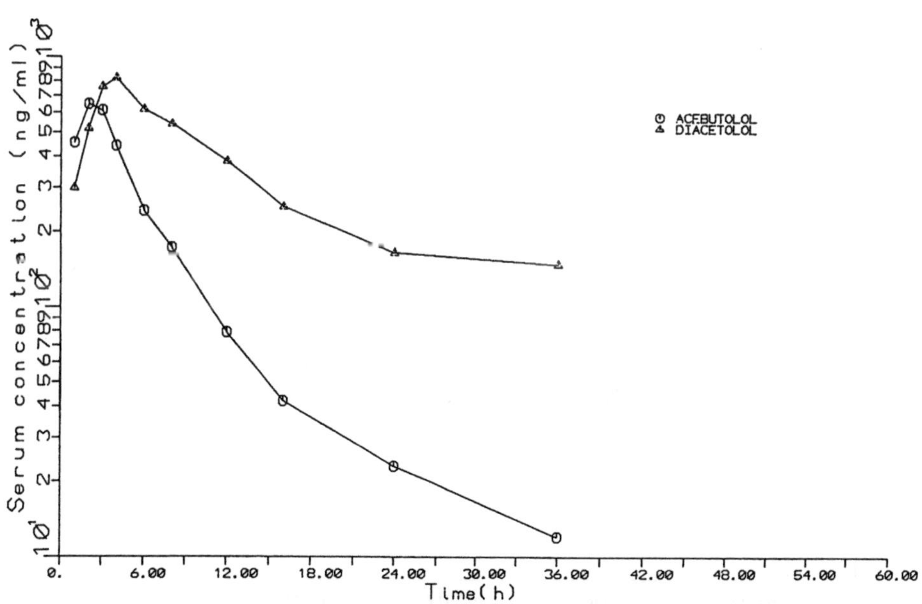

Fig. 4. Mean serum levels of acebutolol and diacetolol in 8 young volunteers after a single oral dose of 400 mg acebutolol

Table 1. Pharmacokinetic parameters of acebutolol (A) and diacetolol (D) in ten male and ten female elderly patients and young healthy volunteers after a single oral administration of 400 mg acebutolol

Population	C_{max} (ng/ml)		t_{max} (h)		AUC (ng/ml h)		$t_{1/2z}$ (h)	
	A	D	A	D	A	D	A	D
Elderly male	1,042	872	3.1	5.3	7,823	19,214	13.1	19.0
±SD	424	296	1.5	1.5	3,183	10,734	7.2	7.3
Elderly female	1,340	923	2.3	3.4	8,516	16,105	13.8	16.1
±SD	413	274	1.4	1.5	2,286	6,575	7.4	6.9
Young	720	845	2.5	3.6	4,154	11,173	11.3	13.4
±SD	269	318	0.9	0.5	1,108	4,317	2.3	7.5

Population	Renal elimination (mg)		Renal clearance (ml/min)	
	A	D	A	D
Elderly male	25.4	47.5	59	49
±SD	16.7	35.0	44	34
Elderly female	25.4	40.2	51	44
±SD	8.7	13.2	17	16
Young	39.8	52.4	171	102
±SD	8.1	8.1	80	92

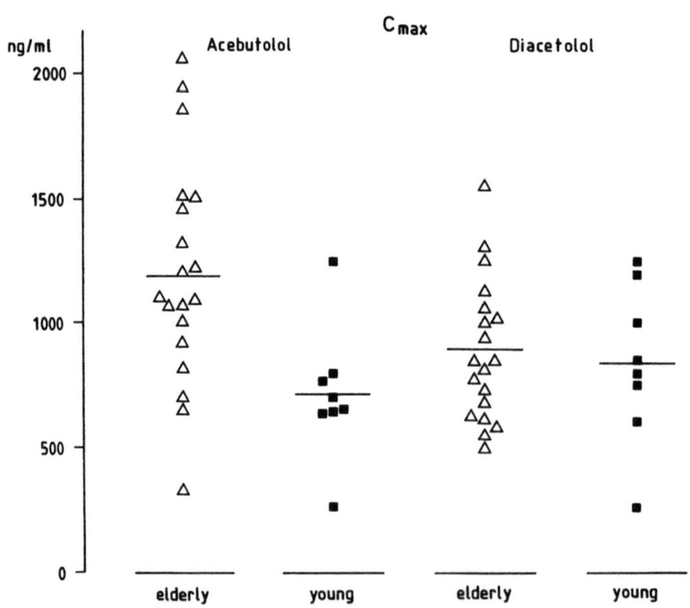

Fig. 5. Maximum serum levels (C_{max}) of acebutolol and diacetolol in 20 elderly patients and 8 young volunteers after a single oral dose of 400 mg acebutolol

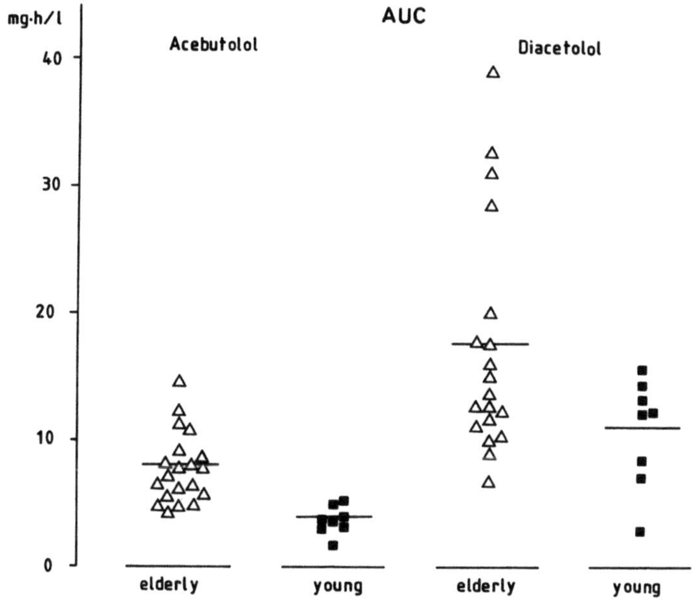

Fig. 6. Areas under the serum concentration time curves (AUC) of acebutolol and diacetolol in 20 elderly patients and 8 young volunteers after a single oral dose of 400 mg acebutolol

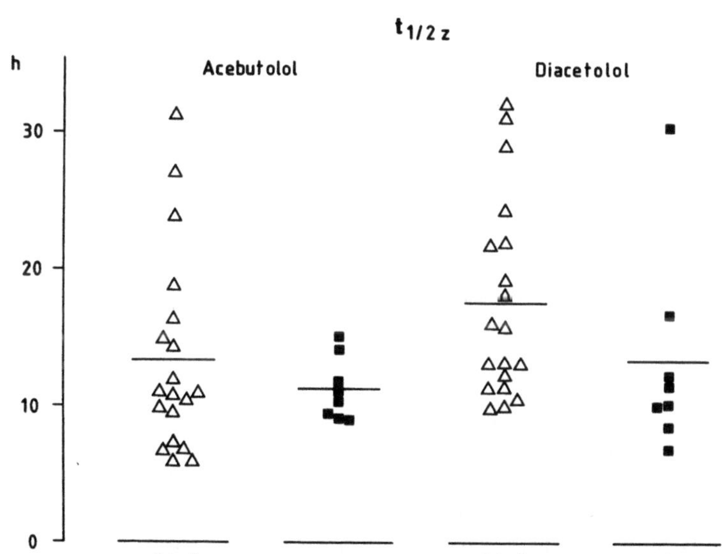

Fig. 7. Terminal half-lives ($t_{1/2z}$) of acebutolol and diacetolol in 20 elderly patients and 8 young volunteers after a single oral dose of 400 mg acebutolol

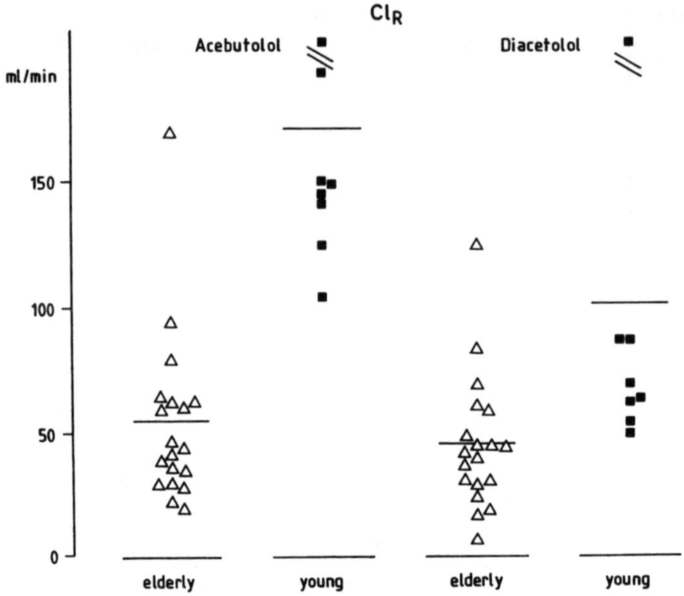

Fig. 8. Renal clearances (Cl_R) of acebutolol and diacetolol in 20 elderly patients and 8 young volunteers after a single oral dose of 400 mg acebutolol

statistical significance ($P=0.07$). This may have been influenced by the insufficient urine collection time period.

The renal clearances of acebutolol and diacetolol were diminished in elderly patients as a result of a decreased renal function (Fig. 8).

Discussion

The method for the determination of acebutolol and diacetolol is simple and reliable. Its specificity, sensitivity, and accuracy are comparable or superior to other TLC and HPLC methods (Meffin et al. 1977; Roux and Flouvat 1978; Steyn 1976).

Maximum serum levels of acebutolol were higher in elderly patients than in young volunteers, but terminal half-lives were unchanged. Although the elucidation of the underlying mechanism of the elevated serum levels was beyond the scope of this study, it should be discussed whether a reduced first pass effect or a reduced volume of distribution is responsible. The decrease in renal clearance may play just a minor role, as renal clearance is only a small fraction of total clearance of acebutolol. The absorption of acebutolol is nearly 80% in healthy young volunteers; therefore an enhanced absorption of acebutolol cannot account for the raised serum levels.

For diacetolol it was evident that the terminal half-lives were increased in the elderly. The most plausible explanation for this is the decreased renal clearance in older patients. Renal clearance of diacetolol is negatively correlated to serum urea ($r = -0.467$) and the half-life of diacetolol is correlated to serum creatinine ($r = 0.539$). Therefore, impaired renal function is an important factor in the variation of diacetolol pharmacokinetics in the elderly.

The results of the study suggest that the acebutolol dose should be reduced in elderly patients to maintain plasma levels comparable to those in young volunteers. But it has been found that the antihypertensive effect of β-blockers is lowered with increasing age. Therefore, the efficacy of acebutolol should serve as a guide when considering dose reduction in elderly patients.

Acknowledgment. We are greatly indebted to Dr. Dennis for providing us with the data on healthy volunteers. The technical assistance of Mrs. G. Hahn and the secretarial help of Mrs. U. Bauer are gratefully acknowledged. This study was supported in part by the Deutsche Forschungsgemeinschaft and Dr.-Robert-Pfleger Stiftung.

References

Guerin A, Baker PG, Goulton J (1981) Multi-centre study of acebutolol in hypertensive subjects: results for patients from the 50 to 64-years' old and over 65 years' old age groups. Curr Med Res Opinion 7:179–184

Gulaid AA, James IM, Kaye CM, Lewellen ORW, Roberts E, Sankey M, Smith J, Templeton R, Thomas RJ (1981) The pharmacokinetics of acebutolol in man, following the oral administration of acebutolol HCl as a single dose (400 mg), and during and after repeated oral dosing (400 mg, b.d.). Biopharmac Drug Disp 2:103–114

Kirch W, Köhler H, Berggren G, Braun W (1982) The influence of renal function on plasma levels and urinary excretion of acebutolol and its main N-acetyl metabolite. Clin Nephrol 18:88–94

Meffin PJ, Harapat SR, Yee Y-G, Harrison DC (1977) High pressure liquid chromatographic analysis of drugs in biological fluids. V. Analysis of acebutolol and its major metabolite. J Chromatogr 138:183–191

Roux A, Flouvat B (1978) Méthode sensible de dosage de l'acebutolol et de son métabolite N-acétylé dans les milieux biologiques par chromatographic liquide haute performance avec détection de fluorescence. J Chromatogr 166:327–332

Roux A, Henry JF, Fouache Y, Chan NP, Hervy MP, Forette F, Boudaris JP, Flouvat B (1983) A pharmacokinetic study of acebutolol in aged subjects as compared to young subjects. Gerontology 29:202–208

Steyn JM (1976) A thin-layer chromatographic method for the determination of acebutolol and its major metabolite in serum. J Chromatogr 120:465–472

Wagner JW (1975) Fundamentals of clinical pharmacokinetics. Drug Intelligence Publications, Hamilton

Pharmacodynamics of Acebutolol in Geriatric Patients with Multiple Diseases

W. MÜHLBERG [2], D. PLATT [1,2] E. MUTSCHLER [3], and W. MÖHRKE [4]

Introduction

Möhrke and co-workers (1986) have demonstrated some significant changes in the pharmacokinetics of acebutolol in elderly patients as compared with young healthy volunteers. The question arises as to whether these pharmacokinetic differences are of clinical importance for the treatment of geriatric patients. Some authors have suggested that the antihypertensive effect of β-blockers may be reduced with increasing age. So far, it cannot be excluded that the affinity of β-receptor antagonists to β_1- and β_2-receptors and the number of these receptor subtypes are age dependent.

Investigations of hypertensive patients after administration of a single dose of acebutolol showed correlations between drug concentration and β-blocking (assessed as a percentage reduction in exercise tachycardia) as well as between these two parameters and the fall in postexercise systolic blood pressure (Martin et al. 1978). The degree of β-adrenoceptor blocking and the plasma level of acebutolol were also well correlated in healthy volunteers (Cuthbert and Collins 1975). Therefore, we investigated the relationship between the plasma level and pharmacodynamics of acebutolol in our geriatric patients.

Materials and Methods

The characteristics of the 20 geriatric patients as well as the pharmacokinetics found in these patients have already been described by Möhrke and co-workers (1986). The diagnoses made in the patients are shown in Table 1. All patients were given a single dose of 400 mg acebutolol. We investigated the relationship between the pharmacodynamics and pharmacokinetics (or the effect kinetics) of acebutolol and its pharmacologically active metabolite diacetolol by means of linear regression analysis. When analyzing the data of the geriatric patients, one of the main difficulties in our study was the lack of a direct comparison with pharmacodynamic data from young healthy volunteers. Usually the measurement of β-adrenoceptor blocking of acebutolol and other β-blockers is done by determin-

[1] Institut für Gerontologie der Universität Erlangen-Nürnberg und
[2] 2. Medizinische Klinik, Klinikum Nürnberg, D-8500 Nürnberg/F.R.G.
[3] Pharmakologisches Institut für Naturwissenschaftler der Johann-Wolfgang-Goethe-Universität, D-6000 Frankfurt/Main/F.R.G.
[4] Röhm Pharma, D-6108 Weiterstadt/F.R.G.

Drugs and Aging
Ed. by D. Platt

Table 1. Diagnoses in the 20 geriatric patients (patients 1–10 female, patients 11–20 male)

Patient No.	Diagnoses
1	Hypertonia, carcinoma of the breast
2	Hypertonia, obstructive jaundice, chronic pyelonephritis
3	Diabetes mellitus, hypertonia, polyneuritis, cardiac insufficiency
4	Diabetes mellitus, hypertonia, coronary artery disease
5	Diabetes mellitus, hypertonia
6	Coronary artery disease
7	Hypertonia, coronary artery disease
8	Coronary artery disease, renal insufficiency
9	Hypertonia, cardiac insufficiency, urinary tract infection
10	Coronary artery disease, cardiac insufficiency
11	Coronary artery disease, cachexia
12	Angina pectoris, cardiac insufficiency
13	Cardiac infarction, hypertonia, cardiac insufficiency, diabetes mellitus
14	Diabetes mellitus, hypertonia, coronary artery disease
15	Cardiac arrhythmia, angina pectoris, diabetes mellitus
16	Hypertonia, transitional ischemic attack
17	Diabetes mellitus, cardiac insufficiency, angina pectoris
18	Hypertonia, diabetes mellitus, transitional ischemic attack, cardiac insufficiency
19	Coronary artery disease, cardiac arrhythmia, pulmonary emphysema
20	Cardiac insufficiency, coronary artery disease, cardiac infarction

ing the reduction of an isoprenaline-induced tachycardia. This method, as well as the measurement of systolic and diastolic blood pressure and heart rate during and after exercise, cannot be applied to elderly patients who are hospitalized and forced to stay in bed. For this reason, only systolic and diastolic blood pressure and heart rate under resting conditions could be determined at the various blood sampling times.

Results and Discussion

1. Relationship Between Plasma Level and Pharmacodynamic Action Including All Measurements During the First 8 h After Administration of 400 mg Acebutolol

As shown in Fig. 1, the reduction of heart rate (in comparison to the mean value before administration of acebutolol) was directly correlated with the plasma levels of acebutolol ($r=0.23$; $n=116$; $P<0.05$) as well as with the plasma levels of diacetolol ($r=0.263$; $n=114$; $P<0.01$; Fig. 2).

In some of our geriatric patients the reduction of heart rate amounted to 52 beats per minute. It is remarkable that this reduction of heart rate in correlation with plasma concentrations was found under resting conditions. However, in the upper range of plasma concentrations of diacetolol (900 + ng/ml) we observed a rapid decrease in the reduction of heart rate.This is in good accordance with results of Bilski et al. (1979), who found a dose-dependent reduction of heart rate after administration of acebutolol in animals; however, an increase of heart rate can be observed with increasing concentrations of acebutolol and diacetolol due

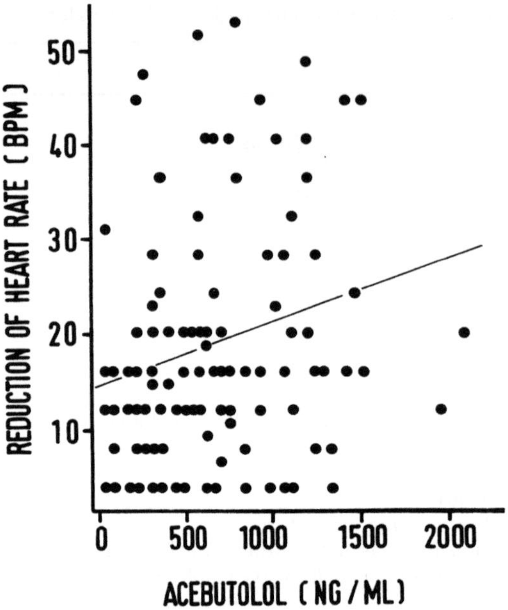

Fig. 1. Relationship between concentrations of acebutolol (ng/ml) and the reduction of heart rate (beats/min): $r = 0.23$; $n = 116$; $P < 0.05$

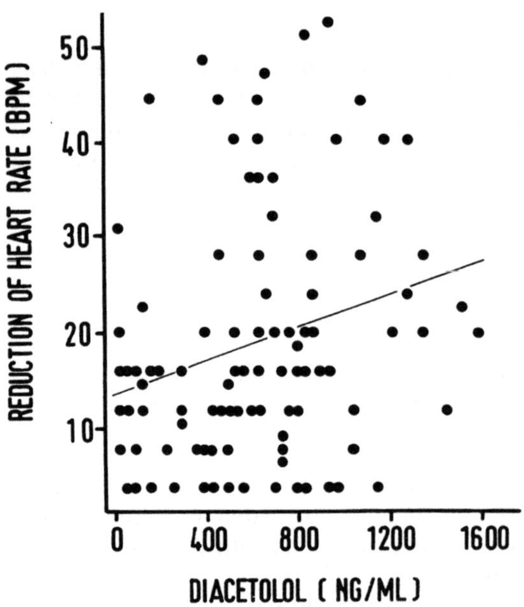

Fig. 2. Relationship between concentrations of diacetolol (ng/ml) and the reduction of heart rate (beats/min): $r = 0.263$; $n = 114$; $P < 0.01$

to the intrinsic sympathomimetic activity of these drugs. We further observed a statistically significant correlation between the heart rate itself and the plasma concentration of the active metabolite diacetolol ($r = -0.189$; $n = 123$; $P < 0.05$; Fig. 3).

Plasma levels of acebutolol – but not those of diacetolol – were closely correlated with the diastolic blood pressure itself ($r = -0.198$; $n = 127$; $P < 0.05$; Fig. 4)

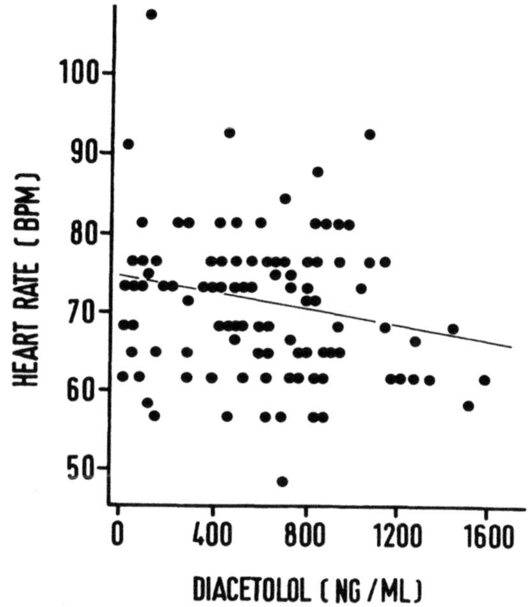

Fig. 3. Relationship between concentrations of diacetolol (ng/ml) and the heart rate (beats/min): $r = -0.189$; $n = 123$; $P < 0.05$

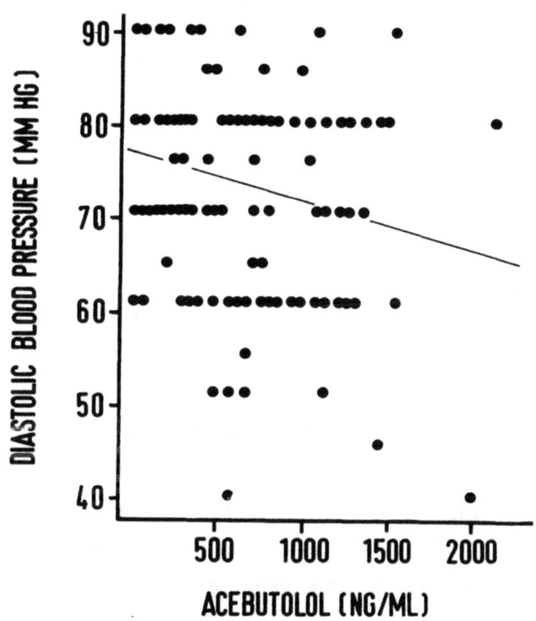

Fig. 4. Relationship between concentrations of acebutolol (ng/ml) and the diastolic blood pressure (mmHg): $r = -0.198$; $n = 127$; $P <= 0.05$

and with the reduction of diastolic blood pressure ($r = 0.314$; $n = 66$; $P < 0.025$; Fig. 5). On the other hand, only the plasma levels of the metabolite diacetolol – not those of acebutolol – showed a statistically significant correlation with the reduction of systolic blood pressure ($r = 0.207$; $n = 98$; $P < 0.05$; Fig. 6).

These results are somewhat surprising for two reasons. First, the results of comparative pharmacological studies (Mougeot et al. 1981) and studies in pa-

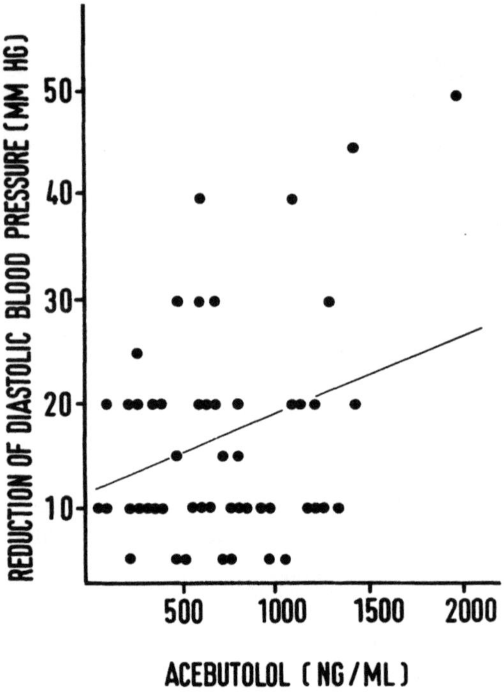

Fig. 5. Relationship between concentrations of acebutolol (ng/ml) and the reduction of diastolic blood pressure (mmHg): $r=0.314$; $n=66$; $P<0.025$

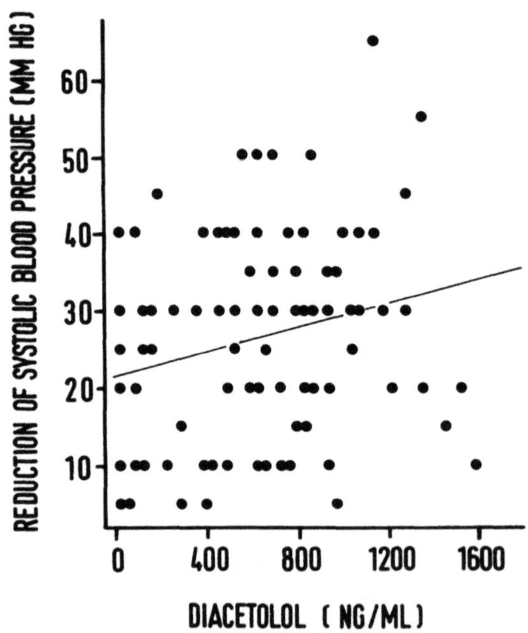

Fig. 6. Relationship between concentrations of diacetolol (ng/ml) and the reduction of systolic blood pressure (mmHg): $r=0.207$; $n=98$; $P<0.05$

tients (Ireland et al. 1981; Holti 1982; Wollam et al. 1979) indicate that in resting subjects vascular responses mediated via the β-adrenergic system are largely unaffected by acebutolol. In contrast to these findings, depending on the plasma concentration of acebutolol we observed a reduction in diastolic blood pressure in resting patients of up to 50 mmHg, and, depending on the plasma concentration of diacetolol, a reduction in systolic blood pressure of up to 65 mmHg.

Secondly, other authors suggest that the pharmacological properties of acebutolol and its active metabolite diacetolol show no or only minor differences, especially with regard to their β-receptor selectivity (Ohashi et al. 1981; Basil et al. 1982). While our results suggest that this is indeed true for the β_1-receptors of the heart (and for the heart rate), there are differences between acebutolol and diacetolol with regard to their pharmacodynamic action on the systolic and diastolic blood pressure.

2. Relationship Between Plasma Level and Pharmacodynamic Action 2 and 6 h After Administration

Two hours after administration the plasma concentration of diacetolol showed a statistically significant positive correlation with systolic blood pressure ($r = 0.458$; $n = 20$; $P < 0.05$). The same relationship was observed for acebutolol ($r = 0.504$; $n = 20$; $P < 0.05$; Fig. 7). Looking at the plasma concentrations of acebutolol in the geriatric patients it is easy to see that most of them exceeded the value of 720±95.2 ng/ml, i.e., the mean peak concentration of acebutolol in healthy young volunteers. We consider this an almost classical example of how elevated

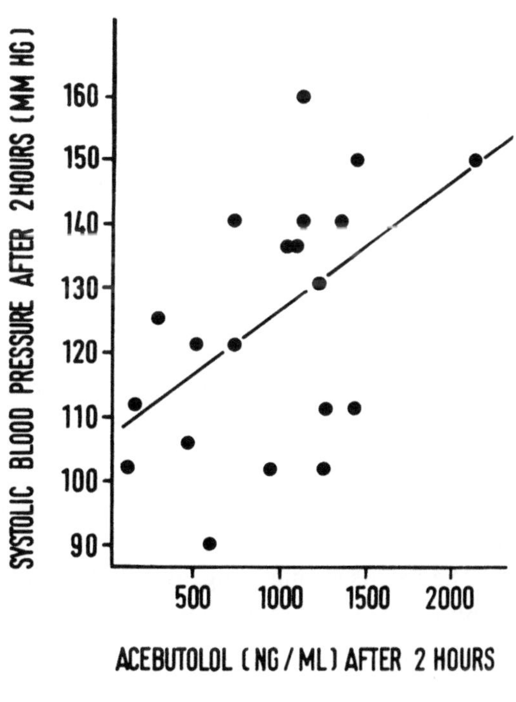

Fig. 7. Positive correlation between concentrations of acebutolol (ng/ml) after 2 h and systolic blood pressure (mmHg): $r = 0.504$; $n = 20$; $P < 0.05$

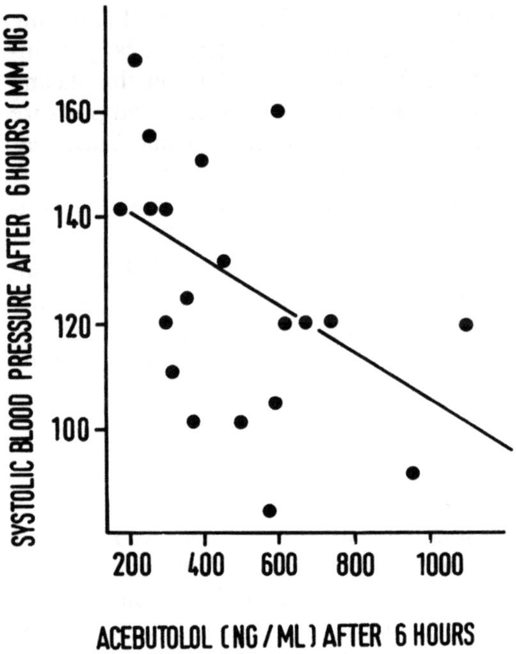

Fig. 8. Inverse correlation between concentrations of acebutolol (ng/ml) after 6 h and systolic blood pressure (mmHg): $r = -0.46$; $n = 19$; $P < 0.05$

plasma levels in old age may lead to an altered or (as in our study) even completely antagonistic pharmacological response to the same drug.

Four hours later (6 h after administration), just the opposite effect could be demonstrated: the plasma concentrations of acebutolol, now in a lower range, showed a statistically significant *negative* correlation with systolic blood pressure ($r = -0.46$; $n = 19$; $P < 0.05$; Fig. 8). The reason for these concentration-dependent antagonistic effects of the same drug has already been mentioned: with increasing plasma levels of acebutolol its intrinsic sympathomimetic action dominates its other effects, i.e., its β-adrenoceptor blocking action.

3. Relationship Between Pharmacodynamics and Pharmacokinetic Parameters of Acebutolol and Diacetolol

The importance of altered pharmacokinetic parameters for changes in pharmacodynamic action can be confirmed by some additional results: the peak time of acebutolol ($r = 0.537$; $n = 20$; $P < 0.025$; Fig. 9) as well as the peak time of diacetolol ($r = 0.58$; $n = 20$; $P < 0.01$; Fig. 10) were closely correlated with the time of maximal reduction of heart rate. In addition, a statistically significant positive relationship could be demonstrated between the AUC (area under time–concentration curve) of acebutolol and the maximal reduction of heart rate ($r = 0.499$; $n = 20$; $P < 0.05$; Fig. 11).

The results strongly suggest that altered pharmacokinetics may indeed play a major role in changes of pharmacodynamics.

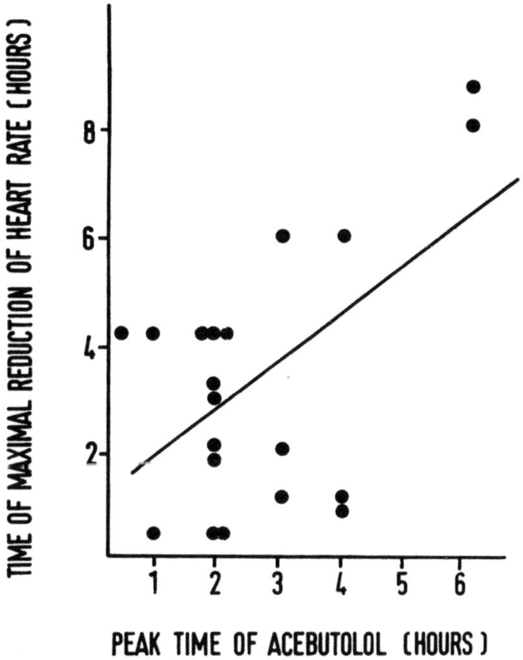

Fig. 9. Relationship between peak time of acebutolol (hours) and the time of maximal reduction of heart rate (hours): $r = 0.537$; $n = 20$; $P < 0.025$

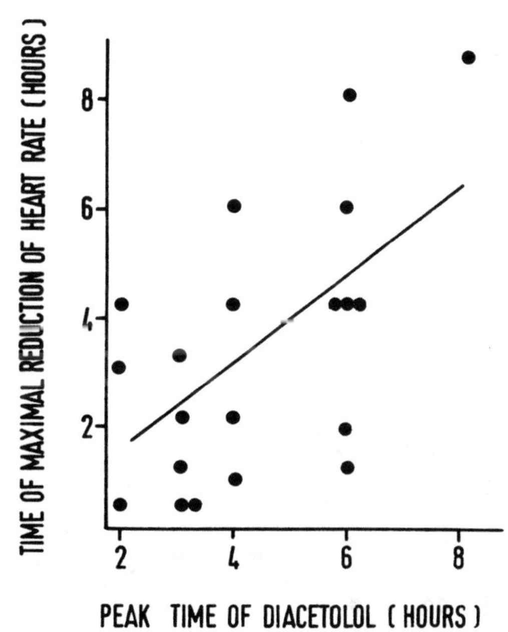

Fig. 10. Relationship between peak time of diacetolol (hours) and the time of maximal reduction of heart rate (hours): $r = 0.58$; $n = 20$; $P < 0.01$

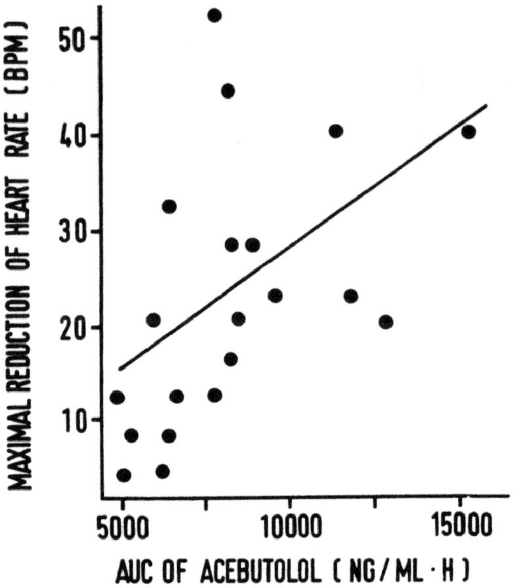

Fig. 11. Relationship between the AUC of acebutolol (ng/ml·h) and the maximal reduction of heart rate (beats/min): $r=0.499$; $n=20$; $P<0.05$

4. Correlations Between Pharmacokinetic Parameters and Biochemical Data in Our Geriatric Patients

The pharmacokinetics of diacetolol seem to be influenced merely by the renal function: we found a statistically significant relationship between the half-life of diacetolol and the serum creatinine ($r=0.539$; $n=20$; $P<0.05$) as well as between

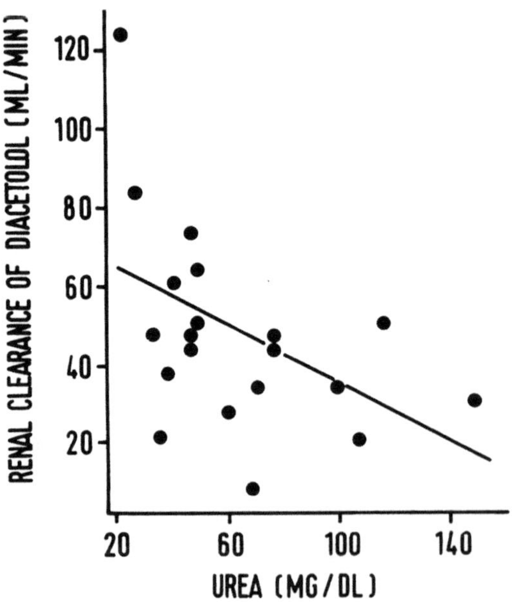

Fig. 12. Relationship between urea (mg/dl) and the renal clearance of diacetolol (ml/min): $r=-0.467$; $n=20$; $P<0.05$

the renal clearance of diacetolol and urea in plasma ($r = -0.467$; $n = 20$; $P < 0.05$; Fig. 12). A close correlation between the volume of urinary excretion during the first 2 h after administration and age also indicates that this means of elimination may be especially age dependent, even in the geriatric group alone.

The elimination and metabolic breakdown of acebutolol is rather complex: acebutolol as well as its active metabolite diacetolol are eliminated via the kidneys, bile, and feces. Looking for other factors which may influence the pharma-

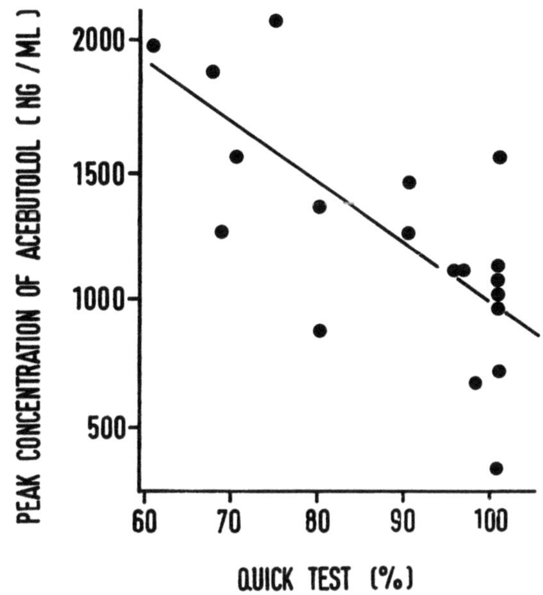

Fig. 13. Relationship between Quick test (%) and the peak concentration of acebutolol (ng/ml): $r = -0.706$; $n = 20$; $P < 0.001$

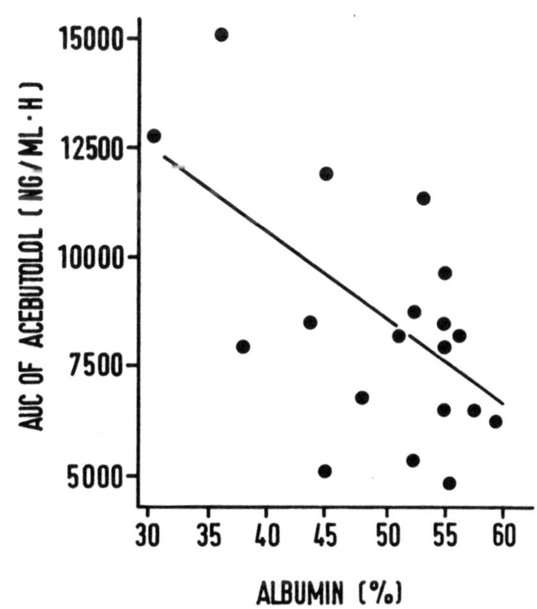

Fig. 14. Relationship between albumin (%) and the AUC of acebutolol (ng/ml · h): $r = -0.577$; $n = 19$; $P < 0.01$

cokinetics of acebutolol in geriatric patients, we found the function of the liver to play a major role too: A parameter of the liver function, the Quick test (prothrombin index), showed a significant inverse relationship with the peak concentration ($r = -0.706$; $n = 20$; $P < 0.001$; Fig. 13) and with the AUC of acebutolol ($r = -0.694$; $n = 20$; $P < 0.001$). The AUC of acebutolol was also closely correlated with the albumin content in the plasma ($r = -0.577$; $n = 19$; $P < 0.01$; Fig. 14) and with the cholinesterase ($r = -0.549$; $n = 20$; $P < 0.05$; Fig. 15), both indicators of the hepatic synthesizing function.

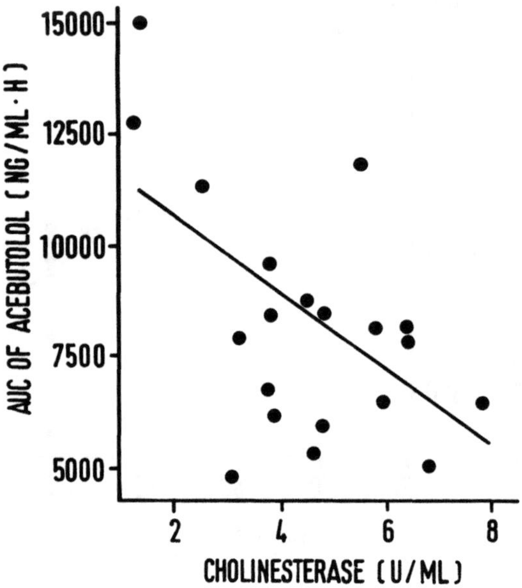

Fig. 15. Relationship between cholinesterase (U/ml) and the AUC of acebutolol (ng/ml·h): $r = -0.549$; $n = 20$; $P < 0.05$

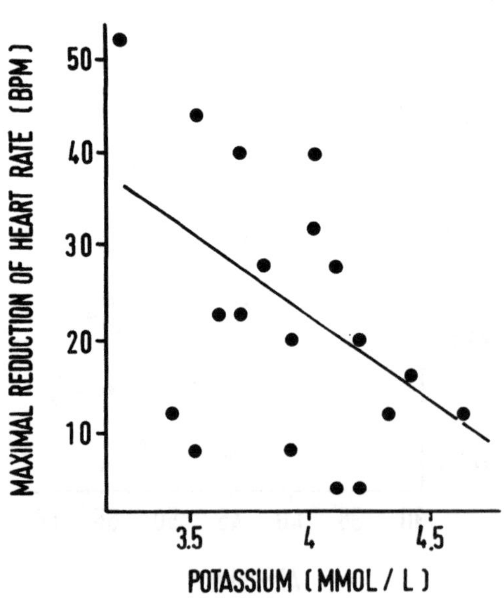

Fig. 16. Inverse correlation between potassium concentration (mmol/liter) and the maximal reduction of heart rate (beats/min): $r = -0.46$; $n = 20$; $P < 0.05$

5. Other Influences on the Pharmacodynamics of Acebutolol

One factor that seems to be of importance is serum potassium. In our geriatric patients it was closely correlated with the observed maximal reduction of heart rate ($r = -0.46$; $n = 20$; $P < 0.05$; Fig. 16). This relationship is interesting from a theoretical point of view since acebutolol is known to produce a slight but significant inhibition of the Na^+-K^+-ATPase activity in the rat heart sarcolemma (Dhalla and Lee 1976). It may, however, also be of interest for the clinician because lowered potassium levels are very frequent in geriatric patients.

References

Basil B, Jordan R (1982) Pharmacological properties of diacetolol, a major metabolite of acebutolol. Europ J Pharmacol 80:47–56

Bilski A, Robertson HH, Wale JL (1979) A study of the relationship between cardiac beta-adrenoceptor blockade and intrinsic sympathomimetic activity in rats depleted of catecholamines. Clin Exp Pharm Physiol 6:1–9

Cuthbert MF, Collins RF (1975) Plasma levels and β-adrenoceptor blockade with acebutolol, practolol and propranolol in man. Br J Clin Pharmac 2:49–55

Dhalla NS, Lee SL (1976) Comparison of the actions of acebutolol, practolol and propranolol in calcium transport by heart microsomes and mitochondria. Br J Pharmac 57:215–221

Holti G (1982) A comparison of two beta-blocking drugs in patients with Raynaud's phenomenon. The Practitioner 226:781–783

Ireland MA, Littler WA (1981) The effects of oral acebutolol and propranolol on forearm blood flow in hypertensive patients. Br J Clin Pharmac 12:363–368

Martin MA, Phillips FC, Tucker GT, Smith AJ (1978) Acebutolol in hypertension: relationships between drug concentration and effects. Europ J Clin Pharmacol 14:383–390

Möhrke W, Mutschler E, Mühlberg W, Platt D (1986) Pharmacokinetics of acebutolol in the elderly. In: Platt D (ed) Drugs and Aging. Springer, Berlin, Heidelberg

Mougeot G, Hugues FC, Julien D, March J (1981) Influence of propranolol and acebutolol on isoprenaline-induced changes in heart rate and peripheral blood flow in man. Archives internationales de pharmacodynamie et de thérapie, vol 251, 1:116–125

Ohashi K, Warrington SJ, Kaye CM, Houghton GW, Dennis M, Templeton R, Turner P (1981) Observations on the clinical pharmacology and plasma concentrations of diacetolol, the major human metabolite of acebutolol. Br J Clin Pharmac 12:561–565

Wollam GL, Cody RJ, Tarazi RC, Bravo EL (1979) Acute hemodynamic effects and cardioselectivity of acebutolol, practolol, and propranolol. Clin Pharmacol Ther, vol 25, 6:813–829

Age-Dependent Pharmacokinetics of Atenolol in Patients with Multiple Diseases

H. SPAHN [1], W. MÜHLBERG [3], E. MUTSCHLER [1], and D. PLATT [2,3]

Introduction

Physiological changes accompanying old age are nowadays well known, especially the reduction in renal function, i.e., in glomerular filtration rate, which is reflected by a decrease of creatinine or inulin clearance. One of the compounds whose pharmacokinetics are correlated with renal function is the relatively cardioselective, hydrophilic β-receptor antagonist atenolol (Fig. 1), which is widely used in the treatment of hypertension. It was shown to be effective in elderly patients; therefore the pharmacokinetic behavior and the corresponding effects of the drug should be known in old age.

Atenolol is only poorly protein bound and is almost entirely eliminated unchanged by the kidneys. In man it is not metabolized to a significant extent; less than 10% undergoes biotransformation and biliary excretion. The elimination half-life is about 7 h in healthy volunteers, and 50%–60% reaches the systemic circulation after oral administration.

The elimination half-life of atenolol was found to increase as the degree of renal insufficiency increases. Significant correlations were shown to exist between the elimination rate constant of atenolol and inulin clearance (McAinsh 1980) or creatinine clearance (Warren et al. 1980) and between the total body clearance and the glomerular filtration rate (Kirch et al. 1981 a).

In a group of five elderly patients (66–72 years) Barber and co-workers (1981) found a significant increase in the area under the plasma concentration time curve

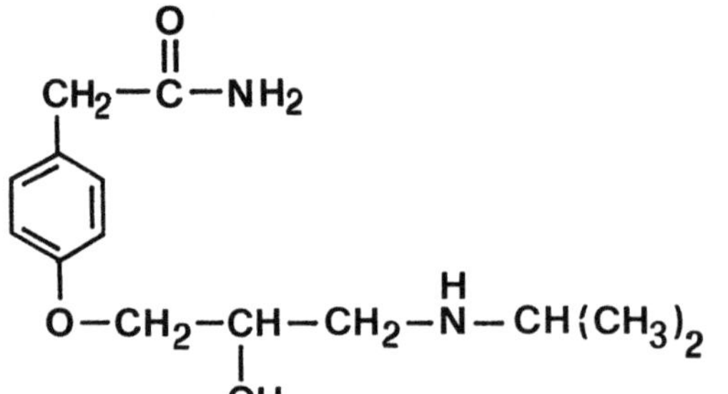

Fig. 1. Structural formula of atenolol (2-[4-(2-hydroxy-3-isopropylamino-propoxy)-phenyl]acetamine)

[1] Pharmakologisches Institut für Naturwissenschaftler der Johann-Wolfgang-Goethe-Universität, Theodor-Stern-Kai 7, D-6000 Frankfurt/Main/F.R.G.
[2] Institut für Gerontologie der Universität Erlangen-Nürnberg und
[3] 2. Medizinische Klinik, Klinikum Nürnberg, D-8500 Nürnberg/F.R.G.

Drugs and Aging
Ed. by D. Platt

(AUC) and a decrease in total body clearance following 8 days of oral treatment, whereas Rubin and co-workers (1982) found no age-related changes of any of the pharmacokinetic parameters in seven old patients (66–78 years). Therefore, the pharmacokinetic parameters of atenolol were investigated in a group of elderly multimorbid and in a group of young hypertensive patients, and these patients were compared with a group of young healthy volunteers. Concomitantly, pharmacodynamic effects on, for example, blood pressure were measured in the patient groups over a period of at least 24 h. Furthermore, we looked for correlations between plasma levels, pharmacokinetic parameters, effects, plasma creatinine, urea, and proteins.

Patients and Methods

In order to perform this study 25 hypertensive patients were selected, 11 of them aged between 20 and 30 years (22.7 ± 2.3; $\bar{x} \pm SD$) and the other 14 aged between 60 and 85 years (71.1 ± 6.2). The patients had given their informed consent.

Patients with a history of renal insufficiency or with severe hepatic disease or a systolic blood pressure of less than 140 mmHg were excluded. All suffered from mild to moderate hypertension, except for three of the elderly patients, who had a systolic blood pressure above 185 mmHg.

Plasma creatinine, plasma urea and total proteins of each patient were determined. Plasma creatinine values did not exceed 1.4 mg/100 ml except in one elderly patient. The plasma level time curve of this patient was not complete. Therefore he was excluded from the data analysis.

The plasma levels and pharmacokinetic parameters of young healthy volunteers (20–35 years) after single dose administration of 50 mg atenolol orally were taken from previous studies. Twenty persons were included in the control group.

After determination of blood pressure and heart rate under placebo and collecting blank plasma, one tablet containing 50 mg atenolol (Tenormin) was administered to each patient.

Blood samples were taken 2, 4, 8, 12, and 24 and in most patients also 26 and 34 h after application. Plasma was separated and the samples frozen until analysis.

At the times of plasma sampling, systolic and diastolic blood pressure and heart rate were measured.

Determination of atenolol plasma levels was performed by quantitative TLC (Schäfer and Mutschler 1979). To 1 ml plasma 1 ml of 1 N sodium hydroxide solution and 5 ml dichlormethane/butanol (95:5, v/v) were added. After shaking and centrifugation, 4 ml of the organic phase was evaporated under nitrogen (60 °C). The residue was dissolved in methanol (50 µl). 40 µl of the resulting solution was applied to a silica gel TLC plate. The plate was developed in chloroform, methanol, and acetic acid (75:20:5, v/v) and then dipped in a solution of paraffin (2%) in cyclohexane.

After chromatography and fluorescence enhancement, the native fluorescence of atenolol was measured on the TLC plates (excitation wavelength: 265 nm, emission wavelength: 313 nm). The variation coefficient was about 5%.

From the plasma level time curves the terminal half-life ($t_{1/2}$), the maximal plasma concentration (C_{max}) and the corresponding time (t_{max}), the area under the plasma level time curve (AUC), and the oral clearance (CL_{oral}) were calculated. The AUCs were determined using the trapezoidal rule.

Statistical analyses were performed with the nonparametric rank sum test of Wilcoxon, Mann, and Whitney, the Wilcoxon test, and the t-test for paired values. Variances were tested as described by Levene (1960) (in Sachs 1978).

Results

Complete plasma level time curves were available from eight elderly patients (68.1 ± 4.9 years, range 61–75 years). The mean plasma levels of the three groups (elderly and young patients and healthy volunteers) are shown in Fig. 2 over a period of 34 or 36 h.

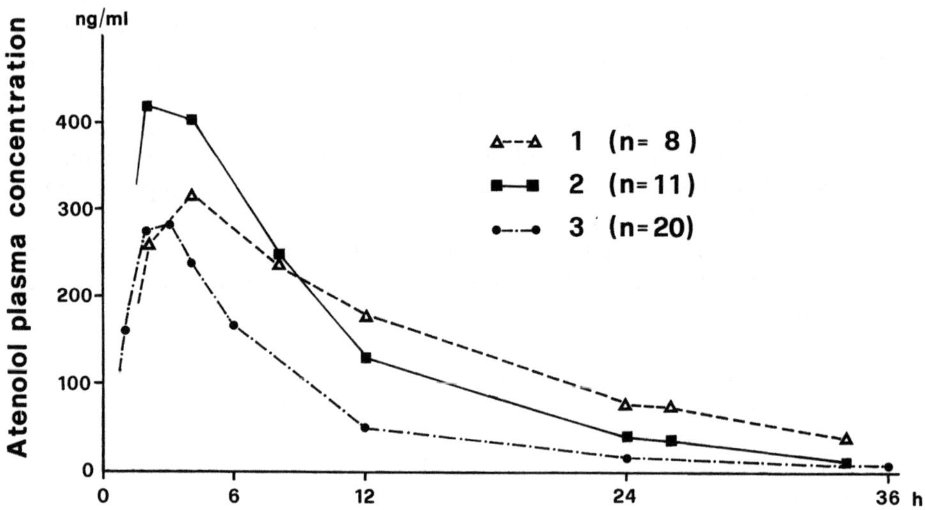

Fig. 2. Mean plasma level time curves of the elderly (*1*) and young patients (*2*) and of healthy volunteers (*3*) after oral administration of 50 mg atenolol

Table 1. Pharmacokinetic parameters (arithmetic means ± SD)

	Patients		Healthy volunteers 20–35 years (*n* = 20)
	> 60 years (*n* = 8)	20–30 years (*n* = 11)	
$t_{1/2}$ (h)	10.6 ± 7.3	7.3 ± 1.4	7.4 ± 1.8
C_{max} (ng/ml)	352 ± 160	469 ± 127	344 ± 113
t_{max} (h)	3.0 ± 1.1	3.3 ± 1.0	2.6 ± 1.1
AUC (ng ml^{-1} h)	6109 ± 4544	4810 ± 1264	2782 ± 636
CL_{oral} (ml/min)	244.3 ± 214	184.0 ± 46	315.6 ± 76

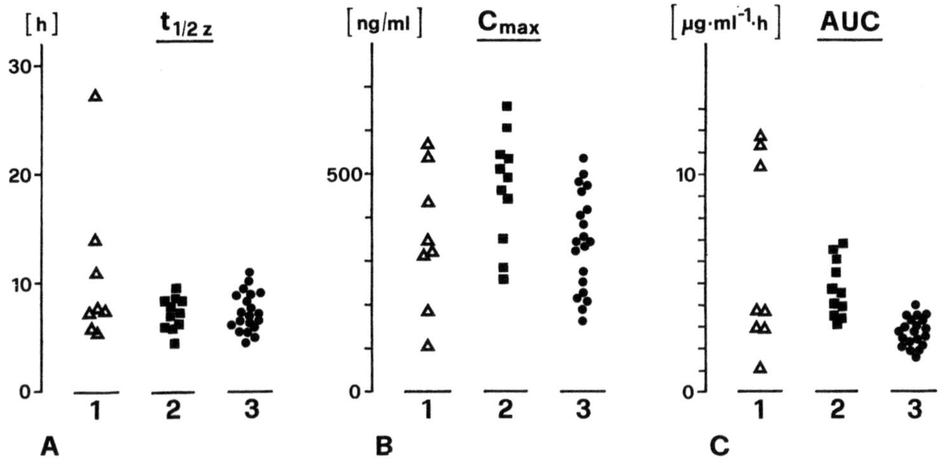

Fig. 3. Comparison of atenolol half-lives (**A**), maximal plasma concentrations (**B**), and areas under the curves (**C**) in elderly (*1*) and young patients (*2*) and in healthy volunteers (*3*)

The pharmacokinetic parameters calculated from the concentration time curves of patients and volunteers are given in Table 1.

The arithmetic mean of the terminal half-lives is enhanced in the group of elderly patients. No difference can be seen between the atenolol half-life in the younger patients and that in volunteers. The standard deviation in the elderly patients is rather high. The $t_{1/2}$ values range from 5.2 to 27 h (75-year-old patient), whereas those of the younger individuals do not exceed 11 h (Fig. 3 A). In the elderly the standard deviation of $t_{1/2}$ is 69%, compared to 19% and 24% in the other groups.

The mean maximal plasma concentration is higher in the younger patients than in the volunteers and the elderly patients (Fig. 3 B). The standard deviations are 45% for the group of elderly patients, 27% for the younger patients, and 38% for the healthy volunteers.

The mean area under the plasma level time curve extrapolated to infinity is significantly enhanced in the elderly if compared to the control group ($P < 0.05$). Here again, standard deviation is very high, namely 74% compared to 23% for healthy volunteers and 26% for young patients. The values range from 1154 to 12660 ng/ml × h in the elderly (Fig. 3 C). The high AUC values in some of the elderly patients are mostly due to the prolonged half-life in these patients. In the group of young patients AUC is also, but not significantly, enhanced.

The arithmetic mean of the oral clearances is higher in the group of elderly patients than in the younger patients. Values range from 66 to 720 ml/min. But in both groups of patients, the mean oral clearance is lower than the mean value of the control group.

It could be proved that the variance of AUC and oral clearance is significantly higher in the group of elderly patients.

The effects of a single oral dose of 50 mg atenolol on systolic and diastolic blood pressure and heart rate at rest are shown in Fig. 4. Reduction of systolic blood pressure and heart rate was statistically significant in the patient groups

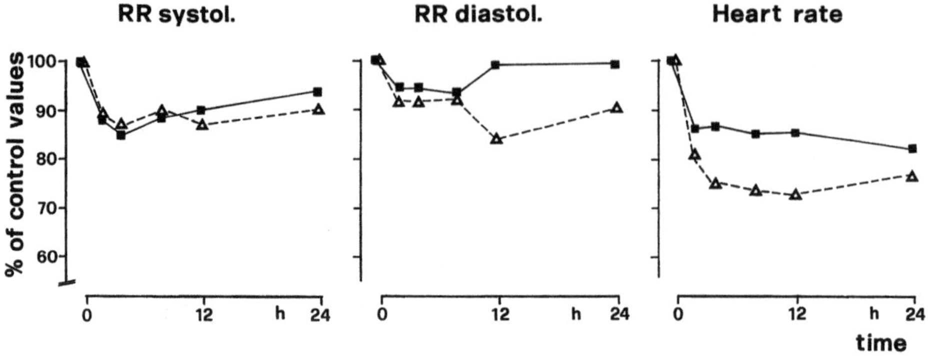

Fig. 4. Reduction of systolic and diastolic blood pressure and heart rate at rest (in % of control value) after a single oral dose of 50 mg atenolol. *Open symbols* patients >60 years old ($n=10$); *closed symbols* patients between 20 and 30 years old ($n=10$)

over a period of 24 h. The differences between the elderly and younger patients were not significant.

If the atenolol plasma levels are correlated with the corresponding systolic blood pressure independently of time, a correlation coefficient of −0.48 is obtained ($P<0.01$).

The reduction of blood pressure after 2 and 4 h seems to be dependent on atenolol levels. (Linear regression analysis gave better correlation coefficients than log linear regression analysis.) The correlation coefficients were 0.68 2 h and 0.63 4 h after administration ($P<0.01$).

Atenolol kinetics did not correlate with plasma creatinine. The plasma creatinine ($\bar{x} \pm SD$) was 0.95±0.25 in the elderly and 1.15±0.19 mg/100 ml in the young patients. Total protein was lowered in the elderly (6.03±0.93 g/100 ml) compared to the younger patients (7.12±0.99 g/100 ml).

Plasma urea was significantly higher in the geriatric (47.3±20.6 mg/100 ml) than in the young group (30.9±6.1 mg/100 ml) ($P<0.05$), possibly reflecting impaired kidney function.

The terminal half-life of atenolol seems to be correlated with plasma urea (the correlation coefficient is 0.74). But there are only a few plasma urea values above 45 mg/100 ml and just one higher than 60 mg/100 ml (87 mg/100 ml).

Discussion

It has already been shown for several other drugs [e.g., cefotaxim, piracetam (Platt 1984), and the β-antagonist acebutolol and its metabolite diacetolol (Möhrke et al. 1984)] that the variance of pharamacokinetic parameters increases with old age.

Although in the case of atenolol there is one main route of elimination and the drug is only poorly protein bound, there is no uniform effect on kinetic parameters in old age; however, the variations in half-life, AUC, and oral clearance are very high.

In one of the elderly patients low plasma levels of 100 ng/ml at the maximum were observed. This might be explained by differences in bioavailability. Melander et al. (1979) was able to show that atenolol plasma levels are markedly reduced by food in healthy volunteers. They found a food-induced reduction of bioavailability. It remains to be investigated whether the atenolol bioavailability in geriatric patients shows the same or a higher sensitivity toward food.

The lower levels in one of the elderly patients could also be explained by impaired absorption in this patient, as, for example, the absorbing surface and gastrointestinal perfusion are known to be reduced in old age. In spite of the low concentrations found in this patient, 50 mg atenolol orally did reduce blood pressure and heart rate, as in all the other patients. Thus it can be concluded that atenolol is effective in old as well as in younger patients.

In previous pharmacokinetic studies it could be shown that atenolol does not interact with several drugs, e.g., furosemide (Kirch et al. 1981), acetylsalicylic acid, allopurinol (Schäfer-Korting et al. 1983), and cimetidine (Kirch et al. 1982). Recently Kendall et al. (1984) were able to demonstrate that there is no pharmacokinetic interaction between atenolol and nifedipine. In addition, chronic liver disease does not influence atenolol kinetics if renal function remains normal (Kirch et al. 1983). An explanation for this behavior is the hydrophilic property of the drug and the fact that it is not metabolized to a relevant extent. Therefore it seems advantageous to use nearly unmetabolized substances in patients who need several drugs because of several diseases, i.e., in multimorbid patients. As the pharmacokinetic behavior of atenolol cannot be predicted in the elderly except when severe renal dysfunction is present, the drug should be administered carefully and in low doses, especially at the beginning of antihypertensive therapy, in order to avoid a hypotonic crisis, severe bradycardia, or other side-effects. Normally, 50 mg should not be exceeded in the elderly.

Summary

Plasma levels and pharmacokinetic parameters of atenolol were compared in young and elderly hypertensive patients and young healthy volunteers. There was no uniform effect of age on the kinetic parameters. C_{max} and t_{max} remained in the normal range. The mean AUC increased with age, but there were also normal and even lower values in the elderly patients. $t_{1/2}$ remained unchanged and increased in some of the elderly patients. Atenolol reduced blood pressure and heart rate at rest in both groups of hypertensive patients. The differences between the groups were not statistically significant.

References

Barber HE, Hawksworth GM, Petrie JC, Rigby IW, Robb OJ, Scott AK (1981) Pharmacokinetics of atenolol and propranolol in young and elderly subjects. Br J Clin Pharmacol 11:118–119

Kendall MJ, Jack DB, Laugher SJ, Lobo J, Smith R (1984) Lack of pharmacokinetic interaction between nifedipine and the β-adrenoceptor blockers metoprolol and atenolol. Br J Clin Pharmacol 18:331–335

Kirch W, Köhler H, Mutschler E, Schäfer M (1981 a) Pharmacokinetics of atenolol in relation to renal function. Eur J Clin Pharmacol 19:65–71
Kirch W, Schäfer-Korting M, Axthelm T, Köhler H, Mutschler E (1981 b) Interaction of atenolol with furosemide and calcium and aluminium salts. Clin Pharmacol Ther 30:429–435
Kirch W, Spahn H, Köhler H, Ohnhaus EE, Mutschler E (1982) Interaction of metoprolol, propranolol and atenolol with concurrent administration of cimetidine. Klin Wochenschr 60:1401–1407
Kirch W, Schäfer-Korting M, Mutschler E, Ohnhaus EE, Braun W (1983) Clinical experience with atenolol in patients with chronic liver disease. J Clin Pharmacol 23:171–177
McAinsh J (1980) Pharmacokinetics of atenolol. In: Cruickshank JM, McAinsh J, Caldwell ADS (eds) Atenolol and renal function. Academic Press, London, p 9–19
Melander A, Stenberg P, Liedholm H, Scherstén B, Wåhlin-Boll E (1979) Food-induced reduction in bioavailability of atenolol. Eur J Clin Pharmacol 16:327–330
Möhrke W, Mutschler E, Mühlberg W, Platt D (1984) Pharmacokinetics of acebutolol in the elderly. (this meeting)
Platt D (1984) Pharmakotherapie im Alter. Internist 25:491–500
Sachs L (1978) Angewandte Statistik, 5th ed. Springer, Berlin Heidelberg New York
Schäfer M, Mutschler E (1979) Fluorimetric determination of atenolol in plasma and urine by direct evaluation of thinlayer chromatograms. J Chromatogr 169:477–481
Schäfer-Korting M, Kirch W, Axthelm T, Köhler H, Mutschler E (1983) Atenolol interaction with aspirin, allopurinol and ampicillin. Clin Pharmacol Ther 33:283–288
Warren DJ, Hood D, Smith S, McAinsh J (1980) Atenolol in subjects with renal failure – a dose finding study. In: Cruickshank JM, McAinsh J, Caldwell ADS (eds) Atenolol and renal function. Academic Press, London, p 41–45

Long-Term Effects of Heterologous Fetal Testis Material on the Biological Age of the Male Rat

G. Hofecker, M. Skalicky, H. Niedermüller, and A. Kment[1]

Introduction

Studies into the mechanisms of biological aging are, for the most part, motivated by the desire to manipulate the aging process. Intervention into the aging process may be aimed at different but somehow related goals, e.g., prolonging mean and/or maximum life span, lowering the rate of aging, extending the vigorous years of life, or alleviating the deficiencies of old age. However, the type of study needed for assessing the effect of intervention into the multicellular aging process is in contrast to the usual pharmacological test procedures since the complex process to be measured does not at present allow for the development of simple, well-defined models. Obviously, the normal aging[2] of the organism does not simply emerge from changes in a particular type of molecule, cell, organ, or functional system, but is probably a systemic process shaped by numerous interactions in a biological hierarchy (Witten 1983). If we use a comparatively simple, well-defined test model, like collagen aging or the clonal aging of mitotically active cells, we will see the effects of intervention on the molecules or cells but we will not be able to predict what consequences this will have on the aging pattern of the organism as a whole. However, it is this complex pattern of effects that will determine the medical success of intervention.

On the other hand, a model at a high level in the biological hierarchy (e.g., behavioral model) will not solve the problem either, for two reasons: (1) Uncontrollable normal variations in the internal status of the organism (e.g., in motivation) are frequently much more pronounced than the gradual change with age and may either obscure or simulate a drug effect. (2) An improvement in the function of a complex system may also be obtained without any interference with the aging process.

A more promising solution to the problem of objectivation of influences on multicellular aging can be obtained by models of *biological age* which make use of a larger number of significantly age-related parameters at various levels of the biological hierarchy. This approach is based on the idea that (a) multicellular aging is characterized by the unidirectional, progressive change in a large number of age parameters, which are interlinked to various degrees, and (b) successful intervention into the aging process should consequently shift the values of the over-

[1] Abteilung für Experimentelle Gerontologie des Instituts für Physiologie der Veterinärmedizinischen Universität Wien, Linke Bahngasse 11, A-1030 Wien/Austria

[2] The aspects of pathology, however important, shall be excluded in this paper since illness does not meet the basic criteria (Strehler 1977) for the identification of aging processes

Drugs and Aging
Ed. by D. Platt

whelming majority of age parameters toward a state of lower age (Hollingsworth et al. 1965; Heikkinen et al. 1974; Ries et al. 1975; Furukawa et al. 1975; Webster and Logie 1976; Pöthig 1984). This type of phenomenological approach provides a means of estimating the age of organisms from the actual values of their age parameters, this estimate being representative of their biological age. According to this definition, the average biological age of an orthologically aging population should be identical with its chronological age, whereas the desirable type of intervention should lead to lower values. It must be added that we may attribute such a change to a retardation of the aging process only if this effect outlasts the end of treatment for a considerable length of time. Effects which are dependent on a continuous medication will rather point to compensation for deficiencies in the aged organism.

For the study of potential influences on the biological age of the rat, we designed a *multivariate model* which was based on data of a long-term cohort study using a series of age parameters from various levels of organization. By means of a *multiple regression analysis,* constants were calculated which give a certain weight to any parameter of the model in estimating the biological age of each individual (Skalicky et al. 1980). In this study, performed with an initial number of 1100 male Sprague-Dawley rats, we also tested experimental influences starting after the attainment of maturity. The influences were moderate dietary restriction, regular physical training, a combination of both dietary restriction and exercise, and as a test of the well known revitalizing effects described by Brown-Sequard in 1889, the parenteral administration of heterologous testis tissue material. The present paper will, in particular, refer to the results obtained with the "testis group" as compared with the "normal aging" controls. In addition, it will be shown by means of a *discriminant analysis* which parameters of the model are the most effective in separating the groups. In the course of the discussion, reference will also be made to a study which was designed to test the reproducibility of the results concerning the physical performance of the rats (Hofecker et al. 1981). Finally, the results of a survival study (unpublished data) will be introduced.

Materials and Methods

Animals

A total number of 1100 male Sprague-Dawley SPF rats (Mus-Rattus AG, Munich, F.R.G.), all born within 1 week, were purchased at an age of 6–7 weeks and housed under thoroughly controlled conventional conditions. The rats were kept in groups of six animals in Macrolon-IV cages at a temperature of 26 °C and 12-h light–dark alternation. Tap water and food (Altromin-R) were accessible ad libitum. The weight and state of health were regularly checked, and animals with obvious clinical symptoms were eliminated. At the age of 6 months the animals were randomly assigned to five groups, one control group (C) (reference population for the assessment of "normal aging") and four groups to be submitted to the experimental influences cited above. The initial number of rats in the control (C) and testis group (T) was 240 and 140 respectively.

Heterologous Testis Material

Lyophilized fetal sheep testis homogenate (Siccacell-testis, Cybila, Heidelberg, F.R.G.) was suspended in Ringer's solution and injected subcutaneously in a dose of 6 mg/animal at the ages of 9, 15, and 24 months. The testosterone content of the lyophilisate, as measured by the competitive protein binding assay, was in the range of 4 ng/mg. The age tests with group T were performed 6–9 months after the last injection. In this way we intended to rule out short-term effects of the injectional procedure and also the effects of the small amounts of androgens in the material.

Age Tests

We used a age test program which has been described previously in more detail (Hofecker 1976; Hofecker et al. 1980). It consisted of parameters of the neurosensomotor system of function (running capacity, motor activity, lipofuscin content of the brain), of the connective tissue (chemical contraction–relaxation of tail tendons, soluble collagen and hexosamine content of the corium), of the circulatory system (ECG, lipofuscin content of the heart, succinate dehydrogenase activity and minerals and trace elements in the heart, stress–strain parameters of the aorta), and of the blood (triglycerides and total cholesterol in the plasma). In addition, the activity of succinate dehydrogenase was also measured in the liver, as well as minerals and trace elements in the kidney. The tests were performed in four age groups of the average ages of 10, 17, 25, and 30 months. In the statistical calculations the actual age of any individual at the time of sacrifice was used. The total number of animals from each group which were tested at the given ages is shown in Table 1.

Table 1. Number of animals in the age groups and experimental groups

Age in months ($\bar{x}$)	C (control)	T (fetal testis)
10	36	–
17	36	24
25	36	24
30	28	19
Total	136	67

Multiple Regression Analysis

A stepwise multiple regression analysis was performed by an SPSS-computer program (Nie et al. 1976). The estimates of biological age were calculated by the linear combination of selected variables according to the equation

$$y = a_0 + \sum_{i=1}^{k} a_i x_i$$

where y equals the estimate of biological age, x_i is the respective variable (age parameter), and a_0 and a_i are constants evaluated by the multiple regression analysis. Since our age parameters revealed a nonlinear relation to the chronological age, which could be accounted for by exponential or logarithmic functions (Skalicky et al. 1978), we also used a modified equation in which y was replaced by its natural logarithm. The significance of difference between the aging curves of the testis group and the control group was tested by means of a discriminant analysis (Nie et al. 1976).

Discriminant Analysis

It was shown by Skalicky et al. (1981) that discriminant analysis provides a useful tool in studies of the assessment of biological age. This type of statistics shows which variables of an age test program are most effective in separating (a) various age groups in a population and (b) experimental groups from the orthologically aging controls. Discriminant analysis attempts to do this by forming one or more linear combinations of the discriminating variables (Klecka 1976). These *discriminant functions* are of the form

$$D_i = d_{i1}Z_1 + D_{i2}Z_2 + \ldots d_{ip}Z_p$$

where D_i is the score of the discriminant function i, the d's were weighting coefficients (standardized discriminant function coefficients), and the Z's are the standardized values of the p discriminating variables used in the analysis. The coefficients obtained by the analysis reflect their value for the separation of the groups. The analysis was also performed by an SPSS-computer program.

Results

Evaluation of "Normal Aging"

The evaluation of *"normal aging"* (group C) started with a total of 42 variables of the age test program. This number was systematically reduced to 23 (Table 2) for four reasons: (1) A high sensitivity of a model to influences on biological age can only be expected if its parameters change sufficiently with age (see also Comfort 1979). Consequently, we selected only parameters with an age change of at least 10% between 10 and 30 months. (2) Variables which did not further improve the multiple correlation were eliminated by the computer program. (3) Variables with an unclear behavior during senescence (like succinate dehydrogenase) were eliminated. (4) Parameters which could not be measured in all age groups had to be eliminated. This was necessary, for instance, with the ECG parameters since in the 25- and 30-month-old rats up to 90% of the ECGs were irregular and could not be quantified.

Using the remaining 23 variables, the constants and the biological age were calculated for those 71 animals of the control group C for which a complete set of data was available (occasional sample losses responsible for the reduction in animal number were regarded as being randomly distributed over all groups). It

Table 2. List of variables used in the multiple regression analysis and discriminant analysis

V2	Running capacity[a]
V4	Hexosamine, corium
V6	Magnesium, heart
V7	Copper, heart
V8	Zinc, heart
V10	Magnesium, kidney
V13	Calcium, heart
V15	Iron, kidney
V18	Tendon y_0 ("cross-links")[b]
V19	Tendon k_1 ("stability")[b]
V20	Tendon k_2 ("permeability")[b]
V26	Aorta b ("elastic fibers")[c]
V27	Aorta c ("collagen fiber spiral")[c]
V28	Aorta d ("collagen stability")[c]
V29	Aorta K_3t (maximum load, transverse extension)[c]
V30	Aorta K_3l (maximum load, longitudinal extension)[c]
V31	Triglycerides, plasma
V32	Cholesterol, plasma
V38	Lipofuscin, heart
V39	Lipofuscin, brain
V40	Spontaneous motor activity[d]
V41	Reactive locomotion[b, e]
V42	Reactive activity[a, b, e]

[a] Treadmill endurance (in meters), 20 m/min, 15° ascent
[b] Parameters from chemical contraction–relaxation of tail tendon fibers (Hofecker et al. 1979)
[c] Parameters from stress–strain hysteresis loops (Pav et al. 1981)
[d] Animex Activity Meter, 45 µA (Hofecker et al. 1978)
[e] Cinematographic method. Activity grades: 0 (rest or sleep), 1 (partial movements), 2 (locomotion) (Hofecker et al. 1978)

turned out that the *exponential* approach to the assessment of biological age was more appropriate than the linear one (for details see Skalicky et al. 1980). As can be seen in Fig. 1 the age curve of group C is practically identical with the predicted 45° line (biological age = chronological age). Its deflection toward lower values of biological age between 25 and 30 months seems to represent the well-known age selection effect.

Testis Group

The estimates of the biological age of the rats of group T were calculated using the constants of the logarithmic model described above. The resulting aging curve of the testis group (37 animals with a complete set of data) shifted clearly toward a lower biological age. A discrimination analysis including all variables showed the groups C and T to be distinct with a $P<0.001$.

A *stepwise discriminant analysis* (Table 3) provides an insight into which of the parameters were the most significant in bringing about this difference. The analysis was performed with two sets of data, one covering the whole age range

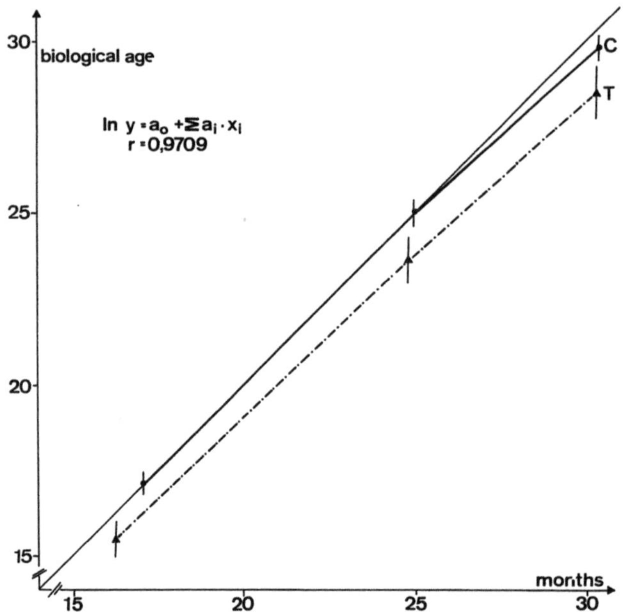

Fig. 1. Estimates of the biological age ($\bar{x} \pm$ SEM) of group T (fetal testis) as compared with the curve of "normal aging" (group C)

depicted in Fig. 1 (Table 3 a), the older using only the data of the age groups 25 and 30 months (Table 3 b). Only those parameters are listed which are, according to their coefficient, significantly ($P < 0.05$) involved in separating the groups. It turned out that, with increasing age, the number of significantly discriminating variables increased. This is in agreement with the slight divergence of the curves

Table 3. Standardized discriminant function coefficients of the function separating the groups C and T

a) *Age groups:* 17, 25, and 30 months

Variable number	Parameter	Coefficient	Direction
V20	Tendon k_2	−0.5589	−
V2	Running	−0.5142	−
V7	Cu, heart	−0.5101	−
V38	Lipof., heart	0.3755	−
V19	Tendon k_1	0.3554	−
V13	Ca, heart	−0.3323	+
V31	Triglyc.	0.3106	−
V10	Mg, kidney	0.2929	+
V29	Aorta K_3t	−0.2488	−
V41	React. locomot.	−0.2210	−

[a] The symbols "+" and "−" indicate that in group T the $\bar{x}$ (all ages) shifted toward "older" or "younger" values, whereas 0 indicates that the discriminating characteristics are not expressed by the arithmetic mean

b) *Age groups:* 25 and 30 months

Variable number	Parameter	Coefficient	Direction[a]
V41	React. locomot.	−0.7293	−
V20	Tendon k_2	−0.6747	−
V19	Tendon k_1	0.6195	−
V39	Lipof., brain	−0.6146	+
V32	Cholesterol	0.4776	−
V2	Running	−0.4562	−
V38	Lipof., heart	0.4406	−
V10	Mg, kidney	0.4309	+
V28	Aorta d	0.3756	0
V30	Aorta K_3l	0.3483	−
V8	Zn, heart	−0.3239	−
V18	Tendon y_0	−0.2958	−
V29	Aorta K_3t	−0.2523	−
V6	Mg, heart	−0.2305	−

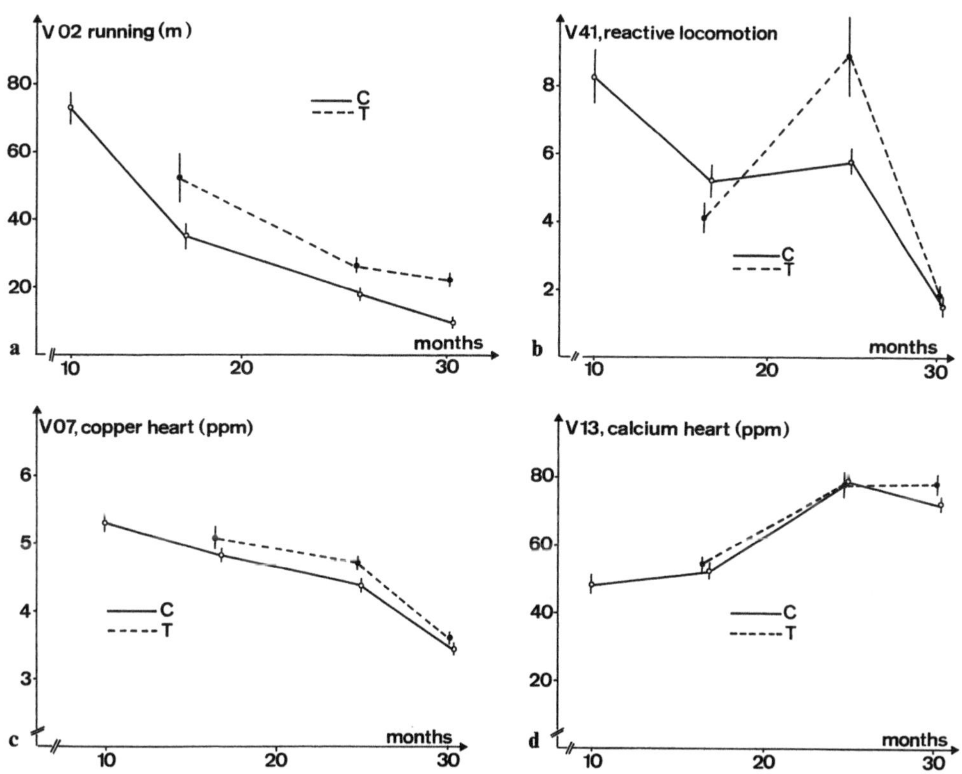

Fig. 2 a–j. Age changes in the parameters listed in Table 3 a ($\bar{x} \pm$ SEM) of the groups C (control) and T (fetal testis). Group T was tested for the first time at the average age of 17 months (first application of fetal testis material at 9 months), whereas the assessment of "normal aging" (group C) started at an average age of 10 months

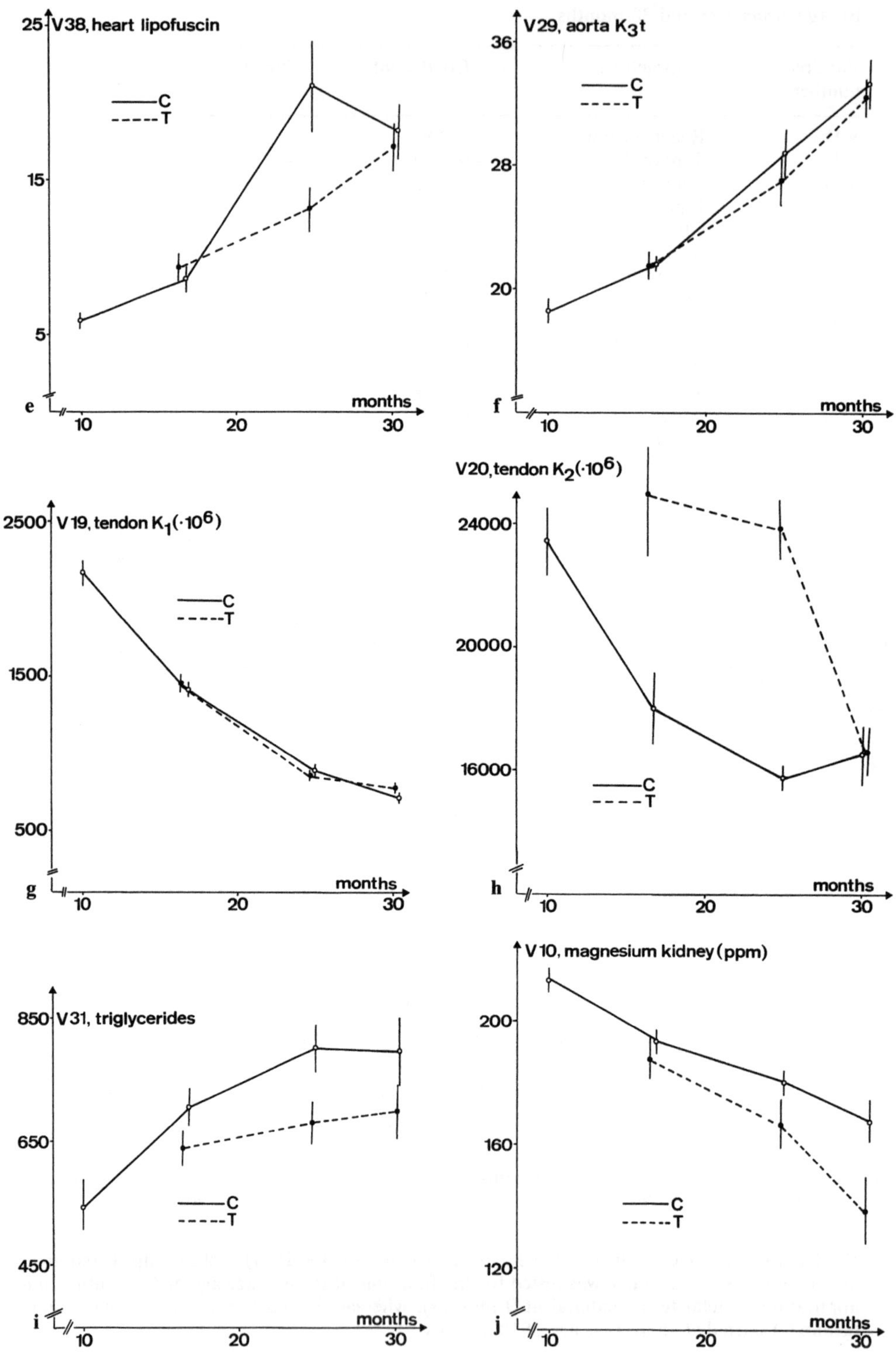
V38, heart lipofuscin
25
15
5
C
T
e
months
10
20
30
V29, aorta K_3t
36
28
20
C
T
f
months
10
20
30
V19, tendon $K_1(\cdot 10^6)$
2500
1500
500
C
T
g
months
10
20
30
V20, tendon $K_2(\cdot 10^6)$
24000
20000
16000
C
T
h
months
10
20
30
V31, triglycerides
850
650
450
C
T
i
months
10
20
30
V10, magnesium kidney (ppm)
200
160
120
C
T
j
months
10
20
30

in Fig. 1. The direction of the changes in the parameter values is indicated by the symbols to the right of the coefficients, where "+" and "−" mean a shift of $\bar{x}$ (all age groups) toward values of higher and lower age, respectively, and 0 express that the change does not appear in the arithmetic mean. With the exception of the variables 10, 13, and 39 (marked with a +) and variable 28 (marked with 0), the overwhelming majority of listed variables point toward a lower biological age (marked with −).

That this effect is obviously not due to the selection of the animals which were considered in the multivariate analysis is shown in Fig. 2. In this set of diagrams, the age course of the parameter values is represented as calculated from all available data from all the animals. The visual impression is, for the most part, in very good agreement with the directions and the coefficients in Table 3a, though there is no simple 1 : 1 relationship between these measures, which are both relevant for the distinction between the groups.

Discussion

The concept of biological age is based on the hypothesis that age-dependent changes in the state of the multicellular organism as a whole can be described by a single complex variable as a function of time (Beier et al. 1973). Since at present no absolute measure for biological age is available, this concept can only be applied to comparative studies which are orientated to the aging of a "normal population." Consequently, we regard models of biological age mainly as a tool for the assessment of intervention into the aging process.

According to the basic ideas of this approach, the validity of multivariate models of biological age depends strongly on the number of body systems and parameters involved. However, a larger number of parameters will also increase the probability that a greater number of individuals will be eliminated from the analysis because of the loss of one or more samples. For this reason, there is a need for a systematic preselection of parameters. We proposed in a previous paper (Hofecker et al. 1980) that this could probably be done by *factor analysis*.

In their present state, the models of biological age may be regarded as a "hypothesis-finding instrument" for testing possible ways of intervention into the aging process. If an effect on aging is indicated by the model, a discriminant analysis can point to variables which bring about the changes in biological age. This may enable us to formulate hypotheses which can be tested by means of more basic and better defined models.

Effects of parenterally applied heterologous fetal testis material on functional parameters of aged rats have already been investigated by Kment (1963). Fetal testis tissue seemed to be of interest because it is built up of incompletely differentiated cells with a high division potential and a close relation to the "immortal" germ line. One would expect these cells to contain substances which can restore the impaired functions of aged cells. This idea was supported by Kment's studies: parameters of memory, tendon collagen, tissue respiration, and mechanical properties of skin and aorta showed significant shifts toward the values of younger animals.

Our present long-term study showed analogous effects of the application of the same material. Since this effect appeared in a larger number of parameters and could be demonstrated even 6–9 months after application (a period that represents about one-third of the average life span of the rat), it is reasonable to assume that at least some processes of aging were influenced. The increase with age in the number of parameters involved in separating the groups C and T (Table 3) allows us to speculate that this effect of the treatment is somehow related to the progressive loss of function in an increasing number of cells. This would mean that certain parts of the material could have been used by aged cells to substitute for losses in certain elements or factors.

However, the purely phenomenological analysis provided by this study can give no insight into the real mode of action. Furthermore, it cannot be deduced from this first step in the investigation of the "Brown-Sequard phenomenon" whether the effect of intervention is specific to the applied material. In addition, we have to consider that there are also a few parameters which shifted toward the values of older animals (e.g., the Mg content of the kidney). These open problems remain to be investigated for each parameter in particular studies, which will also serve to test the reproducibility of the effects.

In a follow-up longitudinal study (covering the age range from 9 to 24 months) of the effects of fetal testis tissue material on the running performance and motor activity of the male rat, the previous results could be confirmed (Reisinger 1980; Hofecker et al. 1981). Since one possible explanation of these results and others from the long-term cohort study (e.g., the effect on tendon collagen) pointed to an involvement of sexual steroids, we measured the plasma testosterone levels of the 2-year old rats, 4 months after the last application of testis material. Testosterone levels were found to be significantly higher in the "testis group" (Table 4). Since testosterone levels decrease with age in the rat (Miller and Riegle 1977; Steger et al. 1979), this may be interpreted as an effect on the secreting cells in the testes or adrenal cortex. It can be ruled out that the small amounts of testosterone injected with the lyophilisate can be detected in the plasma 4 months after application. The importance of this finding is being subjected to further studies.

Testosterone is believed to have a life-shortening action in the male. Asdell et al. (1967) have shown that in rats androgens shorten life whilst estrogens prolong it. This seems to be in contradiction to our own findings of increased testosterone levels accompanied by lower values of biological age. The question arose as to whether the shift in biological age would be reflected in survival curves. To investigate this problem, we designed a survival study, the results of which are given

Table 4. Plasma testosterone levels (ng/ml)

	Control	Fetal testis
n	27	22
$\bar{x}$	0.52	0.77
SEM	0.07	0.08
$P<0.025$		

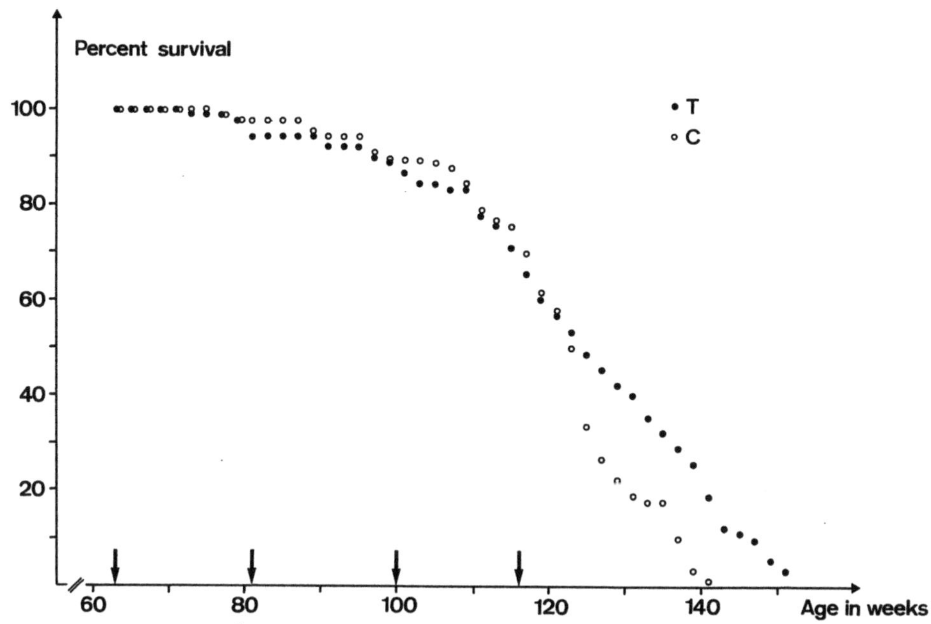

Fig. 3. Survival curves of two groups of 90 male rats: group T (fetal testis) and group C (control). *Arrows* indicate the time of injection of testis material (*T*) and Ringer's solution (*C*)

in Fig. 3. Two groups of 90 male Sprague-Dawley rats were used. The animals of group T were injected with lyophilized fetal testis (6 mg/rat) in Ringer's solution at the points of time indicated by the arrows, the control animals (C) receiving Ringer's solution at the same time. At the age of 50% survival, the curves separated, showing a slightly better characteristic for the "testis group." At present, three animals of the "testis group" are still alive, outliving the last rat of the controls by 2 months. The effect on intervention on the survival curve seems to be in good agreement with the effect we measured by means of our model of biological age. Therefore, we believe that in fact aging processes were influenced by the application of the heterologous fetal testis material. However, it has not been established whether this was the result of a general impact on basic processes or was brought about by an improvement of the functions of either a single system or a few of them. In addition, it is not possible to talk of *rejuvenation* since this would imply a general reversal of those processes which lead to a decrease in vitality during senescence. No evidence of such an effect on highly developed multicellular organisms has been provided up to now. It seems to be more appropriate to describe this kind of effect as *revitalization* according to the definition given by Kment (1978), as "a prolonged maintenance or recovery of a vitality level appropriate to a significantly lower biological age than is in accordance with the chronological age of the organism."

References

Asdell SA, Doornenbal H, Joshi SR, Sperling GA (1967) The effects of sex steroid hormones upon longevity in rats. J Reprod Fertil 14:113

Beier W, Brehme KH, Wiegel D (1973) Biophysikalische Aspekte des Alterns multizellulärer Systeme. Thieme, Leipzig

Brown-Séquard CE (1889) Des effects produits chez l'homme par des injections sous cutanées d'un liquide retiré des testicles de cobaye et de chien. C R Soc Biol 41:415

Comfort A (1979) The biology of senescence. Churchill Livingstone, Edinburgh London

Furukawa T, Inoue M, Kajiya F, Inada H, Takeda H, Abe H (1975) Assessment of biological age by multiple regression analysis. J Geront 30:422

Heikkinen E, Kiiskinen H, Käythy B, Rimpelä M, Vouri I (1974) Assessment of biological age. Gerontologia 20:33

Hofecker G (1976) Messungen des biologischen Alters im Tierversuch. Akt Gerontol 6:103

Hofecker G, Kment A, Niedermüller H (1978) Die motorische Aktivität als Altersparameter der Ratte. Akt Geront 8:271

Hofecker G, Niedermüller H, Skalicky M, Jahn J (1979) Die chemische Kontraktion von Schwanzsehnenfäden der Ratte: mathematische Analyse der Kontraktions-Relaxationskurven. Akt Gerontol 9:469

Hofecker G, Skalicky M, Kment A, Niedermüller H (1980) Models of the biological age of the rat. I. A factor model of age parameters. Mech Age Dev 14:345

Hofecker G, Niedermüller H, Skalicky M (1981) Der altersbedingte Leistungsabfall und seine Beeinflussung im Tierexperiment. Akt Gerontol 11:188

Hollingsworth JW, Hashizume JW, Hablon S (1965) Correlations between tests of aging in Hiroshima subjects: an attempt to define "physiological age". Yale J Biol Med 38:11

Klecka WR (1975) Discriminant analysis. In: Nie HN, Hull CH, Jenkins JG, Steinbrenner K, Bent DH (eds) Statistical package for the social sciences. McGrew-Hill, New York

Kment A (1963) Die tierexperimentelle Objektivierung des Revitalisierungseffektes nach Zellinjektionen. In: Schmid F, Stein J (Hrsg) Zellforschung und Zellulartherapie. Huber, Bern

Kment A (1978) Altern und Geriatrica aus der Sicht der experimentellen Gerontologie. Akt Gerontol 8:241

Miller AE, Riegle GD (1977) Aging and testosterone secretion in the male rat. Fed Proc Am Soc Exp Biol 36:612

Nie NH, Hull CH, Jenkins JG, Steinbrenner K, Bent DH (1976) SPSS, statistical package for the social sciences. McGraw-Hill, New York

Pav E, Hofecker G, Skalicky M (1980) A mathematical model of mechanical properties of the rat's aorta. Adv Physiol Sci 34:37

Pöthig D (1984) Experimentelle Entwicklung eines klinischen Diagnostikmodells zur Objektivierung des biologischen Alters des Menschen. Med Dissertation (B), Leipzig

Reisinger E (1980) Das Verhalten der Altersparameter motorische Aktivität und Laufleistung der Ratte nach Verabreichung von Testislyophilisat. Veterinärmed Dissertation, Wien

Ries W, Sauer I, Junker B, Pöthig D, Schwerdtner U (1975) Untersuchungen zur Erfassung des biologischen Alters. In: Schulz FH, Schmidt UJ, Brüschke G (Hrsg) V. Kongreß der Gesellschaft für Gerontologie der DDR, Berlin-GDR

Skalicky M, Hofecker G, Niedermüller H, Kment A (1978) Zeitlicher Verlauf von Altersparametern der Ratte. Akt Gerontol 8:281

Skalicky M, Hofecker G, Kment A, Niedermüller H (1980) Models of the biological age of the rat. II. Multiple regression models in the study on influencing aging. Mech Age Dev 14:361

Skalicky M, Hofecker G, Kment A, Niedermüller H (1981) Diskriminanzanalyse von Altersparametern der Ratte. Akt Gerontol 11:4

Steger RW, Peluso JJ, Bruni JF, Hafez ESE, Meites J (1979) Gonadotropin binding and testicular functions in old rats. Endokrinologie 73:1

Strehler BL (1977) Time, cells and aging. Academic Press, New York

Webster IW, Logie AR (1976) A relationship between functional age and health status in female subjects. J Gerontol 31:546

Witten M (1983) A return to time, cells, systems and aging: Rethinking the concepts of senescence in mammalian systems. Mech Age Dev 21:69

Drug Albumin Binding Kinetics in the Aged: Conformational Changes and the Effect of Fatty Acids

G. MENKE [1], P. PFISTER [1], A. H. STAIB [1], B. G. WOODCOCK [1], and I. RIETBROCK [2]

Introduction

The binding of drugs to biological macromolecules is not simply the attachment of a ligand at a fixed preformed binding site. There is much experimental evidence to show that binding is often accompanied by conformational changes (changes is shape) of the macromolecule. This has been well demonstrated for the glycolytic enzyme hexokinase and its substrate glucose, where binding induces the movement of large regions of the protein molecule for a distance of 0.8 nm (Bennett and Steitz 1978).

Human serum albumin (HSA) is an important carrier protein for drugs in the vascular system and interstitium. The tertiary structure is not fully known, but the molecule seems to consist of three domains with several independent binding sites (Kragh-Hansen 1981). Albumin can bind numerous endogenous and exogenous substances, some at specific binding sites, others at nonspecific sites. Five specific binding sites are generally recognized. Binding site I (Sudlow et al. 1976; Fehske et al. 1981) is specific for anionic drugs such as warfarin (Garten and Wosilait 1972), phenylbutazone (Brown and Crooks 1976), and azapropazone (Fehske et al. 1980).

Binding site II (Sudlow et al. 1976) is specific for anionic drugs including benzodiazepines (Kragh-Hansen 1981; Fehske et al. 1981; Müller and Wollert 1973) and carboxylic acid drugs such as ibuprofen (Whitlam et al. 1979; Fehske et al. 1981). Dansylsarcosine (DS) is bound with high specificity at site II and has been used as a binding probe (Sudlow et al. 1976).

A separate binding site seems to exist for various digitalis glycosides (Brock 1976; Fehske et al. 1980) and at least two different classes of specific binding sites are known for endogenous substances (Kragh-Hansen 1981). One of these, the bilirubin site, has a very high affinity for this ligand (Jacobsen 1969; Kuenzle et al. 1976).

Free fatty acids are strongly bound at two different sites on albumin which do not overlap with those mentioned above (Goodman 1958; Spector et al. 1973).

The number of nonspecific binding sites available on albumin varies from ligand to ligand (Kragh-Hansen 1981).

---

[1] Abteilung für Klinische Pharmakologie am Klinikum der Johann-Wolfgang-Goethe-Universität Frankfurt, Theodor-Stern-Kai 7, D-6000 Frankfurt 70/F.R.G.

[2] Klinik für Anästhesiologie und Intensivmedizin, Klinikum der Landeshauptstadt Wiesbaden/F.R.G.

Of the drug binding sites on HSA, that for benzodiazepines is the most specific. The binding characteristics of this site are sensitive to physiological and pathological changes. Thus, binding is reduced in sera from patients with uremia (Reidenberg and Drayer 1984) and hepatic disease (Kober et al. 1978). These reductions may involve competitive interactions but recent studies in this laboratory show that site II is sensitive to allosteric interference when the two fatty acid sites are occupied. The kinetics of binding, and the effects of allosteric interference arising from conformational changes, can be studied by the stopped-flow method (Laßmann and Rietbrock 1983). In this technique the time course of the change in a physical parameter, e.g., fluorescence, is used to measure the rate of the process. In our work the fluorescence of dansylsarcosine is used to follow the kinetics of human serum albumin–drug binding at the benzodiazepine binding site (binding site II).

Earlier studies from our laboratory, comparing binding kinetics in serum and solutions of purified serum albumin, have demonstrated that the binding of DS to albumin can be followed even in the presence of other serum proteins (Ulrich et al. 1983). This observation has enabled us to carry out studies on the binding properties of serum albumin without the need for prior purification of the binding macromolecule and to investigate, using serum from newborn infants and adults, whether a relationship exists between drug albumin binding kinetics and age.

Methods

Sera for dansylsarcosine–albumin binding studies were obtained from newborn infants (umbilical cord blood; $n=14$) and adults in the age groups 22–65 years ($n=16$) and >65 years ($n=18$), including two centenarians. Blood chemistry parameters showed no evidence of any underlying hepatic or renal pathology. Six of 18 subjects in the age group >65 were receiving medication which included nitroglycerin, digitalis, theophylline, glibenclamid, and doxycycline, but not anionic drugs binding at site II. The protein content of the sera was measured by the Biuret method. HSA concentrations were determined by electrophoresis. With the exception of the two centenarians, in whom the concentrations were 4.8 and 4.0×10^{-4} M (3.3 and 2.8 g/100 ml), there were only minor differences between newborn infants (mean value $5.8 \pm 0.5 \times 10^{-4}$ M or 4.0 ± 0.3 g/100 ml), adults aged 22–65 years (mean value $6.9 \pm 1.0 \times 10^{-4}$ M or 4.8 ± 0.7 g/100 ml), and adults >65 years (mean value $6.3 \pm 0.5 \times 10^{-4}$ M or 4.3 ± 0.4 g/100 ml).

The free fatty acid concentrations were determined using the method of Trout et al. (1960).

Binding Kinetics

1. Measurement

The binding experiments were carried out in a Durrum-Gibson apparatus as described by Laßmann et al. (1983). The signals were stored on a digital oscilloscope. The best fitting biexponential function for each signal was determined by on-line computation giving the constants k_{obs1} and k_{obs2} (relaxation constants), which were then used to calculate kinetic parameters for the chosen model by iteration (Laßmann et al. 1983).

2. *Reaction Mechanism*

Coupled equilibria are assumed to be involved in the binding reaction such that dansylsarcosine and HSA associate to form an unstable complex (DS–HSA #). The unstable complex rearranges to a more stable state (DS–HSA) involving specific binding forces:

$$DS + HSA \underset{k_{-1}}{\overset{k_1}{\gtrless}} DS - HSA \underset{k_{-2}}{\overset{k_2}{\gtrless}} DS - HSA \quad \text{(I)}$$

k_1, k_{-1}: velocity constants for step 1
k_2, k_{-2}: velocity constants for step 2

Using this model a linear relationship between k_{obs1} and k_2, k_{-2}, $k_2K_{A'}$, K_A, and the equilibrium concentrations c_{DS} and c_{HSA} can be obtained where:

$$\frac{1}{k_{obs} - k_{-2}} = \frac{1}{k_2} + \frac{1}{k_2 K_{A'} (c_{DS} + c_{HSA})} \quad \text{(II)}$$

$K_{A'}$: binding constants of the preequilibrium
K_A: binding constant for the specific binding equilibrium of DS and HSA

and

$$K_A = K_{A'} \frac{k_2}{k_{-2}} \quad \text{(III)}$$

Step 1 is controlled by the diffusion of the ligand and binding at the surface of the albumin (Fig. 1). The rate of this nonspecific binding process is exceedingly

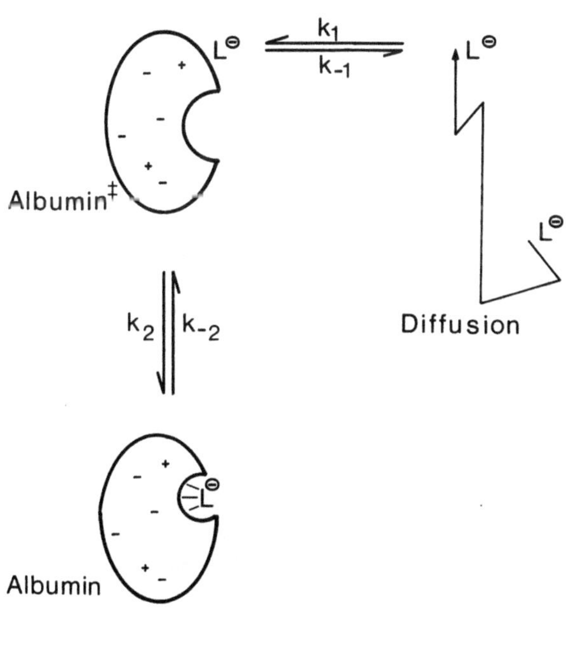

Fig. 1. Schematic illustration of the nonspecific and specific binding of a small ligand (*L*) on human serum albumin (albumin). *Albumin –L* is the primary complex (nonspecific binding); *Albumin–L* is the stable complex (specific binding). k_1,k_{-1}: velocity constants for step 1 [Eq. (I)]; k_2,k_{-2}: velocity constants for step 2 [Eq. (I)]

rapid, with a half-life time of approximately 2 ms. Thus a preequilibrium state is established at the moment the reactants enter the measuring cell. The time course of the observed fluorescence change reflects the step 2 (k_2,k_{-2}) conversion into the stable state with accompanying concomitant conformational changes on the albumin molecule. This rearrangement is therefore the rate-limiting step, is sensitive to allosteric perturbations, and is for these reasons of particular clinical and pharmacological interest.

Results and Discussion

Stopped-flow measurements on sera from 49 healthy newborn infants and adults showed that the protein binding kinetics of dansylsarcosine may be age dependent. Rearrangement into the stable complex, given by the association velocity

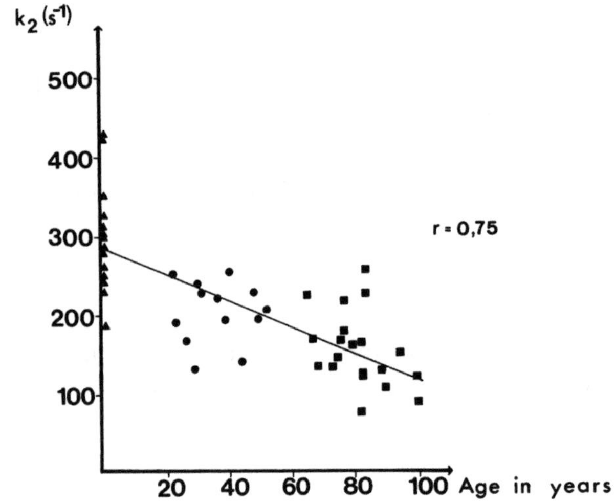

Fig. 2. Association rate constant k_2 (s^{-1}) obtained with serum for dansylsarcosine–albumin binding (DS–HSA) as a function of age

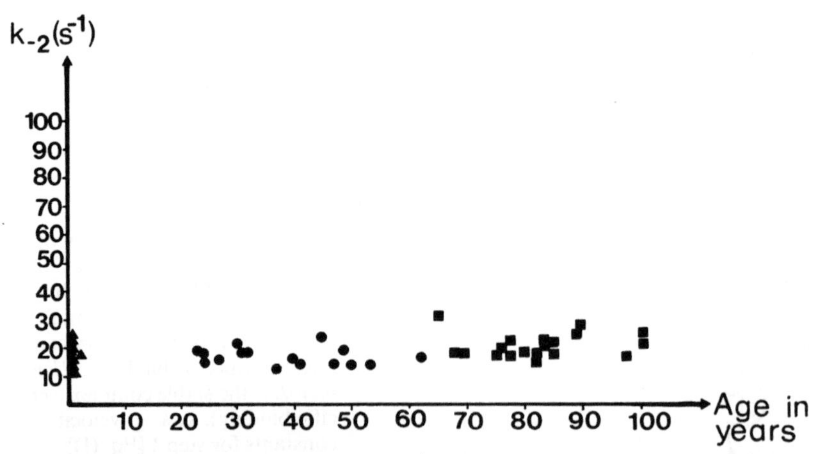

Fig. 3. Dissociation rate constant k_{-2} (s^{-1}) obtained with serum for dansylsarcosine–albumin binding (DS–HSA) as a function of age

constant k_2, was fastest in serum from newborn infants ($k_2 \cong 300 \pm 71\ s^{-1}$; adults aged 22–65 years $k_2 \cong 200 \pm 34\ s^{-1}$). Furthermore, of the 13 subjects examined who were older than 75 years, the rate of rearrangement in six cases was slower ($k_2 < 120\ s^{-1}$) than observed in all other subjects investigated (Fig. 2). In contrast, there is no relationship between the dissociation constant k_{-2} and age, where $k_{-2} \cong 20\ s^{-1}$ in all age groups (Fig. 3). In agreement with these findings, it was observed that with the decrease in k_2 with increasing age, the percentage of dansylsarcosine bound, as reflected in the calculated value for K_A (Eq. III), tended to fall. Studies have been published in which a relationship between the percent-

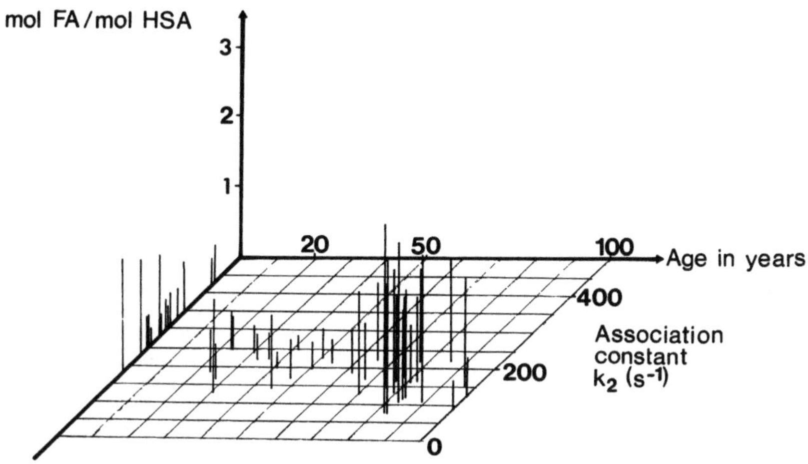

Fig. 4. Three-dimensional plot of the relationship between the free fatty acid–albumin molar concentration ratio c_{FA}/c_{HSA}, age, and the association constant k_2 (s^{-1}) for DS–albumin binding

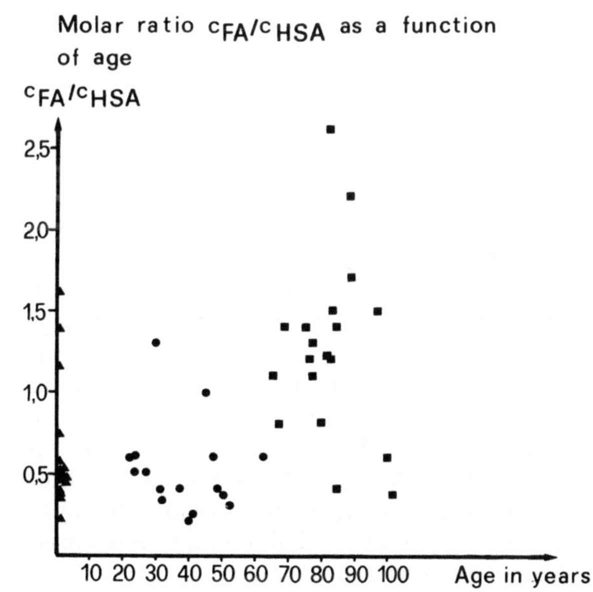

Fig. 5. Relationship between the free fatty acid–albumin molar concentration ratio c_{FA}/c_{HSA} and age

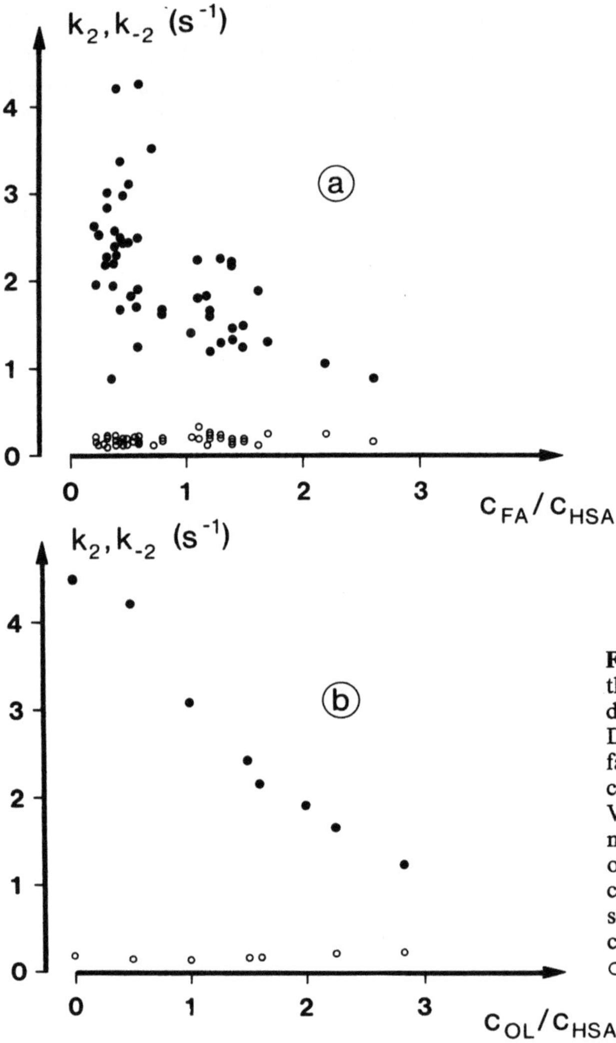

Fig. 6 a, b. Relationship between the association constant k_2 and dissociation constant k_{-2} for DS–albumin binding and the free fatty acid–albumin molar concentration ratio c_{FA}/c_{HSA}. **a** Velocity constants obtained with native sera; **b** velocity constants obtained with a synthetic system consisting of purified human serum albumin and varying concentrations of oleate. ●, k_2 (s^{-1}); ○, k_{-2} (s^{-1})

age binding of benzodiazepines and age could not be demonstrated (Klotz et al. 1975; Kraus et al. 1978); however, the observations of these authors were confined in the main to adults below 70 years of age.

Comparison of the relationship between k_2, the free fatty acid concentration, and age (Fig. 4) shows that the lower DS binding in the aged subjects is associated with a high fatty acid–albumin molar concentration ratio (c_{FA}/c_{HSA}). Thus it can be shown that the free fatty acid–albumin molar concentration ratio increases with increasing age (Fig. 5). Since it is known that free fatty acids can bind to serum albumin, and thus have the potential to produce allosteric changes in the albumin molecule, they may be the cause of the lower dansylsarcosine k_2 values in the aged. This interpretation is supported by the finding that in a synthetic system consisting of purified albumin, k_2 is decreased up on the addition of increasing amounts of oleic acid (Fig. 6).

In conclusion, our results demonstrate that with the stopped-flow method useful information can be obtained on the nature of drug–protein binding in patients. In addition to the thermodynamic binding constant, it is possible to determine values for the velocity constants not obtainable by conventional binding experiments based on the equilibrium state and the law of mass action. Velocity constants are indices of the dynamics of drug–protein binding and may be important determinants of disposition characteristics, e.g., tissue uptake and elimination, of drugs in the body.

A decreased association velocity at the benzodiazepine binding site on albumin is evident in the sera of aged subjects and this is due, at least in part, to the presence of higher free fatty acid–albumin molar concentration ratios. It has been shown here that the free fatty acids produce these effects even at very low molar ratios, suggesting that allosteric interactions are more important than competitive inhibition.

Our observations suggest that, where liver metabolism and albumin concentration are reduced in the aged, the slower association rate may enhance the effect of the low albumin concentration (Woodford-Williams et al. 1964), leading to accumulation of drug in the blood and a rise in the unbound drug concentration. The presence of multiple morbidity and multiple drug therapy, not uncommon in the aged, might be expected to further modify drug binding kinetics, but investigations on these aspects have not yet been reported.

References

Bennet WS, Steitz TA (1978) Glucose-induced conformational change in yeast hexokinase. Proc Natl Acad Sci USA 75:4848–4852

Brock A (1976) Binding of digitoxin to human serum albumin: influence of free fatty acids, bile acids, and protein unfolding on the digitoxin–albumin interaction. Acta pharacol et toxicol 38:497–507

Brown KF, Crooks MJ (1976) Displacement of tolbutamide, glibenclamide and chlorpropamide from serum albumin by anionic drugs. Biochem Pharmacol 25:1175–1178

Fehske KJ, Jähnchen E, Müller WE, Stillbauer A (1980) Azapropazone binding to human serum albumin. Naunyn-Schmiedeberg's Arch Pharmacol 313:159–163

Fehske KJ, Müller WE, Schläfer U, Wollert U (1981) Characterisation of two important drug binding sites on human serum albumin. In: Rietbrock N, Woodcock BG, Laßmann A (eds) Progress in drug protein binding. Vieweg, Braunschweig/Wiesbaden, p 5–15

Garten S, Wosilait WD (1972) An analysis of the binding of coumarin anticoagulants by human serum albumin. Comp Gen Pharmacol 3:83–88

Goodman DS (1958) The interaction of human serum albumin with long chain fatty acid anions. J Am Chem Soc 80:3892–3898

Jacobson J (1969) Binding of bilirubin to human serum albumin. Determination of the dissociation constants. FEBS Letters 5:112–114

Klotz U, Avant GR, Hoyumpa A, Schenker S, Wilkinson GR (1975) The effects of age and liver disease on the disposition and elimination of diazepam in adult man. J Clin Invest 55:347–359

Kober A, Jenner A, Sjöholm I, Borga O, Odar-Cederlöf I (1978) Differentiated effects of liver cirrhosis on the albumin binding sites for diazepam, salicylic acid and warfarin. Biochem Pharmacol 27:2729–2735

Kragh-Hansen U (1981) Molecular aspects of ligand binding to serum albumin. Pharmacol Rev 33:17–53

Kraus JW, Desmond PV, Marshall JP, Johnson RF, Schenker S, Wilkinson GR (1978) Lorazepam elimination in liver disease. Clin Pharmacol Ther 24:411–419

Kuenzle CC, Gitzelman-Cumarasamy N, Wilson KJ (1976) Affinity labeling of the primary bilirubin binding site of human serum albumin. J Biol Chem 251:801–807

Laßmann A, Rietbrock N (1983) Insight into drug protein binding obtained by stopped-flow measurements. In: Wyn-Jones E, Gormally J (eds) Aggregation processes in solution. Studies in physical and theoretical chemistry 26, p 383–409

Laßmann A, Kratzer W, Rietbrock N (1983) Kinetik der Bindung von Dansylsarkosin (DS) zur Spezifizierung von Humanalbumin (HSA) in Serumkonserven. Fresenius Z Anal Chem 314:487–490

Müller WE, Wollert U (1973) Characterization of the binding of benzodiazepines to human serum albumin. Naunyn-Schmiedeberg's Arch Pharmacol 280:229–237

Reidenberg MM, Drayer DE (1984) Alteration of drug–protein binding in renal desease. Clin Pharmacokin 9:18–26

Sudlow G, Birkett DJ, Wade DN (1976) Further characterization of specific drug binding sites on human serum albumin. Mol Pharmacol 12:1052–1061

Trout DL, Estes EH, Friedberg SJ (1960) Titration of free fatty acids in plasma: a study of current methods and new modifications. J Lipid Res 1:199–202

Ulrich R, Laßmann A, Kaufmann R, Rietbrock N (1983) Stopped-flow und fluorescenzspektrometrische Untersuchungen des Bindungsverhaltens von Dansylsarkosin an Albumin in Nativserum. Fresenius Z Anal Chem 315:534–538

Woodford-Williams E et al. (1964) Serum protein patterns in normal and pathological ageing. Gerontol Clin 10:86

Drug Interactions in Geriatric Patients

M. R. P. Hall [1]

Introduction

It has long been recognized that the incidence of adverse drug reactions increases with age (Seidl et al. 1966; Hurwitz 1969). Moreover, the more drugs being taken, the greater the likelihood of an adverse reaction (Williamson and Chopin 1980; Williamson 1984). It was suggested in the report of a Working Party of the Royal College of Physicians of London (1984) on "Medication for the Elderly" that the incidence of adverse drug reactions was the direct result of disproportionate prescribing. Indeed, 80% of the subjects studied by Williamson (1984) were taking prescribed drugs. These were people being admitted to hospital. However, elderly people living at home have a similar pattern, for in a random sample Moir and Dingwall-Fordyce (1980) found that 56% were taking one to three preparations, 15% had four or more, and only 28% had no prescribed medication. Our own findings in Southampton (Table 1) are similar, for in a randomly selected sample of elderly living at home, 61% were taking one to three preparations, 19% four or more, and 20% none. Our sample, however, was structured to contain a larger proportion of elderly (aged 75 years or more) (Table 2), and we also included self-prescribed drugs in our analysis. This may account for the smaller percentage tak-

Table 1. Number of preparations being taken at start of study

No. of preparations being taken[a]	Total percentage
0	20%
1, 2, 3	61%
4, 5, 6, 7–12	19%
Total 673	100%

[a] Average: two preparations per subject

Table 2. Age spectrum of subjects studied for 2 years

No. taking drugs	No. not taking drugs
Males 65+69	Males 65+16
Males 75+48	Males 75+13
Females 65+57	Females 65+13
Females 75+46	Females 75+ 1

[1]University of Southampton, Faculty of Medicine, Southampton General Hospital, Southampton SO9 4XY, Great Britain

Drugs and Aging
Ed. by D. Platt

Table 3. Preparations being taken during 2-year observation period of 263 subjects

No. of preparations being taken	Percentage at start	Percentage at finish
0	24	16
1–3	64	62
4 or more	12	22
	Average: 1.7/subject	Average: 2.1/subject

ing no drugs and it was interesting to find that only one woman over 75 years was taking no drugs. It should also be recognized that as people age, the number of drugs taken increases. We were able to study 263 of our original sample over a period of 2 years and found that the number of preparations taken increased from 1.7 per subject to 2.1, an increase of 20%. Since many of these elderly take more than one preparation, the risk of drug interaction must increase (Table 3).

Types of Interaction

The British National Formulary (1984) describes drug interactions as being of three types – pharmaceutical, pharmacokinetic, and pharmacodynamic.

Pharmaceutical Interactions

Pharmaceutical interactions occur when two drugs are given together, e.g., in an infusion, or when a drug reacts with the infusion solution. While it is necessary to be aware of this type of interaction, it is relatively uncommon and will not be considered in this paper.

Pharmacokinetic Interactions

Pharmacokinetic interactions may be defined as those interactions in which the disposition of the first drug, sometimes called the object drug (Aronson and Graham-Smith 1981), is altered by the second drug or precipitant drug. As a result, the effect of the first (object) drug is either diminished or increased. Interference with absorption, distribution, metabolism, or excretion can give rise to an increase or decrease in drug effect, and the precipitant drug may cause the interaction by more than one mechanism.

Absorption

Interactions relating to absorption are not very important since most drugs are absorbed by passive diffusion. Alterations in gut motility have comparatively little effect, though anticholinergics may cause increased absorption of some drugs. Tetracyclines tend to chelate calcium, aluminum, magnesium, and iron, so that lower blood levels of tetracycline will be found. Consequently antacids should be given at a different time to tetracyclines.

Metabolism

Several drugs, however, may undergo sulfoxidation or sulfate conjugation in the gut wall and this renders them inactive. Isoprenaline and chlorpromazine are examples. Vitamin C undergoes sulfate conjugation and can inhibit sulfate conjugation of other drugs metabolized in this way, e.g., paracetamol, hence raising drug level (Houston and Levy 1976). It is unlikely, though, that this mechanism is of clinical importance. Of much greater importance is first pass metabolism in the liver. Many drugs are metabolized by hepatic microsomal oxidation, and if these enzymes have already been induced enzymatic action may be increased, and drug effect reduced. The more lipid-soluble β-blockers, such as propranolol and metoprolol, are extensively metabolized and have a high first pass clearance. Enzyme-inducing drugs will, therefore, increase clearance and reduce bioavailability. The clearance of propranolol is also affected by hepatic blood flow, and other drugs which alter this may increase plasma concentrations of β-blocker, e.g., hydralazine. In some hypertensives this is a useful interaction. However, in the case of lignocaine, propranolol will produce toxicity (Graham et al. 1981) and will also increase the blood concentrations of chlorpromazine (Peet et al. 1981).

Distribution

Interaction may result from alteration in tissue binding and transport mechanisms. Highly protein bound object drugs may be displaced by precipitant drugs so that more object drug is available in active form. This may account for the interactions which may occur between oral anticoagulants, such as warfarin, and nonsteroidal anti-inflammatory drugs (NSAIDs) or hypoglycemic agents such as the sulfonylureas. Similarly, drugs such as the tricyclic antidepressants are bound within nervous tissue and will block the effect of adrenergic blocking agents, e.g., guanethidine.

Excretion

Renal excretion is of vital importance, particularly when this applies to drugs which are mainly eliminated by the kidneys, such as digoxin and antibiotics. The effect of quinidine, for instance, will increase the plasma concentration of digoxin by, on average, a factor of 2. Phenylbutazone reduces the renal clearance of chlorpropamide and both drugs are excreted by active tubular secretion. Similarly, frusemide and ethacrynic acid decrease excretion of gentamicin.

Pharmacodynamic Interactions

Pharmacodynamic interactions may be either direct or indirect. In the case of direct reactions, the precipitant or object drugs act on the same system, e.g., alcohol and drugs which react on the central nervous system. There are many other examples; for instance, potassium-sparing diuretics may react with each other if given concurrently or with potassium chloride to give rise to hyperkalemia. β-Blockers will potentiate the effects of many antiarrthymic drugs such as verapamil, disopyramide, and lignocaine, increasing the risk of myocardial depression, cardiac failure, hypotension, bradycardia, and asystole (Beeley 1984).

Indirect reactions are of two kinds: Firstly, the interaction in which the precipitant drug causes some alteration of fluid or electrolyte balance which influences the effect of the object drug, for instance, diuretics causing hypokalemia enhancing a cardiac glycoside. Secondly, the precipitant drug alters the structure of the organ; for instance, drugs which give rise to gastrointestinal erosion or ulceration will enhance bleeding if an anticoagulant is given concurrently.

Discussion

There is no doubt that drug interactions occur in old people; we have only to look at some of their drug regimes to see how these may occur (Table 4). Williamson (1984) showed that the principal groups of drugs which give rise to reactions were diuretics; antidepressants, tranquilizers, and psychomimetics; digitalis; hypnotics, sedatives, and anticonvulsants; analgesics and antipyretics; hypotensives; and tremor and rigidity controllers, in that order, though a relatively greater proportion of reactions occurred in the last two groups.

How big is the potential risk? In our group of 263 subjects (Table 5) we find that the greatest potential risk lies in the group of cardiovascular drugs with in-

Table 4. Patient drug regimens

Patient A	Patient B
Warfarin[a]	Cimetidine[a]
Thyroxin	Triamterene[a]
Phenytoin[a]	Frusemide[a]
Frusemide[a]	Digoxin[a]
Mianserin[a]	Chlormethiazole[a]
Temazepam[a]	Ferrous sulfate
Paracetamol	Paramol 118[a]
	Calcium *c* vit D

[a] Drugs likely to interact

Table 5. Drugs most likely to cause adverse reaction

Drugs	Percentage ($n=263$ subjects)
Digitalis	7
Diuretics	35
Antidepressants, tranquilizers, psychotropics; Hypnotics, sedatives, anticonvulsants	27
Analgesics	40
Hypotensives	6
Rigidity and tremor controllers	–
Antibiotics	–
Corticosteroids	3
Insulin and hypoglycemics	5

Table 6. Number of drugs taken at the start and end of the study

Drugs or drug group	Total subjects at start of study T (1)	Total subjects at end of study T (2)
Cardiovascular drugs	159	195
Digoxin	18	18
Inderal or other β-blocker	23	22
Diuretics $\pm$K	67	91
K salt	17	20
Vasodilator	16	25
Hypotensive	15	16
Other cardiovascular drug	3	3

Table 7. Number of drugs taken at the start and end of study

Drugs or drug group	Total subjects at start of study T (1)	Total subjects at end of study T (2)
Analgesics	107	106
Paracetamol	18	14
Aspirin	17	22
NSAIDS	30	31
Distalgesic	17	14
Other	25	25

Table 8. Number of drugs taken at the start and end of study

Drugs or drug group	Total subjects at start of study T (1)	Total subjects at end of study T (2)
Psychotropics	73	71
Sedatives and antipsychotics	30	32
Antidepressants	18	17
Hypnotics	25	22

teractions possible between β-blockers and hypotensives (Table 6). Similarly, other potential common interactions may occur with NSAIDs (Table 7), the psychotropic group (Table 8), and the bronchodilators.

However, while we must be aware of the action of drugs and the interaction which may take place between them, we must remember that the elderly suffer from multiple pathology and may need several drugs to maintain their health and independence. We should not let our fear of interactions prevent us from prescribing appropriate drugs. Nevertheless, when doing this we must remember how each drug is handled by the body and use as few drugs as are absolutely necessary.

Acknowledgment. Part of the material presented in this paper was obtained while undertaking a Study for Schwarzhaupt (Cologne). This support is acknowledged.

References

A Report of the Royal College of Physicians (1984). J Roy Coll Phys Lond 18:7–17
Aronson JK, Graham-Smith DG (1981) Clinical pharmacology. Adverse drug interactions. Brit Med J 282:288–291
Beeley Linda (1984) Drug interactions and beta-blockers. Brit Med J 289:1330–1331
Graham CF, Turner WN, Jones JK (1981) Lignocaine-propranolol interactions. N Engl J Med 304:1301
Houston JB, Levy G (1976) Drug biotransformation interactions in man. VI. Acetaminophen and ascorbic acid. Pharmacol Sci 65:1218–1221
Hurwitz N (1969) Predisposing factors and adverse reactions to drugs. Brit Med J 1:536–539
Moir DC, Dingwall Fordyce I (1980) Drug taking in the elderly at home. J Clin Exp Gerontol 2:329
Peet M, Middlemiss DN, Yates RA (1981) Propranolol in schizophrenia. II. Clinical and biochemical aspects of combining propranolol with chlorpromazine. Br J Psych 139:112–117
Seidl LG, Thornton GF, Smith JWW, Cluff LU (1966) Studies on the epidemiology of adverse drug reactions. Bull J Hopk Hosp 119:299–315
Williamson J (1984) Epidemiological consideration of adverse reactions to drugs. In: Barbagello-Sangiorgi G, Exton-Smith AN (eds) Aging and drug therapy. Plenum Press, New York London, p 41–49
Williamson J, Chopin JM (1980) Adverse reactions to prescribed drugs in the elderly. A multicentre investigation. Age & Aging 9:2, 73–81

Plasma Concentration Measurement and Clinical Parameters in a Geriatric Population Treated for Cardiac Insufficiency Using the Nonrenal-Dependent Cardiac Glycoside Pentaformylgitoxin (Gitoformate)

B. G. WOODCOCK [1], S. KUBIN [1], and R. SCHMITT-RÜTH [2]

Introduction

Gitoformate, or pentaformylgitoxin, is a semisynthetic cardiac glycoside which, like digitoxin, is nonrenal dependent, cleared by the liver, and suitable for use in patients with decreased or variable renal function (Batz et al. 1983; Rietbrock et al. 1984).

On absorption, via the GI tract and on crossing the liver, gitoformate is hydrolyzed quantitatively to 16-formylgitoxin, which carries the greater part, if not all, of the pharmacological activity. Gitoformate appears in plasma, therefore, as 16-formylgitoxin, and small quantities of gitoxin can also be detected. 16-Formylgitoxin is a naturally occurring glycoside found along with digitoxin in the foxglove, *Digitalis purpurea.*

This paper describes observations, including measurements of plasma drug concentrations, in a multimorbidity geriatric group of patients. The majority of the patients had impaired renal function and were receiving the medication as a combination therapy with a diuretic for the treatment of cardiac insufficiency of diverse etiologies.

Of particular interest were answers to the questions:

1. Is gitoformate well tolerated by these aged patients?
2. Is the relatively low dose, along with a diuretic, effective?
3. Can the clinical findings be related to the plasma drug concentrations?

Methods

A summary of the study protocol and the numbers of patients evaluated are shown in Table 1. Of the 31 patients included, 3 could not be evaluated. In the case of one of these patients, this was due to severe bradycardia and discontinuation of the treatment. The average period of hospitalization was 22 days.

Gitoformate (Dynocard, Dr. Madaus & Co., Cologne) was administered at a dose rate of 0.06 mg daily following a loading dose of 3 × 0.06 mg daily for 3 days. Five patients previously digitalized underwent a 7-day glycoside-free period before taking gitoformate. Drug plasma concentrations, measured as gitoxin

[1] Abteilung für Klinische Pharmakologie, Klinikum der Johann-Wolfgang-Goethe-Universität Frankfurt, Theodor-Stern-Kai 7, D-6000 Frankfurt 70/F.R.G.

[2] Institut für Gerontologie der Universität Erlangen-Nürnberg, Heimerichstr. 58, D-8500 Nürnberg/F.R.G.

Drugs and Aging
Ed. by D. Platt

Table 1. Protocol

Patients included in therapy 31 (m 7, f 24)	
Patients dropped 3[a]	
Patients evaluated 28	
Age of patients (yrs) 79.2±5.9 (range 69–91)	
Days under observation 22±7.5 (range 11–42)	
Patients previously digitalized $n=5$	
Gitoformate dosage:	
Loading 3×0.06 mg (3 days)	
Maintenance 1×0.06 mg daily	

[a] 1 patient (digitalis sensitivity–bradycardia)
1 patient died on day 6 (acute heart failure
1 patient suspected of self-medication with digitalis

Table 2. Renal characteristics of patients

Creatinine clearance below 50 ml/min ($n=17$)	
Serum creatinine (mg/100 ml)	1.66±0.43 (range 1.1–2.8)
$Cl_{(creatinine)}$ (ml/min)	38.47±12.2 (range 15–50)
Creatinine clearance above 50 ml/min ($n=11$)	
Serum creatinine (mg/100 ml)	1.75±0.64 (range 1.0–3.4)
$Cl_{(creatinine)}$ (ml/min)	81.0±31.9 (range 51–136)

Values given are mean ± SD

equivalents (Gitoxitest, A. Christiaens, Brussels), were obtained at intervals during maintenance therapy.

Classification of the severity of symptoms, recorded before and after therapy with gitoformate, was based on three categories – absent, moderate, severe – giving 3×3 contingency tables which could be statistically analyzed using the chi-squared test of Bowker. Details of the renal function for the 28 patients are shown in Table 2. The majority, 17, had measured creatinine clearance values below 50 ml/min at the commencement of treatment and only four of the remainder had values above 85 ml/min.

Results and Discussion

Renal function tests under gitoformate treatment, and measured at the end of hospitalization, showed no significant change, but body weight was decreased by 4 kg on average (Table 3).

Figure 1 shows the results of between one and four drug concentration measurements at different time intervals on a total of 27 patients during maintenance treatment. A concentration above 5 ng/ml was attained by most patients within 2–3 weeks. The therapeutic range for this drug is 5–15 ng/ml (gitoxin equivalents) (Ulbrich et al. 1984). The value in brackets (17 ng/ml was obtained in a noncompensated, digitalis-resistant patient who received twice the protocol dose owing to poor response. This female patient had a body weight of only 54 kg. She ex-

Table 3. Renal function and body weight

Parameter	Before treatment (mean ± SD)	After treatment (mean ± SD)	% change	*P*
Diuresis (ml/day)	1,675 ± 927	1,527 ± 322	− 9	NS
Serum creatinine (mg/100 ml)	1.72 ± 0.51	1.55 ± 0.71	−10	NS
$Cl_{(creatinine)}$ (ml/min)	58 ± 30	59 ± 33	+ 2.6	NS
Body weight (kg)	67.3 ± 13.3	63.4 ± 13.8	− 6	<0.001

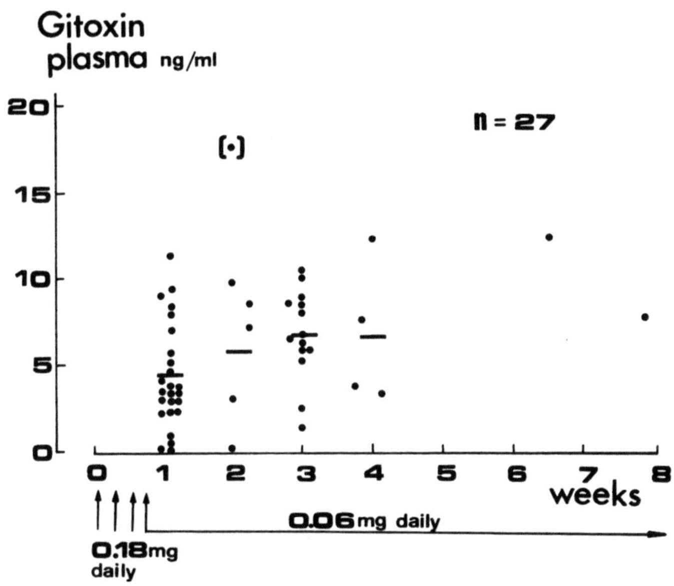

Fig. 1. Gitoformate plasma concentrations (gitoxin equivalents) in 27 geriatric patients (between one and four measurements per patient) during maintenance treatment with 0.06 mg gitoformate daily

perienced frequent nausea. Two of the three patients with the highest concentrations measured at 7 days were also "little old ladies." In contrast, the lowest measurements obtained after 7 and 14 days occurred in a single patient with a body weight of 92 kg. Clearly, some of the variability in concentration is due to the use of a standard dose without correction for body weight differences. Gitoformate should be administered according to body weight.

A global clinical assessment of the success of the treatment based on all clinical findings before and upon discharge is summed up in Table 4. With the omission of one patient dropped because of poor digitalis tolerance (bradycardia; see below), only 2 of 19 patients decompensated at the beginning of therapy showed an unsatisfactory response. One of these was the patient referred to earlier, in whom the doubling of the daily dose produced no improvement. Thus gitoformate diuretic treatment at a daily dosage of 0.06 g was effective in cardiac insufficiency in 26 of the 28 patients evaluated.

Table 4. Global clinical assessment of gitoformate/diuretic treatment in cardiac insufficiency

Before \ After		Compensated −	Compensated +	Total
Compensated	−	2	17	19
	+	0	9	9
Total		2[a]	26	28

[a] Not including one patient dropped because of digitalis sensitivity (bradycardia under therapeutic levels of gitoformate; HR = 48 bpm)

χ^2-test (McNemar):
$\chi^2 = 16.02 > 10.83 = \chi^2_{1,0.001}$

Table 5. Effect of gitoformate/diuretic treatment on the signs associated with cardiac insufficiency

Sign[a]	χ^2 [b]	*P*
Dyspnea (rest)	17.20	<0.001
Dyspnea (exercise)	20.18	<0.001
Cyanosis	11.27	<0.05
Edema	19.14	<0.001
Venous congestion	17.10	<0.001
Pulmonary congestion	20.09	<0.001
Hepatomegaly	9.11	<0.05

[a] Evaluation on 28 patients. Classification as (−) absent, (+) moderate, (++) severe
[b] Calculated using Bowker's χ^2-test with 3 degrees of freedom

The effect of gitoformate/diuretic treatment on the signs associated with cardiac insufficiency, including those obtained by objective X-ray investigations, are given in Table 5. The effects on dyspnea at rest and under exercise, edema, and the venous and pulmonary congestion were highly significant. Adverse reactions were seldom seen, although not absent, in this multimorbidity population. One patient with bradycardia referred to previously had to be dropped from the group. Serum drug levels were in the therapeutic range and serum potassium was normal. Other than the "little old lady" who received double the dose of gitoformate, only two other subjects reported side-effects. These were nausea in one and nausea and loss of appetite in the other, confined in both cases to the commencement of treatment.

Gitoformate has been credited with having relatively low negative chronotropic activity in comparison with its positive inotropic action (Abate et al. 1980; Ambrosioni et al. 1980). In this study a marked negative chronotropic action was seen only in patients with some degree of tachycardia. In 12 patients with pulse rates in the range 70–80, 0.06 mg gitoformate lowered the pulse rate by 5–6 beats per minute, a difference found to be highly significant using Student's paired t-test. Apart from these changes in rhythm, the ECGs showed no other significant alterations or conduction disturbances which could be associated with digitalis toxicity. The repolarization phase was usually improved, as was the frequency of extrasystoles in the few instances when they were present.

Summary

Gitoformate is a highly effective drug for the treatment of cardiac insufficiency in a multimorbid geriatric population. At a dose rate of 0.06 mg daily given in combination with diuretic therapy the drug was well tolerated even by those aged patients (mean age 79 years) with marked renal function impairment. The occurrence of therapeutic drug concentrations (5–15 ng/ml) and the absence of toxicity is a reflection of the nonrenal dependence of this drug's elimination. Some adjustment of the dose is necessary according to body weight, especially in the case of "little old ladies," in whom 0.03 mg seems adequate. The presence of bradyarrhythmias, is, as for other cardiac glycosides, a contraindication and was seen in one digitalis-intolerant patient out of a total 31 patients treated. A negative chronotropic action was usually only apparent in patients with initial pulse rates above 80 beats/min.

References

Abate G, Polimeni RM, Cuccurullo F, Sollecito AM, Puddu P (1980) Effects of gitoformate on senile heart. Drugs Exptl Clin Res 6:243–246

Ambrosioni E, Magelli C, Boschi S, Pasetti L, Magnani B (1980) Clinical efficacy of gitoformate. Drugs Exptl Clin Res 6:221–231

Batz H, Busanny-Caspari E, Viehmann P (1983) Eine Multicenterstudie mit Gitoformat – dem pentaformylierten Ester des Gitoxins. Med Klin Prax Sondernummer 2:61–65

Rietbrock N, Woodcock BG, Hrazdil U (1984) Gitoformat und Digitoxin als Alternative zu nierenpflichtigen Glykosiden in der Therapie der Herzinsuffizienz. Arzneim-Forsch 34:915–917

Ulbrich M, Alken RG, Belz GG (1984) Pharmakokinetik und Wirkungskinetik von Gitoformat. In: Rietbrock N, Schlepper M, Busanny-Caspari E (Hrsg) Gitoformat – ein nicht-nierenpflichtiges Digitalisglykosid. Vieweg, Braunschweig/Wiesbaden, S 71–80

Pharmacokinetic Studies of Doxycycline in Geriatric Patients with Multiple Diseases

R. Böcker[1], C.-J. Estler[1], D. Platt[2,3], and W. Mühlberg[3]

Doxycycline (Fig. 1) has been used clinically as a broad spectrum antibiotic for about 15 years (Antibiotika-Fibel 1975). Pharmacokinetic analyses have been performed in experimental animals and humans. They have shown that, in comparison to other tetracyclines, doxycycline complexes less readily with bivalent or trivalent cations and therefore is well absorbed from the gastrointestinal tract even when given together with food (Fabre et al. 1966; Böcker and Estler 1981). In blood it is more than 90% bound to serum proteins but may also be bound to cellular components.

According to the literature, the half-life of doxycycline in young subjects ranges from 16 to 22 h, and 30% of a dose is eliminated renally (Fabre et al. 1966; Schach von Wittenau 1968; Rosenblatt 1966). It has been reported that some drugs, such as diphenylhydantoin or carbamazepine or barbiturates, can shorten the half-life of doxycycline by about 50% when they are given simultaneously with it (Neuvonen and Penttilä 1974; Penttilä et al. 1974; Neuvonen et al. 1975). This effect is explained by most of the authors as being a result of an increased rate of biotransformation of doxycycline. But this is only a matter of speculation as the rate of metabolism of doxycycline has never been measured quantitatively. In fact, surprisingly little is known about the biotransformation of doxycycline. Only one metabolite (*N*-demethyl-doxycycline) has been found very recently in our laboratory (Böcker et al. 1982; Böcker 1983), but this metabolite accounts for only a very small fraction of the dose administered (Böcker and Estler 1983). The main metabolites are still unknown, and it should be mentioned that about 20% of the dose cannot be recovered in experimental animals or in humans.

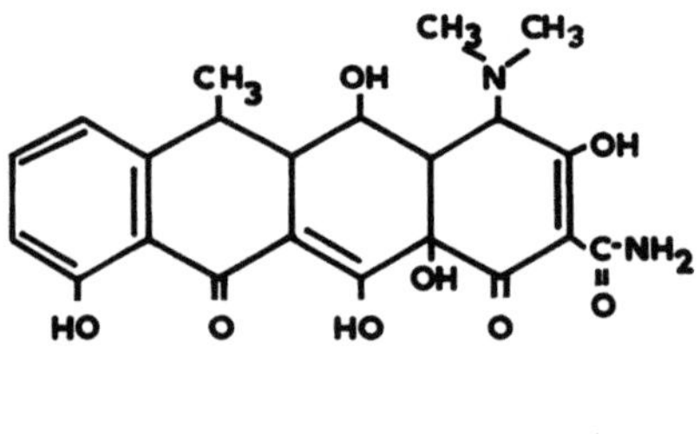

Fig. 1. Structure of doxycycline

[1] Institut für Pharmakologie und Toxikologie der Universität Erlangen-Nürnberg, Universitätsstraße 22, D-8520 Erlangen/F.R.G.
[2] Institut für Gerontologie der Universität Erlangen-Nürnberg und
[3] 2. Medizinische Klinik Nürnberg, Flurstraße 17, D-8500 Nürnberg/F.R.G.

Drugs and Aging
Ed. by D. Platt

Table 1. Basic data regarding the patients included in the study

Number of female patients	15
Number of male patients	10
Age ± SD (years)	76.3 ± 6
Body weight ± SD	65.6 ± 13.8
Creatinine clearance ± SD (ml/min)	42.1 ± 21.1
Total serum protein content ± SD (g/100 ml)	6.4 ± 0.7
Albumin content (% of serum proteins)	51.3 ± 4.7
Serum β-globulin (% of serum proteins)	11.7 ± 2.3
Serum iron content (μg/100 ml)	48.1 ± 23.8

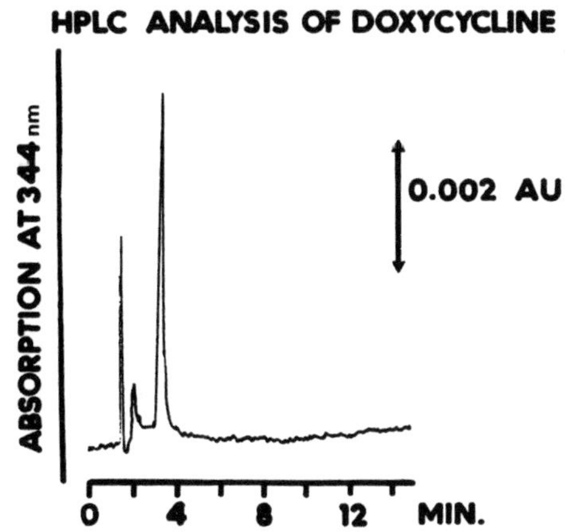

Fig. 2. Chromatographic analysis of doxycycline on RP C_8, 10 μm. Chromatographic conditions: column 25 × 0.4 cm; eluent 3.5 mmol/liter NaH_2PO_4 in water–acetonitrile (68:32), pH 2.5; flow rate 1.9 ml/min; detection at 344 nm

Most studies with doxycycline have been performed on healthy subjects or young and middle-aged patients, and up to now few data are available on the pharmacokinetics of doxycycline in elderly humans (Simon et al. 1975; Hendricks et al. 1982). As, however, animal experiments from our laboratory have shown that the pharmacokinetics of the tetracyclines, and especially their organ distribution, vary with sex and age (Böcker and Estler 1979; Böcker et al. 1984), we tried to investigate the influence of age, sex, disease state, and additional medication on the serum levels and half-life of doxycycline in geriatric patients.

The study was performed at Professor Platt's department in the city hospital of Nürnberg. Twenty-five patients who for medical reasons had to be treated with doxycycline were included in the study. They were informed about the study and consented. The age of the patients ranged from 65 to 90 years, with an average of 76.3 ± 6 years (Table 1).

Doxycycline was given intravenously at a dose of 200 mg. On the first day of treatment the drug concentration in the serum was measured up to 10 h after the initial dose. For each patient an individual standard was prepared by adding doxycycline to serum derived from a blood sample drawn before administration of the antibiotic. The concentration of doxycycline was determined by a high performance liquid chromatographic method, and a typical analysis is shown in Fig. 2 (Böcker 1980). The method yields the same results as conventional micro-

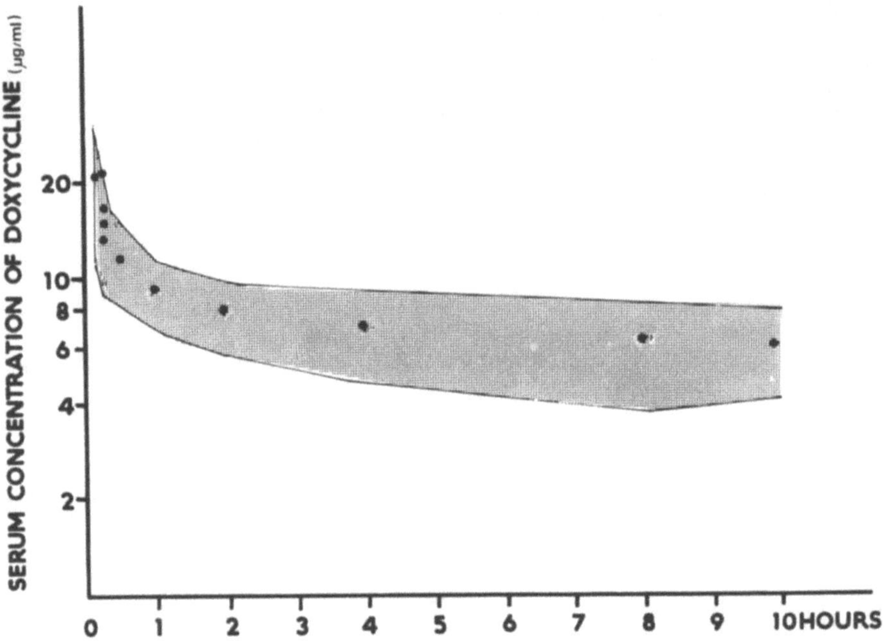

Fig. 3. Mean serum concentration ±SD of doxycycline in geriatric patients after i.v. administration of 200 mg

biological methods (Böcker and Weber 1980): 85%–90% of the doxycycline determined by high performance liquid chromatography is microbiologically active. Blood constituents or drugs given as concomitant therapy do not interfere with the analysis of doxycycline.

The levels of doxycycline found in our study are shown in Fig. 3. During the first 30 min after i.v. administration the concentration of doxycycline declined rapidly. For this phase of distribution the half-life (t/2 α) was 10.1 ± 7.2 min. This rapid decrease was followed by a slower decrease of the serum levels. The apparent half-life during this elimination phase (t/2 β) ranged from 6.5 to 34 h, with an average of 15.1 ± 18.8 h. From the β-phase of elimination the apparent volume of distribution was calculated. It was 24.8 ± 8.9 liters, the range being 15.8–42.9 liters.

As the analytical method is very precise – its potential error being less than 6% – the great variations in the serum levels within the patient group reflect true interindividual variations. We tried to correlate the individual serum levels and half-lives with the patients' age, sex, or concomitant drug use but were unable to find any overt correlation. In particular, no influence of drugs known to induce or inhibit drug metabolism became apparent. Also, the renal function of the patients did not correlate with the interindividual variations in the half-life of doxycycline (Table 1).

Statistical evaluation of the pharmacokinetic data revealed some mathematical correlations with clinicochemical parameters determined prior to the doxycy-

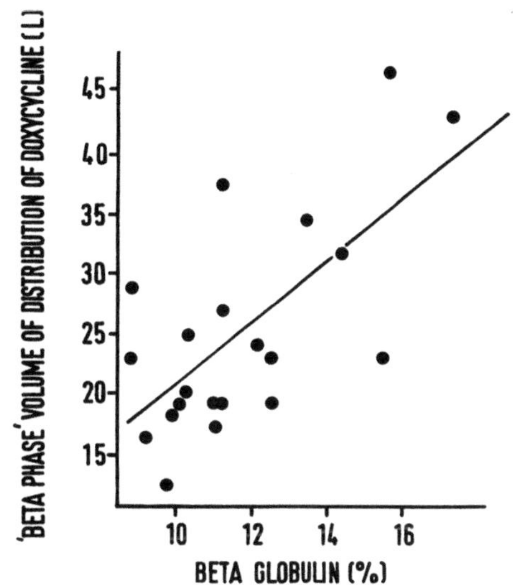

Fig. 4. Correlation between serum β-globulin content (as a percentage of the total serum protein) and the apparent β-phase volume of distribution (liters); $r=0.665$

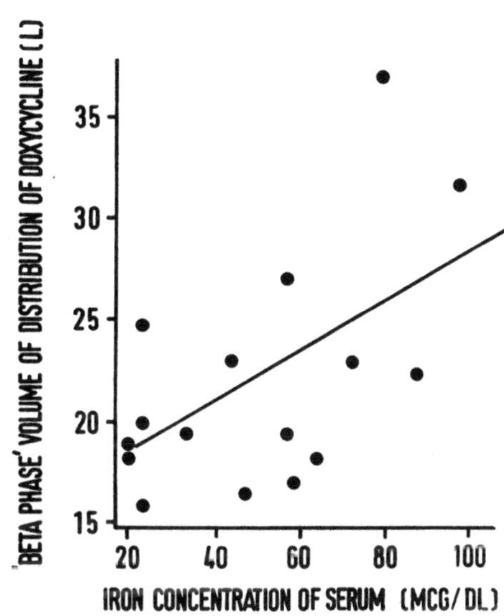

Fig. 5. Correlation between serum iron content (µg/100 ml) and the apparent β-phase volume of distribution (liters); $r=0.571$

cline treatment, e.g., blood pressure or erythrocyte volume, which may or may not correspond to biological correlations. Among these, one finding shall be stressed here because it may be important for the pharmacokinetics of doxycycline: The apparent volume of distribution $V_{D\beta}$ correlates well with the β-globulin concentration of the serum (Fig. 4). A similar correlation can be seen between the $V_{D\beta}$ and the iron content of the serum (Fig. 5). In addition, the steady state volume of distribution also correlates with the β-globulin concentration (Fig. 6) and with the iron content of the serum (Fig. 7). As the β-globulin fraction contains iron binding proteins like siderophilin, these findings indicate that iron-containing proteins may play a role in the binding and distribution of doxycycline.

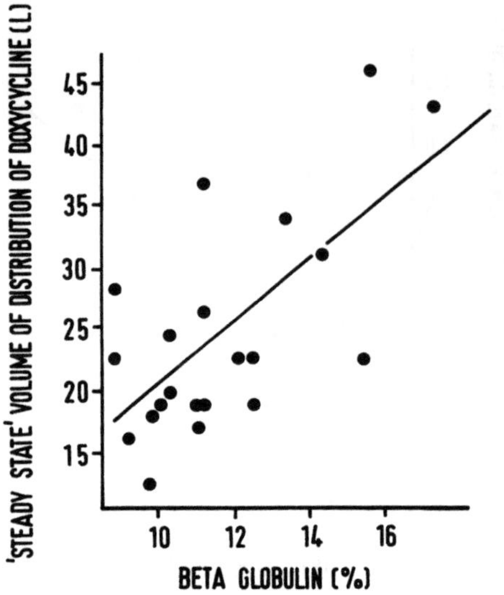

Fig. 6. Correlation between serum β-globulin content (as a percentage of the total serum protein) and the apparent steady state phase volume of distribution (liters); $r = 0.663$

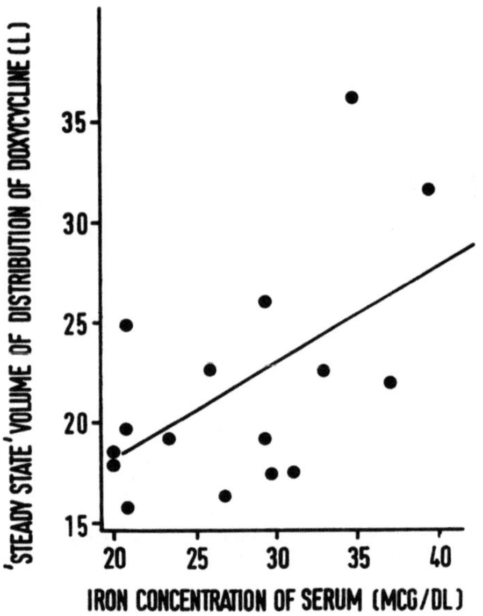

Fig. 7. Correlation between serum iron content (μg/100 ml) and the apparent steady state phase volume of distribution (liters); $r = 0.558$

Though it is well known that doxycycline forms stable complexes with iron salts (Dürckheimer 1975) and that the absorption of doxycycline can be influenced by ferrous ions (Neuvonen and Penttilä 1974), the formation of complexes of doxycycline and protein-bound iron has not yet been studied. The reason is that such studies are difficult to perform since doxycycline in stable complexes is measurable neither by microbiological nor by chemical methods. It seems conceivable that doxycycline bound to iron-containing proteins in the serum escapes detection by conventional methods and that, therefore, its serum concentration appears to be low when the serum iron content is high.

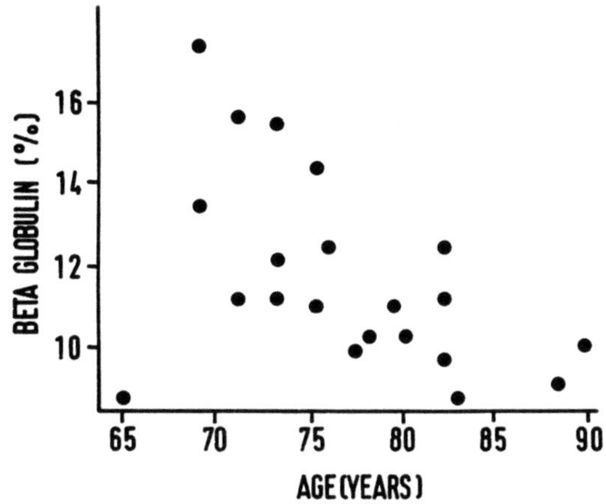

Fig. 8. Serum β-globulin content as a function of age in the geriatric patients included in the study

Table 2. Concentration of doxycycline in various organs of deceased persons (µg/g). The concentration of doxycycline is corrected for the organs' blood content

Patient	B. F.	V. X.	H. K.
Serum (µg/ml)	1.3	–	0.9
Lung	12.2	13.7	7.1
Liver	10.2	14.2	10.1
Kidney	17.5	30.8	7.4
Spleen	20.1	14.6	1.4
Bile (µg/ml)	–	145.9	–
Thyroid gland	22.0	29.7	–

In this way the apparent volume of distribution should become smaller when the serum iron or β-globulin content is reduced. As the β-globulin content decreases with age (Fig. 8), the amount of doxycycline detectable should increase in older persons.

In this connection it is interesting to note that the serum levels of doxycycline are considerably higher in our patients than in younger persons in comparable studies (Schach von Wittenau 1968; Fabre et al. 1971; Füsgen et al. 1977; Malmberg 1984). There were no differences in the apparent half-lives of distribution and elimination.

In three patients who had died from their diseases in spite of the antibiotic therapy, samples of various organs could be obtained 15–20 h after death. The doxycycline levels measured in these organs were essentially higher than those found by other investigators in tissue samples resected during surgical procedures (Table 2) (Fabre et al. 1971; Moorthi et al. 1974; Pelz et al. 1977; Clauberg 1979). For instance, concentrations in lung tissue of deceased persons were twice as high as in lungs of surgical patients. In liver and thyroid glands even 10–15 times higher levels were found. It is not clear whether this great difference is due to post-mortem changes or whether it reflects the in vivo situation in old persons in general.

As these patients had no obvious signs of liver or thyroid dysfunction, the high organ concentration measured appears still to be below the toxic level. This means that after single dose administration there is no compelling reason for a general adjustment of the dose regimen of doxycycline in aged persons.

Summary

1. In geriatric patients the serum concentration of doxycycline in the β-phase of elimination is about twice the concentration found in middle-aged patients or healthy subjects.
2. The higher doxycycline concentrations may be due to the lower iron content of the serum of the geriatric patients and therefore result from a decreased binding capacity for doxycycline.
3. The concentrations of doxycycline in lung, liver, and thyroid glands were found to be much higher than those reported in the literature.
4. The half-life of doxycycline in geriatric patients does not differ from the half-life in middle-aged patients or healthy subjects.

References

Antibiotika-Fibel (1975) Otten H, Plempel M, Siegenthaler W (Hrsg). Georg Thieme Verlag. Stuttgart, S 330

Böcker R (1980) Rapid analysis of doxycycline from biological samples by high-performance-liquid chromatography. J Chromatogr 187:439–441

Böcker R (1983) Analysis and quantitation of a metabolite of doxycycline in mice, rats, and humans by high performance liquid chromatography. J Chromatogr 274:255–262

Böcker R, Estler C-J (1981) Comparison of distribution of doxycycline in mice after oral and intravenous application measured by a high performance liquid chromatographic method. Arzneim-Forsch 31:2116–2117

Böcker R, Estler C-J (1983) Quantitative assessment of a newly detected metabolite of doxycycline. In vitro formation and in vivo distribution of *N*-demethyl-doxycycline in mice. Drugs Exptl Clin Res 9:813–819

Böcker R, Weber A (1980) Vergleichende Untersuchungen zur Bestimmung von Doxycyclin-Konzentrationen in biologischen Proben mit Hilfe der Hochdruck-Flüssigchromatographie und Agar-Diffusionsmethode. Zbl Bakt Hyg, I Abt Orig A 247:276–281

Böcker R, Estler C-J, Weber A (1983) Metabolism of doxycycline. Lancet, November, 1155

Böcker R, Warnke L, Estler C-J (1984) Blood and organ concentrations of tetracycline and doxycycline in female mice. Comparison to males. Arzneim-Forsch 34:446–448

Clauberg C (1979) Doxycyclin-Spiegel in Lungen- und Bronchialgewebe. Münchener Med Wochenschr 121:1469–1470

Dürckheimer W (1975) Tetracycline: Chemie, Biochemie und Struktur-Wirkungsbeziehungen. Angew Chem 87:751–764

Fabre J, Pitton JS, Kunz JP (1966) Verteilung und Ausscheidung von Doxycyclin beim Menschen. Chemotherapia 11:73–85

Fabre J, Milek E, Kalfopulos P, Marier G (1971) Die Kinetik der Tetracycline beim Menschen unter besonderer Berücksichtigung von Doxycyclin. Schweiz Med Wochenschr 101:593–598

Fabre J, Milek E, Kalfopulos P, Marier G (1971) Die Kinetik der Tetracycline beim Menschen unter besonderer Berücksichtigung von Doxycyclin. Schweiz Med Wochenschr 101:625–633

Füsgen J, Summa J-D, Weih H (1977) Serumspiegel von Oxytetracyclin und Doxycyclin unter forcierter Diurese. Med Klin 72:1645–1648

Hendricks W, Hartleb O, Böcker R (1982) Therapie akuter Infektionen mit Doxycyclin bei geriatrischen Patienten. Fortschr Med 100:246–248

Malmberg A-S (1984) Bioavailability of doxycycline monohydrate. A comparison with equivalent doses of doxycycline hydrochloride. Chemotherapy 30:76–80

Moorthi K, Becker WD, Geiss T, Kentner D (1974) Vergleichende Gewebe-, Galle- und Serum-Spiegel nach verschiedenen parenteralen Tetracyclingaben. Therapiewoche 24:3147–3150

Neuvonen PJ, Penttilä O (1974) Interaction between doxycycline and barbiturates. Brit Med J I:535–536

Neuvonen PJ, Penttilä O (1974) Effect of oral ferrous sulphate on the half-life of doxycycline in man. Eur J Clin Pharmacol 7:361–363

Neuvonen PJ, Penttilä O, Lehtovaara R, Aho K (1975) Effect of antiepileptic drugs on the elimination of various tetracycline derivatives. Eur J clin Pharmacol 9:147–154

Pelz K, Herdter F, Marcushen M (1977) Anwendung von Tetracyclinen bei Gallenerkrankungen. Therapiewoche 27:8585–8591

Penttilä O, Neuvonen PJ, Aho K, Lehtovaara R (1974) Interaction between doxycycline and some antiepileptic drugs. Brit med J II:470–472

Rosenblatt JE, Barrett JE, Brodie JL, Kirby WMM (1967) Comparison of in vitro activity and clinical pharmacology of doxycycline with other tetracyclines. Antimicrob Agents Chemother 134:141

Schach von Wittenau M (1968) Some pharmacokinetic aspects of doxycycline metabolism in man. Chemotherapy 13:41–50

Simon C, Malerczyk V, Engelke H, Preuss I, Grahmann H, Schmidt K (1975) Die Pharmakokinetik von Doxycyclin bei Niereninsuffizienz und geriatrischen Patienten im Vergleich zu jungen Erwachsenen. Schweiz Med Wochenschr 105:1615–1620

Subject Index

MIX
Papier aus verantwortungsvollen Quellen
Paper from responsible sources
FSC® C105338

If you have any concerns about our products,
you can contact us on
ProductSafety@springernature.com

In case Publisher is established outside the EU,
the EU authorized representative is:
Springer Nature Customer Service Center GmbH
Europaplatz 3, 69115 Heidelberg, Germany

Printed by Libri Plureos GmbH
in Hamburg, Germany